D0971499

Another Person's Poison

A HISTORY OF FOOD ALLERGY

Matthew Smith

COLUMBIA UNIVERSITY PRESS   NEW YORK

COLUMBIA UNIVERSITY PRESS
Publishers Since 1893
New York   Chichester, West Sussex
cup.columbia.edu

Copyright © 2015 Columbia University Press
All rights reserved

Library of Congress Cataloging-in-Publication Data

Smith, Matthew, 1973–
    Another person's poison : a history of food allergy / Matthew Smith.
      pages   cm. — (Arts and traditions of the table: perspectives on culinary history)
    Includes bibliographical references and index.
    ISBN 978-0-231-16484-9 (cloth : alk. paper)
    ISBN 978-0-231-53919-7 (e-book)
    1. Food allergy—History.   I. Title.
RC596.S39 2015
616.97'5—dc23

                                                                    2014041702

Columbia University Press books are printed on permanent and durable acid-free paper.
This book is printed on paper with recycled content.
Printed in the United States of America

c 10 9 8 7 6 5 4 3 2 1

COVER IMAGE: PEANUT, WHEAT (© SHUTTERSTOCK; TEST TUBES © GETTY/PAUL TILLINGHAST)
COVER DESIGN: MARY ANN SMITH; BOOK DESIGN: VIN DANG

References to Web sites (URLs) were accurate at the time of writing.
Neither the author nor Columbia University Press is responsible for URLs
that may have expired or changed since the manuscript was prepared.

FOR MICHELLE,
whose enduring selflessness reveals the true shape of love

Contents

Acknowledgments

WHEN I BEGAN MY DOCTORAL RESEARCH at the University of Exeter, my supervisor, Mark Jackson, would introduce me as follows: "This is Matt Smith. He's doing a PhD on allergy." At the time, this slightly befuddled me since I thought I was working on ADHD. Ultimately, both of us were correct, but, while writing this book, I have grown increasingly grateful to Mark not only for his peerless supervision but also for steering me toward the fascinating world of allergy. I am very grateful that Jennifer Crewe and Columbia University Press were willing to take this project on board and thank them, as well as the reviewers, for their suggestions.

This book would not have been possible without the generous support of the Wellcome Trust. In addition to a Wellcome Trust postdoctoral fellowship, which allowed me to research and write, the Wellcome Library and its fabulous staff (particularly Ross MacFarlane and Phoebe Harkins) always went beyond the call of duty. I also relied on the Royal Society of Medicine's Library, Harvard University's Francis A. Countway Library, Boston University's Howard Gotlieb Archival Research Center, and, especially, the AAAAI and ACAAI records at the University of Wisconsin–Milwaukee and the University of Wisconsin–Parkside, respectively. I am also grateful to the BBC/AHRC New Generation Thinker scheme for allowing me to reach out to a wider audience.

Although oral history does not feature heavily in this book, I did conduct some interviews and I want to thank my interviewees. I had always thought that there are those who eat to live and those who live to eat; you helped me realize that reality is much more complicated. Your stories informed my approach as much as anything, and I will make more explicit use of them in future. Thanks also to Anne Muñoz-Furlong and FARE for connecting me with interviewees.

I am also grateful for my colleagues at the University of Strathclyde and the Centre for the History of Health and Healthcare. Jim Mills and Arthur McIvor provided me with excellent advice—in addition to weekly squash beatings—and Emma Newlands, John Stewart, Janet Greenlees, Peter Kirby, Vicky Long, and others offered guidance and support. Thanks also to Gayle Davis and the executive committee of the Society for the Social History of Medicine for reminding me that the history of medicine does—and always will—have a purpose in informing medical debate.

Friends and family have also kept me focused. Thanks especially to Stephen Mawdsley for sending me new stories about allergy, which would have passed me by, and Tindy Agaba for putting life in perspective. Mark Doidge, Angus Ferguson, Despo Kritsotaki, Matthew Eisler, Rima Apple, Ali Haggett, Leah Songhurst, Ed Ramsden, Jonathan Reinarz, David Gentilcore, Erika Dyck, and many others all provided advice and friendship along the way. Although I am grateful to all my family and friends back home in Canada for their encouragement (Mom, Dad, Herberts, Burkes, Lentzes, Burnses, Pattersons, all), I am eternally in debt to Michelle and Dashiell for their patience and understanding and—last but not least—little Solveigh, for waiting until the writing was done before making her arrival!

Abbreviations

AAA	American Academy of Allergy
AAAI	American Academy of Allergy and Immunology
AAAAI	American Academy of Allergy, Asthma and Immunology
AAEM	American Academy for Environmental Medicine
AAO	American Academy of Otolaryngology
ABAI	American Board of Allergy and Immunology
ABMS	American Board of Medical Specialties
AC	Anaphylaxis Campaign
ACA	American College of Allergists
ACAAI	American College of Allergy, Asthma and Immunology
ACSH	American Council on Science and Health
ADHD	attention deficit hyperactivity disorder
AMA	American Medical Association
APA	American Psychiatric Association
BHA	butylated hydroxytoluene
BHT	butylated hydroxyanisole
BMJ	*British Medical Journal*
CECU	Comprehensive Environmental Control Unit
CMAJ	*Canadian Medical Association Journal*
DSM	*Diagnostic and Statistical Manual of Mental Disorders*
FAAN	Food Allergy and Anaphylaxis Network

FAI	Food Allergy Initiative
FAN	Food Allergy Network
FARE	Food Allergy Research and Education
FDA	Food and Drug Administration
FPIES	food protein–induced enterocolitis syndrome
FSA	Food Standards Agency
HCFA	Health Care Financing Administration
HiB	*Haemoiphilus influenzae* type b
IFIC	International Food Information Council
IgA	immunoglobulin A
IgD	immunoglobulin D
IgE	immunoglobulin E
IgG	immunoglobulin G
IgM	immunoglobulin M
ILSI	International Life Sciences Institute
JACI	*Journal of Allergy and Clinical Immunology*
JAMA	*Journal of the American Medical Association*
JCAI	Joint Council of Allergy and Immunology
MCS	multiple chemical sensitivity
MMR	measles, mumps, and rubella
MSG	monosodium glutamate
NEJM	*New England Journal of Medicine*
NIAID	National Institute of Allergy and Infectious Diseases
NPCA	National Peanut Council of America
NRA	National Restaurant Association
OIT	oral immunotherapy
P-K	Prausnitz-Küstner
RAST	radioallergosorbent test
SBS	sick building syndrome
SCE	Society for Clinical Ecology
SSAAC	Society for the Study of Asthma and Allied Conditions
USDA	United States Department of Agriculture
WHO	World Health Organization

Another Person's Poison

Introduction

IN AUGUST 2009, the venerable hard rockers AC/DC were scheduled to play the 60,000-seat Commonwealth Stadium in Edmonton, Alberta. A few days before the concert, the *Edmonton Journal* published a list of tips for fans. Concertgoers were encouraged to arrive early, use public transportation, and tread lightly on the local neighborhood. In order to ensure that security procedures ran smoothly, a list of prohibited items was also posted. Included were many of the usual suspects, including guns, knives, drugs, alcohol, pets, and glass containers, but heading the list was a more unexpected hazard: peanuts.[1]

According to another newspaper, the *Edmonton Sun*, the ban on peanuts was instituted after the mother of a young peanut allergy sufferer wrote to complain that her son felt "anxious" about the peanuts consumed at Edmonton Eskimo football matches held at the stadium.[2] Up until the ban, unshelled peanuts were a popular snack at Commonwealth Stadium. Exiting the stadium meant shuffling through millions of peanut shells, which created a low-lying cloud of peanut dust, a daunting prospect for those who might go into potentially fatal anaphylactic shock when exposed to even a few milligrams of peanut. The city of Edmonton, which owned the venue, acted promptly, prohibiting peanuts from not only football games but all other stadium events as well. Expressing his support, Rick Lelacheur, president and CEO of the Edmonton Eskimos, stated that "peanut allergies are a serious medical problem facing a growing number of people. The Eskimos support the City of Edmonton's initiative and we hope our fans will do their part to make Commonwealth Stadium a safe, healthy environment for everyone."

Lelacheur's comments about the seriousness of peanut allergy reflect contemporary statistics about food allergy generally. Allergies occur when the immune system overreacts to a foreign substance, in the case of food allergy, proteins found in food. Although food allergy has been thought to trigger a wide range of symptoms, the most feared reaction to peanuts is anaphylaxis, a sudden, intense immune response characterized by precipitous drops in blood pressure, skin eruptions, and swelling severe enough to block the airway and cause death. Today it is estimated that 4 percent of adults and 8 percent of children in North America are allergic to some food.[3] According to the American Academy of Allergy, Asthma and Immunology (AAAAI), peanut allergy alone affects more than 3 million Americans, and more than 6 million are affected by seafood allergies.[4] While peanuts dominate the headlines, allergies to more ubiquitous foods such as egg and milk are even more common in children, making shopping and meal preparation a time-consuming and worrisome task for parents. Despite the rising awareness of food allergy and preventive strategies, anaphylactic reactions to foods result in between 150 and 200 fatalities per year in North America, with half of those cases being triggered by reactions to peanuts, and a quarter more caused by tree nuts, such as walnuts and pecans. Children, not surprisingly, are disproportionately affected. The fact that the lives of so many young people are put into jeopardy by something as apparently innocuous as a peanut speaks to the frightening and bizarre nature of food allergy, and helps to explain the often draconian approaches to preventing accidental exposure.

Complicating matters is the fact that allergic reactions to food, and especially peanuts, are also on the increase. Between 1997 and 2002, peanut allergy doubled in children, with the number of children being discharged from hospital for serious food allergy reactions trebling from 1998 to 2006.[5] Overall, it is estimated that the annual instances of food anaphylaxis increased from 21,000 in 1999 to 51,000 in 2008.[6] Although many explanations for such increases have been offered, none has proved satisfactory. As a result, food allergy remains, for an increasing number of people, a constant reminder of how vulnerable they are to what should be the most life-giving substances on earth: food.

"WHAT IF I SMELL YOUR PEANUTS AND DIE?"

This does not mean, however, that everyone agrees with the measures to prevent reactions to potent allergens like peanuts. Edmonton's AC/DC fans, for example, were decidedly divided about Commonwealth Stadium's peanut prohibition. In one corner were allergy sufferers, who felt that the risks they faced were unappreciated. In the comments that followed the *Edmonton Journal's* article, one angry fan retorted that those who thought the ban was too drastic

> need to learn about allergies! I am so allergic to peanut products that I will swell up like a balloon. . . . Once on a plane trip to France, some bone head decided to eat a peanut butter sandwich . . . we had to make an emergency landing about 20 minutes later. . . . You know, I could have died on that plane and now these "boneheads" want to bring peanuts to the concert. . . . What if I smell your peanuts and die? Huh what if???[7]

Other sufferers argued that while an allergic reaction could be fatal, the ban certainly did not mean "the end of the world" for those who used to enjoy peanuts at the stadium; fans who did not like the restrictions could simply "stay home" if they wanted peanuts so badly. Another person sensibly asked, "Since when do you need peanuts to enjoy an ACDC concert? I could understand if the[y] banned alcohol, but seriously peanuts?"

Such arguments did not faze those in the other corner. Responding to the claim that peanut allergy could be triggered by smell, one fan retorted: "You can't have a [*sic*] allergic reaction to the smell of peanuts. Go back to your doctor and get the real facts." Another fan questioned why peanut allergy sufferers could not "bring a medical kit to deal with the situation," complaining that he was "so sick and tired of situations where 60,000 people have to change what they do because one person can't be bothered to look after themself [*sic*] and be prepared. Sorry you're allergic but enough already. The world isn't turning only for you." Still others expressed (one hopes on purpose) the decidedly black humor inherent in the situation. While one fan complained dramatically that if "I can't enjoy a good bag of peanuts while I listen to AC/DC then I might as well end it all," another ominously warned, "I'm bringing peanuts in, and nobody can stop me."[8]

Although Commonwealth Stadium has been the most spectacular instances of a peanut ban—perhaps mimicking the overblown, excessive nature of anaphylaxis itself—it is not the only place where peanuts have been banned. The humble peanut has become unwelcome in many public spaces where it was once common if not somewhat integral, sparking controversy about how to balance the rights of the many to eat peanuts with protecting the allergic. Baseball stadiums, where peanuts and Cracker Jack (containing peanuts) are not just commonplace but hailed during the seventh-inning stretch in the ubiquitous anthem "Take Me Out to the Ball Game," have come under particular pressure.[9] While most parks have not banned peanuts outright, many have opted to have peanut-free zones or peanut-free days. Progressive Field, in Cleveland, for example, provides a peanut-free section for certain games and donates some of the proceeds from ticket sales to the Food Allergy and Anaphylaxis Network (FAAN).[10] Peanuts were also recently banned from a section of Boston's iconic Fenway Park, but not all fans heeded the prohibition. One fan purchased a "'small' 48-ounce bag" from a local store and smuggled it into the park. Stating that "peanuts bring people together in a section. It's like glue," the fan proceeded to share his nuts by pouring them into the baseball caps of his fellow—presumably not allergic—fans.[11]

Other susceptible industries have also taken steps to prevent accidental allergic reactions to peanuts.[12] Mars Canada, for instance, decided to ban peanuts from all its factories in 2006 and marketed its Mars bars in television commercials as being completely peanut-free. Many commercial airlines have also stopped serving peanuts during flights. Despite these voluntary measures, the U.S. Department of Transportation recently considered imposing a ban not only on serving peanuts to passengers but also on passengers themselves bringing peanuts on flights. Although the peanut industry understandably felt such measures were too extreme, FAAN argued that on an airplane, where space is confined and air is recycled, it was possible for the peanut dust released when many packages of peanuts are opened to enter the bloodstream and trigger a reaction in a highly sensitive person, something to which the allergic AC/DC fan just mentioned would attest.[13]

In Canada, the Canadian Transportation Agency ruled that Air Canada, the nation's largest carrier, had to provide a buffer zone for passengers with nut allergy. The measure was enforced after complaints from a passenger who claimed that she had to spend forty minutes in a cramped toilet while nuts were being served on a flight. On another occasion, the same passenger stated that the captain forced her to sign a waiver, clearing the airline of liability had she suffered a reaction while on board.[14] Upset about the ban and not being able to eat Air Canada cashews while in flight, an angry respondent argued that "eating nuts on airplanes is a tradition that goes back to the early days of commercial airline service and I think it is a tradition which needs to be defended in the face of an onslaught of anti-nutism." Unimpressed by such historical justification, another retorted that her "4yr. old has a nut allergy (all nuts including cashews) and it is VERY LIFE THREAT-ENING. . . . If you could only feel the fear with your own child you all might be more understanding."[15]

Eating peanuts may be tasty tradition in North American sports culture, and might indeed be a familiar part of the onboard routine during air travel, but despite the comments of peanut aficionados it is difficult to argue that the snack is necessary condition of enjoying a baseball game or getting through a transatlantic flight. Sports stadiums sell plenty of other snacks, and those tasked with sweeping up the stands after games would certainly not miss all those shells. As for airplane nuts, most airline passengers these days should count themselves lucky if they get anything complimentary from an airline. But peanuts have also been banned from spaces where they have served a more vital purpose, specifically, schools and child-care facilities. For much of the twentieth century, peanuts, especially in the form of peanut butter, were a staple of school lunchboxes, providing an excellent and inexpensive source of calories, fat, protein, and dietary fiber. In the last decade, however, an increasing number of schools and child-care facilities have become peanut-free; whereas my mother packed thousands of peanut butter sandwiches into my school lunchbox, my son's nursery is completely nut-free, as are many other child-care facilities. Some schools, such as Edge-water Elementary in Florida, have gone even further. Acting on behalf of the parents of a six-year-old girl with a severe peanut allergy, the school required that all students wash their hands and rinse their mouths before entering the school, and hired a peanut-sniffing dog to ensure that the grounds were completely peanut-free.[16] In protest, parents took to picketing the school with signs that stated messages such as "No Dogs" and "Our Children Have Rights Too!" and suggested that the girl be homeschooled.

Such stories highlight not only the seriousness of peanut allergy but also its divisiveness. Although food allergy has always been controversial, its ability to change public-health policy, the manufacture and marketing of food products, and what we eat at school, on airplanes, and at AC/DC concerts is a much more recent development. Instead of being treated in terms of a public-health risk, for most of the twentieth century, food allergy was considered by many physicians as a condition of dubious validity, a "scrap basket diagnosis" used by misinformed or even unscrupulous food allergists to explain the problems of difficult patients.[17] To many physicians, including most allergists, food allergy was an excellent example of why allergy was considered "witchcraft, a fad, or a racket," and, as such, the condition did little to boost the reputation of allergy as a legitimate medical practice rooted in scientific medicine.[18]

UNDERSTANDING FOOD ALLERGY

Why has food allergy transformed from a questionable medical entity to a condition deemed serious enough to change the ways in which we produce, prepare, and consume food? Why has food allergy always been so controversial? Why have explanations for food allergy been so elusive? And why are more and more children allergic to food? In order to address these questions, this book the describes the history of this complex and troubling condition. And as the history demonstrates, both understandings and experiences of food allergy have been affected by a wide range of factors, some rooted in the inherent difficulties of conceptualizing and treating the condition, but others emanating from the complex political, economic, cultural, and ideological milieu in which food allergy has existed. Food allergy matters a great deal to allergists, who recognize its significance to how the broader field of allergy is perceived, but it matters also to food and pharmaceutical companies, which see it alternatively as either a threat to profits or an opportunity for exploitation. In addition, environmental activists and their opponents regard it as central to their arguments about the health of the planet, and, of course, it is vitally important to patients, who seek to inform the debates about food allergy.

In this way, the history of food allergy is very much a history of how medical knowledge, and particularly controversial medical ideas, has evolved over the course of the twentieth century, adapting and conforming to different pressures and contexts. Determining the facts about food allergy and deciding who is a food allergy expert have always been contentious issues, sparking debate and division among allergists, the food and drug industry, and health-policy makers, often leaving patients at a loss about how to explain and deal with their perplexing symptoms.[19] Although clinical allergists valued the knowledge they acquired inductively from listening to and treating their patients, allergists based in academic and laboratory settings preferred learning about food allergy deductively through the application of immunological theory by means of experimentation.[20] Such differences in how to generate knowledge about food allergy resulted in different conceptualizations of the condition. Whereas food allergists tended to employ a broad definition of allergy, meaning that they believed it was responsible for a wide range of otherwise undiagnosed symptoms, orthodox allergists were more conservative, restricting it to cases in which a clear immunological mechanism could be demonstrated. These differing understandings were also mirrored in the membership and ambitions of allergy associations, particularly the conservative American Academy of Allergy (AAA), the forerunner of the AAAAI, and the more clinically based American College of Allergists (ACA), now the American College of Allergy, Asthma and Immunology (ACAAI).

Since it has been so difficult to resolve many of the debates about food allergy, its study has been characterized by the simultaneous existence of seemingly mutually exclusive ideas that have fed into clinical practices. This has also been the case in other contested areas of medicine, and none more so than psychiatry. Just as a person suffering from anxiety in 1960 might have had his problems interpreted and treated either neurologically or psychoanalytically, depending on which psychiatrist he saw, a contemporary patient's unexplained migraine or hives might now be attributed to food allergy or diagnosed as psychosomatic, contingent on the allergist she visited. Although there have been examples of both psychiatrists and allergists who approached their subject more pluralistically, the majority remained dogmatic in their approach.[21] Again, as with psychiatry, the resolution of such incongruities in allergy have mattered not just in terms of how to treat patients but also with respect to the desire of allergists to have their field perceived as an authoritative medical science. Whereas similar pressures helped to fuel psychiatry's move away from psychoanalysis and toward seemingly more scientific biological approaches during the 1970s, allergy's ambition to be seen as a legitimate medical profession privileged certain understandings of food allergy over others, increasingly so since the emergence of peanut allergy.

Although issues about the veracity of mental illness have mattered in the history of psychiatry, particularly during the height of the anti-psychiatry movement in the 1960s, and are becoming predominant once more, psychiatrists themselves have tended to debate more about how to explain and treat mental illness. For those interested in allergy, however, the greatest challenge in the epistemology of food allergy has been simply defining what it was. Long before the Austrian pediatrician Clemens von Pirquet (1874–1929) coined the term "allergy" as "any form of altered biological reactivity," physicians recognized that foods could cause a wide range of unexpected symptoms in certain people, a phenomenon known as "idiosyncrasy," but they debated about the nature, extent, and meaning of such reactions.[22] An idiosyncrasy to food might have explained mysterious symptoms such as asthma and eczema for some physicians, but others were suspicious of such explanations, arguing that they were overly reliant on the preconceived notions of patients. Von Pirquet might have given physicians a new term to describe such reactions and might have connected such reactions with the functioning of the immune system, but his broad definition of allergy did not resolve debates about how to distinguish food allergy as a pathological immune response to an otherwise harmless foreign food protein from mere intolerance or dislike. Because of this, the meaning of food allergy has been constantly contested, negotiated, and altered, often to reflect clinical observations and laboratory experiments but also to support alternate agendas, such as allergy's claims to be an authoritative medical science or ecological notions about food allergy as a disease of civilization. Often lost in these broader debates were the experiences of patients themselves, despite the fact that their account of the symptoms from which they suffered was often crucial to diagnosing their ailment.

AN UNNATURAL HISTORY OF FOOD ALLERGY

Despite the similarities between allergy and psychiatry in terms of their precarious positions on the medical ladder, the epistemological shifts that have transformed each field, and the controversies that continue to characterize them, the historiographies of allergy and psychiatry have differed markedly. While the history of psychiatry is arguably the most covered territory in the history of medicine, having been explored from countless methodologies and ideological perspectives, allergy's history is only beginning to be examined.[23] Fortunately, many of the initial forays into the history of allergic disease have been particularly instructive, thus providing insights into how best to understand food allergy. Responding to a call made by Warwick Anderson, Myles Jackson, and Barbara Gutmann Rosenkranz in 1994 for critical histories of immunology that went beyond telling a story of scientific advancement, historians, anthropologists, and philosophers such as Kenton Kroker, Ilana Löwy, Emily Martin, Richard A. Cone, Alfred Tauber, and Thomas Söderqvist, among others, began unpacking how and why thinking about immunology has changed over time.[24] Rather than regarding immunology as a science that had successfully answered most of its pressing questions, as pioneering and Nobel Prize–winning immunologists Frank Macfarlane Burnet (1899–1985) and Niels Jerne (1911–1994) had done, such writers interpreted immunology as a field of knowledge imbued by metaphor, politics, nationalism, and the complex personalities of the players involved.[25]

In the case of allergy, an example of a disease where immunity goes awry and the rules of immunology do not seem to apply, such factors have also been at play, but the progressive notions that used to dominate the history of immunology have rarely been present even in the most optimistic and Whiggish accounts.[26] Allergy, the "Strangest of All Maladies," as one early allergist described it, can be more accurately described as a disease about which more questions have been posed than answered.[27] Perhaps because of this intractability, there have been many disparate attempts by a range of theorists to explain the phenomenon of allergy, none particularly satisfactorily. As Mark Jackson describes in his groundbreaking *Allergy: The History of a Modern Malady*, allergy tended to be depicted as a "disease of modern civilization," but the precise nature of the pathology at play was difficult to determine.[28] While affluent, urban lifestyles were targeted by some, others focused on chemical pollutants, infant feeding, dietary change, vaccination regimes, and even psychogenic factors. During the middle of the twentieth century, asthma and hay fever were thought to be caused by anything from emotionally overbearing parents to sibling rivalry and overcrowding.[29]

Jackson also explores how notions of allergy have been shaped by the technologies developed and sold to diagnose and treat allergy, ranging from allergen extracts for testing and desensitization therapy to bronchial inhalers and epinephrine injectors. Gregg Mitman has also recognized the intimate relationship between allergists and the medical–industrial complex, particularly regarding the treatment of hay fever and asthma.[30] This relationship evolved from pharmaceutical companies working with physicians to develop "pollen vaccines" in the early twentieth century to the development of facilities such as Denver's Children's Asthma Research Institute and Hospital where biomedical solutions to asthma were sought.[31] This symbiotic relationship between allergy and the pharmaceutical industry was slow to develop in the case of food allergy, though, separating it and those who treat it from what Jackson has called the "global economy of allergy."[32]

It is quite understandable that Mitman and others working on the history of allergic disease have gravitated toward seeing allergy in broadly ecological terms, encompassing both the physical and the socioeconomic environment. They argue, often in contrast to conventional medical opinion, that environmental explanations of and solutions for allergy should take preference over other rationales and therapies, such as genetic predisposition and pharmaceutical treatments. In the case of asthma, Mitman criticizes the medical community for focusing too much on creating biomedical treatments, such as inhalers, instead of acknowledging and acting on the fact that it and other allergic diseases are "not separate from the complex of environmental relations—physical, social, economic—out of which it came into being."[33] In other words, there is precious little effort to control the environmental and socioeconomic factors, ranging from air pollution and the use of insecticides to socioeconomic and racial inequalities, that are central to rising rates of asthma and the disproportionate effects it has caused to vulnerable populations.

Similarly, Michelle Murphy questions how biomedical notions about sick building syndrome (SBS) have outweighed more ecological and patient-centered interpretations. This syndrome emerged in the 1980s as an affliction affecting primarily female office workers in hermetically sealed buildings designed to conserve energy following the energy crises of the 1970s.[34] The lack of air circulation in such buildings was thought to result in an accumulation of toxic office chemicals from photocopier fluids, cleaning solvents, synthetic carpets, and paint that caused a range of symptoms, including headaches, rashes, and immune system disorders, in addition to allergic disease. Despite the proliferation of anecdotal evidence, it was difficult for physicians to definitively link the chemicals to the symptoms of SBS; even sympathetic toxicologists could not always detect the suspected chemicals on their equipment.[35] In this atmosphere of uncertainty, those afflicted by SBS, some of whom were scientists themselves, became so-called popular epidemiologists and looked to other sources of evidence to back up their claims.[36] Murphy empathizes with SBS sufferers and their conceptualization of environmental illness, despite the uncertainty she describes. Her instinct, as she eloquently explains, is to trust them rather than the medical authorities who doubt the validity of SBS. Other writers who have discussed multiple chemical sensitivity (MCS), such as Peter Radetsky, Steve Kroll-Smith, and H. Hugh Floyd, have gone even further in empathizing with those who claim to suffer from allergic diseases caused by chemicals in the environment.[37]

To an extent, there is nothing wrong with historians taking an environmentalist position on such issues, particularly when ecological viewpoints have been marginalized by physicians, pharmaceutical companies, and chemical producers who have vested ideological and commercial interests. Mitman's heartfelt message about seeking to prevent asthma through targeting socioeconomic inequalities and improving air quality rather than simply focusing on new pharmaceutical treatments, in particular, transcends the specific debates about why rates of asthma are increasing. Surely such measures would be beneficial in a wide variety of ways even if definitively establishing the link between such conditions and allergic disease proved elusive or if social and environmental factors were only a partial explanation.

But by privileging ecological understandings of allergy over other explanations, it is possible that historians are somewhat guilty of a blinkered approach to what is a considerably more complex condition. As tempting as it is to see allergy through the lens of environmentalism, other conceptualizations of the condition have also predominated and deserve consideration. Jackson's approach to allergy, in contrast, unfailingly subjects all understandings of allergy to the same degree of critical analysis, creating histories that may not provide easy answers but do explain a great deal more about both the inherent intricacies of allergy and its many meanings in Western society.[38] Such a methodology can be informed by the history of other divisive and ideologically driven fields of medicine, and psychiatry in particular, a topic that Jackson knows well.[39] The historiography of psychiatry may be characterized by its political zeal, its variety of perspectives, its many debates, and the passion with which it has been told, but it has not always done a good job of simply describing how and why understandings and experiences of mental illness have changed over time. In other words, in the midst of theorizing and politicizing, some historians of psychiatry have lost sight of its subject altogether.[40] This has not quite been the case in histories written about allergic disease—all the works cited earlier are excellent histories characterized by both insight and passion—but in the case of especially controversial conditions such as food allergy, there is a risk of not subjecting attractive explanations to enough scrutiny and analysis.

Of course, some historians of psychiatry have also recognized the risk of letting theory override the actual evidence and have pioneered different ways of interpreting the history of mental illness. Mark Micale's "sociosomatic" approach to the history of hysteria, for instance, marries both the external (social) and internal (biological) etiologies of disease, resulting in a pluralistic interpretation of mental illness.[41] Since the biological and social realities of food allergy have similarly been at odds with one another, resulting in confused, myopic, and rigid thinking about the condition, Micale's framework, in addition to Jackson's nuanced methodology, provide a solid foundation for understanding the history of food allergy. Instead of letting one ideology overshadow another, I hope to describe a history of food allergy that moves beyond dogma, demonstrating that such an approach not only provides more historical insights but is a good starting point for informing contemporary debates about this perplexing condition.

OVERVIEW

Although most of what follows focuses on the twentieth and twenty-first centuries, it is helpful to understand how adverse reactions to food were understood prior to the emergence of von Pirquet's term "allergy" in 1906. Chapter 1 discusses how physicians in previous centuries came to understand and explain the bizarre symptoms that some people experienced after eating particular foods. Although accounts of these reactions, known as idiosyncrasies, were rare, they were nevertheless controversial, showing how many of the debates about of food allergy in the twentieth century had predecessors in previous eras.

Chapter 2 charts the emergence of allergy as a specific field of medical inquiry at the dawn of the twentieth century. The competing theories of allergy that emerged cast a long shadow on how food allergy would be understood. It also quickly became apparent, as chapter 3 discusses, that while food allergy was included in the same family of allergic disease as hay fever and pet dander allergy, it did not always follow the same rules as those conditions. Early food allergists had to diagnose, treat, and classify food allergy differently than orthodox allergists who focused on other allergies. They also relied more on the testimony and cooperation of their patients. The two factions that would emerge within allergy—food allergists, who employed a broad definition of food allergy and thought it was widespread, and orthodox allergists, who employed a narrower definition of food allergy and thought it was rare—would contest how to understand, explain, and treat food allergy throughout the twentieth century.[42]

Despite the fact that many pioneering allergists emphasized the extent of food allergy during the interwar period, the topic became more controversial after the Second World War, as detailed in chapter 4. Some food allergists, such as Theron Randolph (1906–1995), began speculating that food allergy symbolized humanity's increasingly strained relationship with the environment. Soon, food additives—including pesticides, colors, flavors, preservatives, and trace chemicals found in food packaging—were being implicated by food allergists as being particularly allergenic. The environmental message of Randolph and others did little to enamor food allergists to the broader allergy community, particularly the AAA, which was attempting to gain more scientific respectability and was becoming more reliant on the food, chemical, and pharmaceutical industries for financial support. Faced with the derision of their orthodox peers, some food allergists, including Randolph, even abandoned allergy altogether and turned instead to a new discipline: clinical ecology. During this period, ecological theories also had to compete with psychosomatic explanations of allergy, which posited that the ills of many so-called sufferers of food allergy were merely manifestations of psychological problems.

Chapter 5 explains how the schism between food allergists and orthodox allergists was finally made complete by the discovery of immunoglobulin E (IgE) in 1966. For academic immunologists and orthodox allergists, IgE was and is an immunological marker for allergic reactions, proving to them that much of what food allergists had claimed was food allergy was in fact either intolerance or psychosomatic. Although IgE ushered in a new era of scientific respectability for orthodox allergists, it pushed many food allergists to the fringes of medical practice. IgE also made it possible for unscrupulous allergists to market dubious allergy tests, which marginalized food allergists and clinical ecologists even farther.

Although food allergy seemed to be a discredited phenomenon by the 1980s, the unexpected escalation of anaphylactic food allergy, and specifically peanut allergy, thrust it back into the medical and media spotlight during the early 1990s. But while peanut allergy made anaphylactic allergy a major public-health issue, sufferers of chronic food allergy, the patients most often seen by food allergists, continued to be disregarded. Furthermore, instead of sorting through the array of explanations for the recent rash of food allergy diagnoses, allergists concentrated on biomedical treatments, such as desensitization therapy, meaning that the mystery and controversy surrounding food allergy continued to increase, fomenting a host of untested theories. *Another Person's Poison* concludes by suggesting that if the explosion of anaphylactic allergy—and other allergic diseases—is to be explained, food allergists and orthodox allergists should look to reconcile their differences and examine food allergy afresh in a more pluralistic, open-minded, and holistic fashion.

By way of conclusion, it is pertinent to acknowledge an elephant in the room: this is a not only a book about the history of medicine, but also a book about food and the often perplexing relationship between food and health. For people living in the developed world, food is paradoxically seen as much as a threat to as a necessity of life. Overeating, undereating, consuming too much of some foods and not enough of others, and wrestling with how to judge the relative risks of chemicals and organic materials that end up in our food—from the pesticides and hormones that are put there on purpose to drugs and bacteria that are not—these are just some of the vicissitudes of filling one's belly in the twenty-first century.[43] Of course, food has always been a vital element for good or ill in the healing traditions from Hippocrates and Galen on, and adulteration of food has long been a source of concern.[44] Perhaps more important, arguments about the relationship between food and health have always been passionately fought, partly because of the many interests involved, partly because the science involved is complex and often interdisciplinary, but also because we all believe that we are experts about what we eat.[45] As food increasingly became a processed and chemically laden commodity following the Second World War, though, such discussions transcended medicine and became part of broader debates about "pathologies of progress," to use Charles Rosenberg's term, pointing out the negative side effects associated with technological advancement.[46]

The history of food allergy, and those who suffer from it, has a unique role to play in this discourse. This is because food allergy has alternatively been seen as an idiosyncratic immunological dysfunction, meaning that it was the individual patient who was at fault, or instead a heightened protective sensitivity, suggesting that sufferers might be better described as proverbial canaries in the coal mine and demonstrating that something, whether it be in food, in drugs, or in the wider environment, was not quite right and might ultimately prove harmful to all. Lingering not too far below the surface of the chapters that follow is the desire to explore, unpack, and possibly reconcile this dichotomy and, in the end, provide the foundation for better ways to understand and come to terms with food allergy for those who study it and, more important, for those afflicted by it.

ONE

Food Allergy
Before Allergy

DID FOOD ALLERGY EXIST before the term "allergy" was coined by Clemens von Pirquet in 1906?[1] To some medical historians, there is nothing wrong with this question. Diseases, from this perspective, are biological entities that may evolve over time (for example, in the case of antibiotic-resistant superbugs), but that essentially retain the same characteristics. Following an analysis of the available evidence, the insightful historian can match up the descriptions of a historical figure's symptoms with a modern disease. Such retrospective diagnoses have been applied habitually, with the "madness" of King George III (1738–1820) and the fatal illness of Queen Victoria's Prince Albert (1819–1861) being two of many well-known examples.[2]

To a degree, retrospective diagnoses have their purpose. Archaeological investigations into what people suffered and died from in previous eras can provide enormous insights into our understanding of the past.[3] The inevitable debates that rage about what killed Alexander the Great or what caused Charles Darwin's gastrointestinal troubles also raise important issues about how to weigh historical evidence and, at the very least, tend to attract the attention of the media—not always a bad thing.[4] But as many medical historians have argued, applying modern medical categories to historical descriptions of disease can also be misleading because doing so often overlooks the fact that that disease is both a social and a biological phenomenon.[5] As societies change, so do their conceptualizations of disease. Syphilis

transformed from a "carnal scourge," the Great Pox, or the French/Spanish/
Italian/Christian disease, perceived as a foreign threat and best treated with
penance, to a bacterial infection, best treated with penicillin.[6] In contrast,
consumption devolved from a romantic, fashionable disease most likely to
afflict the genteel in the mid-nineteenth century to tuberculosis during the
late nineteenth century, a disease associated with working-class immigrants
in the United States.[7] Along with changes in how diseases are understood
come profound changes in how sufferers experience the disease not only in
terms of diagnosis and treatment but also socially and psychologically. An
investigator might be able to claim that Darwin's gastrointestinal problems
were caused by Crohn's disease, a common twentieth-century condition, but
such a diagnosis, however well defended, does little to tell us about how he
and his family coped with or understood his intestinal troubles, let alone
provide any insight into how stomach pain was interpreted by physicians
during the nineteenth century. The debates over retrospective diagnoses,
therefore, become much sound and fury, signifying nothing.

It has been in the history of psychiatry where retrospective diagnoses
have been most common but also most contentious. In a short publication
from 1958 suitably titled *Retrospective Diagnoses of Historical Figures as
Viewed by Leading Contemporary Psychiatrists*, the pitfalls of the practice
become apparent. In the booklet, figures ranging from Nero to Rasputin
were given psychoanalytically oriented mental disorders based on their reported behaviors; whereas Nero was diagnosed with "sociopathic personality disturbance, dissocial reaction (formerly sociopathic personality with
asocial and amoral trends)," Rasputin was identified as a "psychopath."[8]
The problem with such retrospective diagnoses is that even as early as the
late 1950s, more biologically minded psychiatrists were beginning to reject
disorders that were heavily imbued with psychoanalytic theory, Nero's diagnosis being such an example. By 1980 and the publication of the *Diagnostic
and Statistical Manual of Mental Disorders III* (*DSM-III*), many diagnoses that
psychoanalysts of the 1960s or 1970s would have been comfortable giving
had been expunged. In other words, *Retrospective Diagnoses* tells us more
about the history of postwar psychiatry than it does about key figures in the
Roman or Russian empires.

As the number of psychiatric conditions listed in subsequent editions of
DSM has expanded, and as mental disorder has increasingly been seen in
essential and universal terms that stress its neurological nature, retrospec-

tively diagnosing mental illness has become quite fashionable in both the medical and popular media.[9] A book by the Dublin psychiatrist Michael Fitzgerald, for example, posits that the creativity of figures ranging from Socrates and Darwin to William Butler Yeats and Andy Warhol was due to autism spectrum disorder.[10] Attention deficit hyperactivity disorder (ADHD) has also been foisted on figures ranging from Lord Byron and Mozart to Winston Churchill.[11]

Although there must be a certain thrill in retrospective diagnosis for the historically inclined psychiatrist, the practice does lead to both historical and medical problems. From a historical perspective, such present-centeredness obscures the impact that a whole range of social forces have had in shaping ideas about mental illness across various times and places.[12] The rise and decline of past mental disorders, such as hysteria and neurasthenia, have largely been due to underlying cultural and political changes rather than to psychiatrists simply determining that they did not exist.[13] Even understandings of the most common of today's psychiatric disorders—for example, depression and ADHD—have varied considerably in different parts of the world and will continue to do so.[14]

Retrospectively diagnosing mental disorders also poses problems for both psychiatrists and their patients. By emphasizing that today's mental disorders are both timeless and universal, in other words, biological phenomena that can be applied to people from any period and any place, psychiatrists assume that current conceptualizations of mental illness are without fault and that they always will be so. Such rigid and myopic thinking contributes to a lack of creativity and flexibility in psychiatric practice, which helps explain why mental illness not only is seen to be on the increase but also is dreadfully difficult to treat or explain.

FOOD ALLERGY AS A RETROSPECTIVE DIAGNOSIS

What bearing does the retrospective diagnosis of mental disorders have on the "prehistory" of food allergy, the period before the term "allergy"? It is tempting to delve into historical medical literature to uncover hidden cases of allergy, but similar problems emerge. First and foremost are difficulties related to the changing definitions and use of the term "allergy," debates that have been present ever since von Pirquet coined the word. Von Pirquet's definition of allergy as "any form of altered biological reactivity" encompassed not only dysfunctional immune reactions, for instance, when an individual broke out in hives after eating strawberries, but also normal immune function, such as the building of antibodies after exposure to a virus. Making matters more complicated is that von Pirquet's term did not become the preferred word for reactions we would now call allergic until the 1920s.[15] Before then, physicians preferred Charles Richet's (1850–1935) term "anaphylaxis," which the French physiologist coined in 1902 to describe cases in which repeated exposure to foreign proteins caused an increase, rather than a decrease, in sensitivity. Since the 1920s, though, anaphylaxis has been used only to describe certain types of allergic responses, such as the sudden, intense, and often life-threatening reactions to bee stings, medication, latex, and, of course, peanuts and other foods.

The word "allergy" has also been used liberally in common speech, to express a pronounced distaste for something instead of a genuine allergic reaction: "I'm allergic to onions, plastic pillows, and Sam," or "I'm allergic to poetry."[16] Some basketball players are "allergic to the paint," meaning they like to shoot from the outside rather than muscle in close for a layup. Employing the word in this way resembles the loose use of psychiatric terms today, when someone is described as a "little autistic" or a "little ADHD." Although some people might bristle at such casual use, the very applicability of these terms indicates how behavior characterized in mental disorders exists on a continuum stretching from the fairly normal, if a little odd, to the pathological, where it severely affects an individual's ability to cope in society or form functional relationships. Loose use of the word "allergic" also highlights debates about the term itself. While orthodox allergists have restricted their definition of allergy to pathological immune responses to foreign proteins, typified in anaphylaxis, others have applied the term more broadly, encompassing reactions that do not seem to involve the immune system. When it comes to retrospective diagnosis of food allergy, the definition of allergy has long been contentious, but it has also been fluid in both medical and popular contexts and will likely remain so.[17]

All this is not to say that there is no point to investigating how physicians and patients explained strange reactions to food in the centuries before the word "allergy" entered the lexicon. In contrast, doing so can be extremely useful both as a historical enterprise in itself and in terms of setting the stage for the history of food allergy in the twentieth century. In what follows, I do not engage in the practice of retrospective diagnosis, but investigate the

prehistory of food allergy, which is quite a different task. Instead of attempting to prove that reports of bizarre food reactions were what we would now
call food allergy, I hope to show how such responses were understood prior
to the emergence of allergy as a medical and cultural phenomenon. How
did physicians interpret strange responses to food before 1906? Were they
common explanations for otherwise unexplained symptoms? If they were
not a regular feature of medical practice, does this mean that reactions to
food were unheard of—a conclusion that might support some current theories about the epidemiology of food allergy—or does it mean instead that
compared with the vast amount of endemic infectious disease and nasty
pathogens commonly found in poorly preserved food, they were believed
to be clinically unimportant? Either way, what bearing does the history of
such reactions, the prehistory of food allergy, have on the understandings of
food allergy that emerged after von Pirquet coined his term? While unusual
reactions to food may not have dominated medical discussions prior to the
twentieth century, they have long been recognized and have often triggered
debates, many of which have not been resolved.

BIZARRE REACTIONS TO FOOD IN ANTIQUITY

In an allergy textbook, the Dutch physician W. Storm Van Leeuwen (1882–
1933) wrote:

> Hypersensitiveness to foodstuffs was undoubtedly the earliest recognized form
> of allergy. Nearly everybody knows that the ingestion of strawberries, lobster,
> crab, shrimps, and various fishes, and also meat and eggs, may cause disagree-
> able and even serious symptoms in some people whereas other people are able
> to eat any amount of these foodstuffs without experiencing any such effects.
> With reference to the prohibition in the Hebrew creed against eating pork, it
> is interesting that this meat seems more apt to induce allergic symptoms than
> any other meat which is generally eaten.[18]

As Van Leeuwen hinted, there is a rich history of different groups across
time and place avoiding foods for a variety of cultural, economic, and, especially, religious reasons. Although some have argued that associating
the consumption of particular foods with ill health helps to explain some
such aversions—for instance, linking pork consumption with trichinosis—
there is little evidence that idiosyncratic reactions, despite Van Leeuwen's

musings, have influenced such dietary practices to a great degree.[19] One exception to this, however, is found in Ponape, one of the Caroline Islands of
the South Pacific, where symptoms similar to those associated with food allergy (diarrhea, hives, dermatitis, and asthma) occur in people who eat food
that is considered taboo. Many of these foods, particularly fish and shellfish,
are commonly associated with food allergies.[20] Such an example might be
unique or at least have an underlying psychosomatic explanation, but it
does point to the possibility that idiosyncratic responses to certain foods
may have influenced how such foods were perceived at certain times and
places.

More generally, dietary advice, including advice about bizarre reactions
to particular foods, was certainly central to many ancient medical philos-
ophies, including traditional Chinese medicine and the humoral medicine
of Hippocrates (460–370 B.C.E.) and Galen (ca. 130–210).[21] Dietary remedies
were common in ancient Chinese medicine, and the quasi-mythical Chinese
emperor Shen Nung is also said to have urged pregnant women to avoid fish,
shrimp, chicken, and horse meat in order to prevent skin ulcerations.[22] For
the followers of Hippocrates and Galen, diet played a pivotal role in balancing the four humors (blood, black bile, yellow bile, and phlegm), which, in
turn, represented combinations of the four qualities of hot, cold, dry, and
wet. Although there were some general rules in terms of the humoral ten-
dencies of particular people—men were usually hot and dry (yellow bile),
women were usually cold and wet (phlegm), and children were warm and
wet (blood)—each individual had his own specific humoral constitution,
meaning that a dietary regimen that was healthy for one person would not
necessarily be healthy for another.[23]

The individualized nature of humoralism suggests that bizarre, idiosyncratic reactions to foods would not be terribly difficult to incorporate into
the overarching medical philosophy. Suitably, one of the first known discussions of such reactions is associated with Hippocrates. In a discussion
of how "knowledge about the physical sciences can be acquired from medicine," Hippocrates highlighted how food and drink can have remarkably
diverse effects on different people.[24] His specific example was cheese: "For
there are many other bad foods and bad drinks, which affect a man in different ways. . . . To take my former example, cheese does not harm all men alike;
some can eat their fill of it without the slightest hurt, nay, those it agrees
with are wonderfully strengthened thereby. Others come off badly."[25] Al-

though Hippocrates did not specify what it meant to "come off badly," he did hypothesize about the mechanism behind such reactions:

> So the constitutions of these men differ, and the difference lies in the constituent of the body which is hostile to cheese, and is roused and stirred to action under its influence. Those in whom a humour of such a kind is present in greater quantity, and with greater control over the body, naturally suffer more severely. But if cheese were bad for the human constitution without exception, it would have hurt all.[26]

Hippocrates's description of the "constituent of the body which . . . is roused and stirred to action," is particularly evocative of what we might today describe as an overactive immune system. Stating that the "humour" may be present in varying quantities also suggests that the reaction portrayed by Hippocrates was not an either/or phenomenon but one that may have existed on a continuum, which fits in neatly with other aspects of Hippocratic medicine that emphasize the importance of balancing humors through a regimen that includes diet, exercise, rest, bathing, and emetics.[27]

The other famous classical reference to bizarre food reactions may not become quite so evocative of allergy on close examination but nonetheless has become the food allergist's aphorism. The saying "one man's food is another man's poison" is attributed to Lucretius (98–55 B.C.E.), a Roman poet, philosopher, and Epicurean, and is found in his didactic poem *De Rerum Natura* (*On the Nature of Things*). Although the adage has been adopted by allergists (and me in the title of this book), the context of the quotation indicates that Lucretius was not describing the same kinds of idiosyncratic somatic reactions that Hippocrates depicted, but rather how individuals and, specifically, animals may differ markedly with respect not only to taste but also to the digestibility of certain foods:

> *And now why different creatures need a different kind of food*
> *I will explain;*
> *And why what seems to one most sweet,*
> *Seems to another evil, noisome, bad.*
> *The difference is very great.*
> *That which is food to one to others proves*
> *A biting poisonous curse.*
> *There is a snake you know, which only touched with human spit,*

Must straightaway die, itself devour itself.
The too the hellebore, to men a biting, poisonous curse
Makes goats and quails grow fat.[28]

In this translation, Lucretius appears to be discussing differences between species rather than differences between individual humans: "That which is food to one to others proves / A biting poisonous curse," given the context of "why different creatures need a different kind of food," does not seem to emphasize humans at all. Other translations, however, have interpreted the same passage as "one man's meat is not another's, and what is bitter and unpalatable to one may strike another as delicious," which does suggest that Lucretius was thinking about the ways humans differ significantly with respect to taste.[29] While the former translation does not lend itself well to notions of allergy that would follow, the latter certainly does, indicating both the complexities of classical translation and how a phrase uttered in one context (and in one language) can be adopted for quite different purposes in another. In this way, Lucretius's aphorism mirrors the ways in which the term "allergy" itself has been reshaped and adapted during the twentieth century.

Likewise, Lucretius's explanation for this peculiar phenomenon foreshadows some of the metaphors that have been used to describe the mechanism of allergy and, more broadly, immunity:

That atom shapes are mingled in all different things,
Quite differently.
All living things that feed on food are outwardly unlike,
A different shaping of the limbs encloses them,
Kind after kind.
So they are made of varying atom shapes.
And as the atom seeds are all unlike
So are the intervals, the passages, the pores—
Different in all their limbs and in the mouth and palate too.
Some must be small, some great;
For certain creatures they must be triangular;
For others square, for many round,
For some with many angles variously arranged.
For as the motion and the shape of atom stuff demands

The passages must vary too,
Just like the texture of the stuff enclosing them.
And so, when bitter food seems sweet to some,
For him to whom the food tastes sweet,
The smoothest atom shapes
Must enter in the pores caressingly.
For him to whom it's sour
The rough and jagged atoms enter in the pores.[30]

Lucretius's description of atoms and passages of different shapes resembles how mid-twentieth-century immunologists, notably the Australian Nobel laureate Frank Macfarlane Burnet, explained the production of antibodies.[31] According to Burnet, the body identifies substances to which it came into contact as either "self" or "non-self."[32] When antigens—for example, foreign bacteria or viruses—are identified as non-self, the immune system creates matching antibodies in order to protect itself in the future.

In most cases, food is seen as "self," so no immune response is necessary; food allergies occur when the body mistakenly perceives a particular food as "non-self" and launches an excessive, potentially fatal immune response in a Pyrrhic attempt to protect the body. As an Epicurean, Lucretius advocated atomic theory, so his idea of "mouth and palate" acted as a kind of atomic immune system, demonstrating through taste which foods and, by extension, which food atoms should be consumed, and attesting that "there must be atomic differences in the different organs of taste."[33] While foods that contain atoms that a body recognizes as "self" taste sweet, other substances are identified as "non-self" through their bitter taste and are rejected.

Although Lucretius (again, depending on the translation) did not suggest as explicitly as Hippocrates that individual constitutional differences could drastically alter responses to particular foods, he did indicate that illness could alter the way in which the body perceived the atoms entering it as food:

When raging fever has attacked a man
Or bile flows high,
Or when the violent onset of disease is roused in other ways
Why then the body as a whole is disarrayed.
And what before suited his taste

Suits it no more;
But other atoms shapes are better suited now
To penetrate, excite a bitter taste.
Now in the taste of honey there are mingled both—
Bitter and sweet.[34]

This description is not particularly suggestive of allergy, but it highlights how the function of Lucretius's atomic system could fluctuate when the body was under duress. Although Lucretius's explanation differed from that of Hippocrates, both acknowledged how foods considered nutritious and tasty to some were the opposite for others.

It is possible to find a handful of other references to strange reactions to food during the classical period, though none are as evocative as the musings of Hippocrates and Lucretius. In the beginning of *On the Properties of Foodstuffs*, Galen described how foods that were easily digestible by some people could be quite unpalatable for others. Some, according to Galen, digested beef more easily than "rock fish," a phenomenon he attributed to a "constitutional peculiarity."[35] The consumption of honey and lentils could also trigger disparate symptoms, depending on one's constitutional peculiarity.

Other anecdotes described by Galen are also reminiscent of food allergy. One such case involved a baby who was covered with sores (or ulcers) after drinking the breast milk of a wet nurse who "lived on a diet of wild vegetables from the countryside, for it was spring time and a food shortage was pressing."[36] Although the sores bring to mind some of the skin conditions that have been associated with milk allergy (for example, eczema), Galen's assertion that the wet nurse and others in the area also suffered from similar sores suggests that the problem lay not with the milk itself but with the wild vegetables. Indeed, strange dermatological reactions to other seasonal fruits and vegetables such as strawberries and asparagus, which are eaten in quantity for a short period of time, have been long cited by other physicians.[37] Nevertheless, many have claimed that this is an instance of Galen describing milk allergy.[38]

Another passage from Galen, which reveals his opinions about eating fresh fruit, showcases the personal connection between food and its effects on health. In a discussion of how Galen gleaned insights about nutrition during his widespread travels, the eminent classicist Vivian Nutton contemplates about whether the physician's "notorious rejection of fresh fruit, which he believes produce bad humours," influenced his theories about the nutritious qualities of other foods.[39] In other words, "How far is Galen generalizing from his own experiences to refute or reject the ideas of others, or to set up his own guidelines for proper diet? This is a major problem, if not *the* major one."[40] It not only is a problem for those who study premodern medicine, given the Galenic dominance of medicine in Europe and the Islamic world until at least the sixteenth century, but also raises questions about the motives and rationales of those who promoted food allergy during the twentieth century. This is because, as discussed later, many food allergists admitted being sufferers of food allergies themselves.

For his part, Nutton discounts the likelihood that an allergy was at the heart of Galen's aversion to fruit. Instead, he contends that fruit's ill effects on Galen were more psychosomatic and linked to Galen's relationship with his father, who was "strongly against fresh fruit."[41] When Galen broke his father's taboo as a young man, eating "a large quantity of autumnal fresh fruits," the result was "an acute illness, cured only by venesection."[42] The illness returned when his father died, and it continued during his eight-year period of study away from home. It disappeared only when Galen gave up fruit altogether, save for small amounts of figs and grapes, and then returned home to Pergamon to resume his familial duties, suggesting a relationship between the illness and Galen's guilt about disobeying his father and leaving home.[43] Whatever the explanation, Galen's attitude toward fresh fruit highlights that ancient physicians believed strongly in the connection between food and health and that their tendency to generalize about diet was often based on their own experiences.[44]

IDIOSYNCRASIES AND DIET

After the classical period, it is difficult to find many examples of strange reactions to food in medical writing or literature until the dawn of the nineteenth century. To a degree, this lacuna is understandable. Western medical thought until at least the sixteenth century was dominated by humoralism, which allowed for a considerable degree of variation with respect to individuals and their constitutions. An individual's aversion to a particular food might be thought necessary to redress a humoral imbalance rather than be indicative of anything peculiar. It is also likely that many untoward reactions to food were due to food poisoning or adulteration—for instance, mixing chalk into flour to stretch it out—both of which practices continue to be causes of ill health.[45] Moreover, the diets of all but the wealthy were relatively restricted compared with those of the present, meaning that the likelihood of an adverse reaction to a particular food was considerably less. Finally, given the number of endemic infectious diseases, ranging from smallpox and tuberculosis to typhoid and diphtheria, combined with widespread malnutrition, vitamin deficiency, and comparatively poor living conditions, it is probable that strange reactions to food were not at the top of many physicians' lists of concerns.

That said, it is possible to find instances where bizarre reactions to foods are described by physicians, usually using the term "idiosyncrasy,"[46] which could apply to any number of singular or unusual predispositions, sometimes connected to health but not always.[47] The Arabic polymath Avicenna or Ibn Sīnā (980–1037), for instance, described how "an idiosyncrasy of the stomach" could lead to diarrhea, adding: "Good and laudable foods may be injurious to some."[48] More generally, Robert James's *Medicinal Dictionary* (1743) defined "idiosyncrasy" as follows: "Every Individual has a State of Health peculiar to himself; and as different Bodies seem to vary from each other, both with respect to the Solids and Fluids, tho' each may, at the same time, be in a sound Condition, this Peculiarity of Constitutions, by which they differ from other sound Bodies, is called Idiosyncrasy."[49] The example James provided of idiosyncrasy underneath his dictionary definition did not involve a food but a drug, specifically a medication used to treat hysteria. Referencing the prominent English physician Thomas Sydenham (1624–1689), James described how "some women, by reason of a certain Idiosyncrasy, or Peculiarity of Constitution, have so great an Aversion to hysteric Medicines, which are so generally serviceable in this Disease, that instead of being reliev'd, they are injur'd thereby. In such, therefore, they are to be wholly omitted; for, as *Hippocrates* observes, it is fruitless to oppose the Tendency of Nature."[50] James proceeded to warn that idiosyncrasy was "so remarkable, and so common, that unless Regard be had to it, the Life of the Patient may be endanger'd," adding that other drugs and plasters could trigger such reactions in susceptible individuals.[51] As far as idiosyncrasies to food, the only one James mentioned involved melons. The sweet flesh of melons may be delicious, but it could also cause fevers and gripes, due to its "cold and humid" quality and tendency "to putrefy in the Stomach."[52] But other symptoms associated with consuming melons, he added, were due to idiosyncrasy rather than their humoral properties.

One of James's contemporaries, the Scottish physician William Cullen (1710–1790), who defined "idiosyncrasy" as "a peculiarity of temperament in a particular part of the system," similarly associated it with unintended reactions to medicine as well as idiosyncrasies to food.[53] In *Lectures on the Materia Medica* (1773), Cullen explained how certain individuals had idiosyncrasies to honey, egg, and crab. In the case of even "a small bit of egg, crab, &c" (sadly, Cullen does not state the foods represented by "&c."), the reactions were described as "spasmodic symptoms . . . which . . . can only be explained from idiosyncrasy."[54] Other eighteenth-century writers wrote about idiosyncrasies to milk, but as with James and Cullen, strange reactions to drugs were more commonly described than those to food prior to the nineteenth century.[55]

During the nineteenth century, however, idiosyncrasy was increasingly associated with diet, in both the medical and the popular literature. Writing in 1884, a London-based emeritus professor of surgery, John Hutchinson (1828–1913), described idiosyncrasy as "a peculiarity of constitutions in some one particular feature developed to a height which at first sight seems inexplicable and possibly almost absurd. It is individuality run mad."[56] Idiosyncrasies were present at birth and tended not to "undergo modification" with age.[57] Hutchinson explained how surgeons, such as himself, were accustomed to idiosyncrasies to particular drugs, such as quinine, bromides, or iodides, but felt obliged to discuss "diet idiosyncrasy," since it was common for patients to inquire about the phenomenon.[58] Eggs were of particular interest to Hutchinson, ever since

several patients consulted me within a short period, who . . . described a liability to attacks of violent vomiting, or of a sense of sinking and abdominal distress which were to them inexplicable. In more than one of these the reason of my being consulted was that the attacks were attended by temporary defect in sight. In one instance the patient was an artist, who declared that frequently he was quite unable, for several hours at a time, to see to paint. . . . It always affected both eyes, and was always attended by a sense of heat at the stomach and abdominal discomfort. I found that these attacks usually occurred within an hour or two of breakfast, and on entering into detail I became convinced that they were due to eating eggs. On telling my patient my conclusion he replied at once that he had always suspected it, yet being very fond of eggs, he had indulged in one once in a month or so. He was quite cured by abstinence. [59]

Other patients experienced symptoms so violent that Hutchinson suspected poisoning. While some reacted to all eggs, even in a small quantity or hidden in a pudding, others reacted only to eggs from certain birds, or those cooked in a particular way.

Although Hutchinson also indicated that tea, fish, lobster, and wine could also cause dietary idiosyncrasies, his focus on eggs is interesting for a number of reasons. First, eggs were frequently cited as a cause of strange reactions and continue to be high on the list of allergens.[60] Second, eggs, specifically egg white or albumen, would commonly be used by early laboratory investigators of allergy in their investigations, hinting that their propensity to sensitize was well known.[61] Third, since eggs were commonly used in cooking and baking, those sensitive to them were liable to consume them without knowing it. One account from a late-nineteenth-century American newspaper, for example, described a young girl who "could not drink coffee that was cleared with an egg" and reacted to the most infinitesimal amount of egg found in baked goods.[62] Because of the ubiquity of eggs in food preparation, egg idiosyncrasies were difficult to identify, meaning that, at least according to Hutchinson, the testimony of patients had to be treated seriously.[63]

Although Hutchinson emphasized egg idiosyncrasies, he acknowledged that "innumerable" examples existed, suggesting that most patients would exhibit some such peculiarity. Hutchinson's acceptance of individual differences, along with his willingness to trust his patients' accounts of their symptoms, marks out one side of a dichotomy that would characterize the way physicians viewed the relationship between food and mysterious symptoms. Specifically, while some physicians put their faith in general principles or theories, which explained most clinical phenomena, others, including Hutchinson, were eager to explore cases, such as those involving dietary idiosyncrasy, in which the rules did not seem to apply. Whether it be migraine headaches, asthma, or skin conditions at issue, the tension between general dietary rules and exceptional nutritional idiosyncrasies was fraught.

SICK HEAD-ACH, OR MEGRIM

In a paper delivered to the Royal Society of Physicians of London in 1778, John Fothergill, a physician, botanist, and Quaker preacher, presented his theories about "sick head-ach," or what other physicians would call migraine, bilious headache, hemicrania, blind-headache, or megrim, headaches that were associated with nausea, vomiting, and visual disturbances.[64] Fothergill, no stranger to such headaches himself, stated that they were common and emphasized that while sedentary individuals were more likely to suffer from them than others, diet was the primary cause. He proceeded to explain:

> There are some things which, in very small quantities, seldom fail to produce the sick head-ach in some constitutions. Such are a larger proportion than usual of melted butter, fat meats, and spices, especially common black pepper. Meat pies often contain all these things united, and are as fertile a cause of this complaint as anything I know; so are rich baked puddings, and every thing of a similar nature. A little error in these things will seldom fail to be attended with much suffering, in many constitutions. . . . Most kinds of malt liquor, taken too liberally, seldom fail to have this effect in particular constitutions, perhaps from the quantity of hops; for most bitters seem rather to increase, than lessen the complaint.[65]

Although emetics, cathartics, and laxatives, along with mineral waters, could help achieve relief, Fothergill warned:

> We are, perhaps, too ready, in chronic cases, where digestion is concerned, to confide in the *materia medica*, and judge it sufficient to select and enjoin such articles in our prescriptions, as are of known use in such cases. But unless the whole plan of diet, both in kind and quantity, are made to conspire with medical prescription, the benefits arising from this are hourly annihilated by neglect or indulgence.[66]

Like many of his contemporaries, Fothergill added that eating slowly and resisting the urge to eat too much (two meals per day was ideal) would not only help to manage "chronic and anomalous diseases" but also preserve health more generally.[67]

On the one hand, Fothergill's advice about sick head-ach amounted simply to general dietary guidance that would be applicable to everyone. As the sociologist Stephen Mennell has observed, dietary advice was proffered in most medical textbooks and primers, in which certain foods were damned and others were praised.[68] The historian Ken Albala and others have also elaborated on the interest in dietary regimens for health during the Renaissance, showcasing the long-standing connection between food and health in Europe.[69] Eminent physicians, such as George Cheyne (1671–1743), writing in his seminal text on nervous disorders, *The English Malady*, argued that

diet was central to health, contending, like Fothergill, that the quality and
the quantity of the foods one ate should match one's lifestyle: robust, active
individuals should not eat a "thin, poor, cool, low Diet;" a "poor, thin, low,
valetudinary Creature" should not eat a gross, full, high Diet."[70] The Scottish politician and agriculturalist Sir John Sinclair (1754–1835), who wrote
a survey of gerontology called *The Code of Health and Longevity*, similarly
agreed with Fothergill that eating in moderation was one of the keys to a
long life.[71] As Fothergill condemned certain foods, such as melted butter,
others heaped praise or scorn on other articles of diet. The nineteenth-century surgeon Edward Jukes, writing about intestinal complaints, described
turnips as "a useless, harmless laxative, affording but little nutrition," and
peas as "extremely indigestible" and to "be avoided by delicate stomachs."[72]
Oysters, uncooked milk, raspberries, and apples fared better in Jukes's esti-
mation. Jukes was particularly concerned about avoiding foods that would
cause flatulence and other embarrassing bodily functions, which were, as
Mennell suggests, a major source of apprehension and even fear for many
people.[73]

On the other hand, Fothergill's discussion of the idiosyncratic aspects of
sick head-ach brings to mind many of the debates that would envelop food
allergy during the nineteenth century. First, the physician's admission that
he himself suffered from such symptoms provides an example of a clinician
who studied a condition from which he suffered, and it also foreshadows
the very intimate relationship that many future proponents of food allergy
had with the disorder. While this personal connection to food allergy often
fostered a relationship of trust and empathy between clinician and patient,
it raised the suspicions of those who downplayed the clinical importance
of the condition. How could the objectivity of clinicians be ensured in such
cases?[74] Second, although Fothergill warned that certain dietary habits,
primarily overeating and eating too quickly, contributed to sick head-ach,
he also emphasized the importance of each person's constitution. In other
words, there was something inherent in the makeup of certain individuals
that made them incapable of consuming rich foods, such as melted butter,
meat pies, and hoppy malt liquors, without suffering dire consequences.
Inactive individuals might be more disposed to such reactions than others,
but at the heart of the condition was a constitutional difference, which de-
manded changes in diet instead of the prescription of medicine.

Fothergill's assertion that errors of diet were largely responsible for sick head-ach would influence both later physicians and popular notions of migraine. In a book on what he termed "megrim," Edward Liveing (1832–1919), who served as the registrar of the Royal College of Physicians, explained how the public was convinced that bilious food was responsible for so-called bilious headaches:

> So deeply rooted with the general public is the notion that most headaches of this class are produced by this cause . . . strengthened as this conviction is in the minds of many sufferers by the retching and consequent discharge of bile which often attends the attacks, that the greatest caution is necessary in accepting statements which such persons make on this subject, and especially the loose and conventional expressions they constantly employ in speaking of their complaints.[75]

One of Liveing's patients believed that bilious food, specifically butter, caused her megrim. After investigating, however, Liveing argued that the headaches were more likely to be hereditary, since her sister also suffered from them, and he hinted that the patient's neuroses might also be partly responsible, something that other physicians, including the Swiss Samuel August Tissot (1728–1797), had also suggested.[76] Dietary explanations were so common that Liveing was surprised when one of his other patients was "never . . . able to trace an attack to any indiscretion in diet or to any particular kind of food."[77] Although Liveing agreed that diet could play a role, it was not always the explanation, and Liveing gently chastised Fothergill for focusing so much on such explanations. While wine, including that of the sacramental variety, and burned pastry had unfailingly triggered megrim in one physician known to Liveing for thirty years, "probably a majority, who, notwithstanding the force of long tradition, unhesitatingly deny the influence for the better or worse of any dietary."[78]

Contemporaries of Liveing also acknowledged that the relationship between diet and migraine was complicated and controversial. In *The Principles and Practices of Medicine*, Charles Fagge and Philip Pye-Smith explained that while popular bilious theories of migraine were a "relic" of humoral medicine, "there is yet no question that some error of diet is often the direct exciting cause of an attack in a person who is liable to it. . . . [S]ome persons at least can always bring on an attack by eating particular articles of diet."[79] Although they argued that mental, physical, or visual fatigue was the most likely cause of such headaches, it was also worthwhile to pay attention to the patient's diet, though restrictions of "bilious" foods, such as butter and cream, were unnecessary.[80] In contrast, the Edinburgh physician Offley Bohun Shore, a cousin of Florence Nightingale, urged migraine sufferers to avoid "rich articles" and "highly-dressed foods," foods that contained a great deal of seasoning and sauce, such as stews and pastries.[81] In the case of migraine, as with other intractable conditions, physicians struggled to reconcile the opinions expressed by both their patients and the general public that blamed "errors in diet" for their sufferings with a theoretical understanding of the underlying mechanism for such symptoms. This balancing act continued to challenge physicians involved in treating food allergy throughout the twentieth century.

ASTHMA

Other chronic, debilitating conditions, which physicians had difficulty explaining and treating successfully, were also commonly attributed to dietary factors. Diet, as Mark Jackson has outlined, has long been thought to be important in controlling asthma, featuring in the theories of writers ranging from the medieval Jewish scholar Moses Maimonides (1138–1204) to the English physician John Floyer (1649–1734), who suffered from it himself.[82] For Maimonides, foods could have both a positive and a negative effect on asthmatic symptoms. While foods ranging from the lungs of foxes to pickled fish were prophylactic, foods that "produced thick or sticky humors" and "increased the accumulation of phlegm"—such as milk, cheese, "juicy fresh fruits," spices, certain types of bread, and the meat of ducks and geese— ought to be restricted. Wine, drunk in moderation, could help some asthma sufferers; excess consumption was likely to trigger an attack.[83] Floyer, who also saw asthma in terms of a humoral imbalance, declared that "no Distemper requires more orderly Diet than Asthma," and, in addition to discouraging the consumption of alcohol, recommended that asthmatics avoid "all that produces a viscid Chyle, thickens the Humours, creates Phlegm and Wind, and stops the Breathing, such is that of Pudding, Crust, and most Meal-meats, of Rice, Peas, Beans; and Milk-meats, as Cream, Cheese, etc., and amongst Flesh-meats as Fish, Eggs, young Creatures, young Pigs, and the Extremity of Animals, and Jelly Broths, Oysters."[84] Although Floyer stated that a number of meats, including mutton, poultry, and pork, were tolerated by asthmatics, sufferers were advised to eat "a very frugal and simple Diet" and to fast regularly.[85]

The humoral conceptualizations of asthma presented by Maimonides and Floyer may have become less influential by the eighteenth century, but many physicians continued to associate particular foods with asthma attacks. Authors of asthma texts, including John Millar (1733–1805), Thomas Withers (1750–1809), and Robert Bree (1759–1839), all indicated that diet played a role in the condition.[86] Asthma was also blamed on other factors, including changes in the weather, "violent exercise," dust, "the fumes of metals and minerals," constipation, anxiety, fatigue, and mental excitement, and, as such, treatments could vary considerably.[87] According to Spencer Thomson, the author of a nineteenth-century dictionary of domestic medicine, the "peculiar" nature of asthma meant that "what gives immediate and full relief to one person totally fails in another."[88] Given that this was the case, and the history of blaming "errors in diet" for asthma, it is not surprising that dietary explanations continued to be cited in medical journals, textbooks, domestic medical manuals, and the writing of the most important authority on asthma during the nineteenth century, Henry Hyde Salter (1823–1871).

Salter was a London physician and, at age thirty-three, the youngest Fellow to be elected to both the Royal College of Physicians and the Royal Society.[89] He was also, as with many physicians who studied asthma, an asthmatic. Along with a slew of journal articles, his chief contribution to the study of asthma was *On Asthma: Its Pathology and Treatment*, first published in 1860.[90] As did Thomson, Salter highlighted the obduracy of asthma, stating that its etiology was the most difficult aspect of the condition for physicians to explain.[91] Reminiscent of Fothergill's and Liveing's discussions of migraine headaches, Salter emphasized that the causes of asthma were twofold: the immediate trigger of an asthma attack, or paroxysm, and the predisposing tendency to have such spasms, which tended to be hereditary.[92] In terms of the former, Salter listed four triggers:

· Irritants admitted into the air passage in respiration
· Alimentary irritants (errors in diet)
· Sources of remote nervous irritation
· Psychical irritants[93]

Despite this rather straightforward list, the causes of individual cases of asthma were stubbornly unique:

> There are probably no two cases alike in the list of things that will bring on an attack; what will be certain to do so in one case will be innocuous in another, and what will be fatal in the other will be innocent in the one. . . . In nothing, I think, does asthma shew its caprice more than in the choice of its exciting causes; every case almost furnishes something new and curious in this respect. The mere enumeration of the whole list would be portentously long.[94]

Underlying all such individual triggers, however, was nothing more definite than "an asthmatic tendency . . . the asthmatic idiosyncrasy with which the individual was born."[95]

Although Salter believed that respiratory irritants, ranging from animal hairs (Salter once described his own affliction as "cat asthma") and pollen to smoke and dust, were the most common triggers, dietary factors were also "a very fruitful source, highlighting an intimate connection between the stomach and the lungs."[96] Food could be pernicious not only if it was "of the wrong quality" but also if it was taken in excess or consumed too late in the day, which was certain to trigger an attack.[97] While the causes of asthma were elusive, Salter did stress that asthmatics tended to be dyspeptic; they were liable to have irritable stomachs and were accustomed to restricting their diets in order to obtain relief. It was highly unlikely to find an asthmatic "with a perfectly sound, strong stomach, about which he has never to think."[98] Short of changing residence to a location where there were fewer respiratory irritants, the best way to prevent asthma was through dietary change.[99]

With respect to the quality of foods, Salter's own attacks were especially triggered by foods "in any way *preserved* . . . such as potted meats, dried tongue, sausages, stuffing and seasoning . . . preserved ginger, candied orange-peel, dried figs, raisins—especially almonds and raisins (a vicious combination)." Cheese, nuts, meat pies, coffee, and malt liquors were also branded as especially "asthmatic."[100] One of Salter's patients claimed that there was "as much asthma in a mouthful of decayed Stilton as in a whole dinner." Another asserted that his asthma was completely dependent on whether he indulged in "the customary post-prandial cup of coffee."[101] Instead of such "unwholesome" victuals, food ought to be plain and well cooked, but also varied; an overly rigid, repetitious, and tedious diet could actually impede proper digestion, resulting in more attacks. Since Salter recommended that asthmatics eat only twice a day, diets also had to be highly nutritious.[102] These general rules, however, could be undermined by the "strongly marked idiosyncrasies in individual cases." While the drinking of Rhine and Bordeaux wines would unquestionably bring about an attack in some of Salter's patients, others reacted only to sherry and port.[103]

Generally speaking, Salter's contemporaries were less likely to stress diet as a cause of asthma. A survey of domestic medical manuals from the mid- to the late nineteenth century indicates that while some works, such as William John Russell's *Domestic Medicine and Hygiene*, were clearly influenced by Salter, nearly quoting him verbatim, others were likely to blame exposure to damp and cold, nervousness, "particular states of atmosphere," or other factors.[104] Nevertheless, diet would continue to be a common, if controversial, explanation for asthma, increasingly so during the twentieth century.

SKIN CONDITIONS

As with migraine and asthma, dermatological complaints were attributed to a wide range of factors during the nineteenth century, including diet. Although the Yorkshire physician Robert Willan (1757–1812) attributed urticaria (nettle rash or hives) to "almonds, mushrooms, herrings, crab-fish, mussels, and lobsters," as early as 1809, William Tilbury Fox's *Atlas of Skin Diseases* blamed the same condition on

> mental emotion, nervous debility, especially from over-work and mental strain, exposure to great alternations of temperature, the circulation of acrid substances, such as uric acid and its allies in gouty and rheumatic subjects and in dyspeptics, or the bile acids, in the blood-current; the action upon the skin of external irritants, such as pediculi [lice]; reflexed irritation from sexual disorder; bad feeding and living in damp tenements.[105]

With respect to diet, Fox stated that shellfish, pork, fruit, mushrooms, and coffee were among the most common triggers of urticaria.[106] The Scottish medical professor McCall Anderson similarly believed that many of these foods could cause nettle rash, and added nuts, onions, garlic, wheat, cocoa, pork, and sausage to the mix.[107] Furthermore, a "medical friend" of Anderson's claimed that hawthorns, raisins, prunes, figs, dates, grapes, peas, beans, oily pastries, tea, and flour dusted onto scones, among other foods, were the cause of his nettle rash. For this sufferer, the only treatment was a brandy or whisky: "[I]ndeed, I can eat most of the above-mentioned articles if I am drinking whisky toddy at the time."[108] A relative of Anderson's also wrote to him, describing that if he consumed "butcher's meat," he would develop a "lump in his stomach," followed by "nettle-rash on my wrists, my arms, my groins, and other tender parts of the skin." Soon, the inside of his throat and nose would swell, his voice would go hoarse, and he would get congested, as if suffering from a cold.[109] Although other family members similarly suffered from nettle rash, they reacted to different foods, including barley meal and oatmeal.[110] In a whimsical conclusion to his missive, Anderson's relative suggested that his meat idiosyncrasy could have a unique scientific function: "If you will make it worth my while, I will come down at the Whitsuntide holidays and be exhibited. I will also eat the Ornithorhynchus paradoxus [duck-billed platypus], if can catch one unstuffed, and finally determine whether it be bird or beast."[111]

The faith of Anderson's relative in the unfailing nature of his idiosyncrasy represents one end of the spectrum by which the relationship between diet and skin diseases could be interpreted. For Anderson, diet was such an important cause of nettle rash that determining the articles at fault through empirical investigation and cooperation with the patient was an essential starting point for every case.[112] Not all physicians, however, embraced this approach, and many questioned the link between skin conditions, such as urticaria, purpura (a purplish rash), pruritis (itching), and eczema, and dietary idiosyncrasy. A number of reasons were cited for such hesitation. Dermatological conditions, as with asthma and migraine, were difficult to treat and explain. Many of them, particularly eczema, were also liable to affect children and infants disproportionately, meaning that there were implications for infant feeding and child nutrition, divisive subjects in their own right. Dermatologists were also often eager to treat eczema with topical medications rather than trying to determine dietary causes, foreshadowing debates between the members of their profession and allergists during the twentieth century.[113] But most important, dietary theories of skin conditions were popular with the lay public, and this made many physicians skeptical. As the London physician Stephen Mackenzie stated in a speech to the Reading Pathological Society about the study of dermatology:

There is probably no subject in which more deeply rooted convictions have been held, not only in the profession but by the laity, than the connection between diet and disease, both as regards the causation and treatment of the latter; and the subject possesses a peculiar fascination for the lay mind. . . . At the same time probably no subject better illustrates the fallacies of reasoning, the binding influence of authority, and the bias of education. In the study of diseases of the skin we have admirable examples of the faulty conclusions that have been drawn and unrivalled opportunities of correcting them by careful observation and unfettered judgement.[114]

For Mackenzie, such misconceptions were most pronounced in the study of infantile eczema, which was "constantly . . . ascribed to faults in diet—too early or excessive use of starchy food, the premature use of meat or gravy, insufficient or deteriorated quality of the mother's milk, or the use of preserved milk. All these no doubt bring evils of their own, but there is no evidence to connect them with eczema as cause and effect."[115] The inevitable result of blaming foods, according to Mackenzie, was not an improvement of symptoms but the inexorable restriction of the patient's diet.

Other physicians concurred with Mackenzie, blaming popular ideas about dermatology and diet and indicting the untested views of physicians. For example, Walter Smith, Fellow of the Royal College of Physicians of Ireland, asked:

Have we any certain or scientific knowledge of the influence of diet in the causation of diseases of the skin? The belief in the potency of this influence is universal with the laity, and widely acknowledged by the profession generally. But the practice of physicians is partly traditional and is, unfortunately, not always based upon real conviction or sound knowledge, and many circumstances conspire to tempt them to give formal advice which rests upon a slender foundation.[116]

Although the Scottish physician W. Allan Jamieson allowed that certain foods, including seasonal strawberries, could cause urticaria and other skin conditions, he was reluctant to give the views of his patients much credence:

We must reject in large measure the statements volunteered by our patients, though we thereby get much information. The former are vitiated by preconceived impressions, or are based on ill-founded deductions; the latter are necessarily imperfect. The patient in nearly all cases ascribes an immediate effect to his diet, though it may be obvious on the least reflection that the action, if exerted at all, must be remote.[117]

In the discussion that followed Jamieson's article, the division between physicians with respect to dermatological conditions and dietary idiosyncrasy was made abundantly clear. While half of the discussants agreed with Jamieson that very few skin diseases could be attributed to diet, others vehemently disagreed. Dr. Morgan Dockerell, for instance, stated that the views of Jamieson and Smith were absurd, arguing that diet was central to many cutaneous diseases. The discussants were also divided on the subject of whether to trust their patients' opinions when it came to diet and dermatology. Dr. Radcliffe Crocker warned that "it was not wise to go in the face of the prejudices of patients in the matter of diet";[118] Anderson disagreed. For his part, the Liverpool physician G. G. Stoppard Taylor "was astonished at the extraordinary differences of opinion that existed."[119]

● ● ●

THE ASTONISHMENT EXPRESSED by Stoppard Taylor is itself surprising, not so much because of the debates about food allergy that would follow but because, as this chapter suggests, physicians found strange reactions to food bemusing, difficult to explain, and a cause for disagreement long before the "birth of allergy" in 1906. Equally, many of the issues surrounding food allergy that would divide twentieth-century physicians were present in discussions of diet and unexplained symptoms centuries before. How were physicians to balance their patients' individual differences—for example, their humoral, constitutional, or idiosyncratic predispositions—with general dietary rules for health?[120] To what extent should a physician's own experiences of suffering from and trying to treat chronic symptoms, such John Fothergill and Henry Salter's respective battles with migraine and asthma, influence their ideas about such phenomena? Similarly, when did the accumulated weight of anecdotal evidence, for instance, McCall Anderson's list of cases, begin to outweigh accepted theories about what caused certain symptoms? Finally, how should physicians view popular and, indeed, their patients' opinions with respect to the relationship between diet and chronic conditions? Were lay ideas about diet and disease enlightening or merely distracting? As the early history of food allergy indicates, pre-twentieth-century physicians struggled with these issues just as their successors would in the twentieth century.

Before leaving the prehistory of food allergy behind, however, a final note on retrospective diagnosis is needed. As stressed earlier, there are many dangers in medical historians performing retrospective diagnoses using anachronistic medical terms. Such attempts are apt to be misleading and present-centered, reading into the past conceptualizations that are only really appropriate for the present, but they also overshadow more useful questions about how physicians in the past actually did try to explain and treat particular conditions. Since one of the burning questions about food allergy today involves its epidemiology and apparent rapid increase in recent decades, it is appropriate to give some consideration to whether food allergy was a common condition prior to the twentieth century. So, was it?

Perhaps the better way to ask this question is to split it into two: Was food allergy common before the twentieth century and, if so, was it a condition that physicians commonly treated? The answer to the first part of the question is most likely a very qualified and cautious yes. Although there is no evidence to suggest that the rates of such strange reactions rivaled that of food allergy in even the first half of the twentieth century, it seems apparent that idiosyncrasies to food were fairly frequent. As mentioned earlier, a whole host of other issues related to diet and health prior to the twentieth century, ranging from the prevalence of pathogens in food to malnutrition, meant that reacting bizarrely to a particular article might not have been a particularly pressing issue for all but the middle and upper classes.

As for the second half of the question, the answer is slightly more complicated. It is clear that many physicians believed that idiosyncratic reactions to certain foods could be manifested in a host of chronic symptoms, including asthma, migraine, and dermatological problems. It is also likely that many people who had unpleasant and even dangerous reactions to certain foods simply avoided them and never sought the assistance of a physician. This is the sense one gets when reading the letter sent to Anderson by his relative, Mr. Duck-Billed Platypus. There is no inkling in the letter that Anderson's relative has required any guidance from a physician regarding his aversion to meat; on the contrary, he seems very much in command of his idiosyncrasy. The apparent proliferation of lay ideas about dietary idiosyncrasy, about which some physicians were apt to complain, also provides evidence for this. During the twentieth century, such self-diagnosis and

self-treatment through restricting one's diet, remained a common occur-
rence, constantly complicating the epidemiology of food allergy.

Leaving the issue of retrospective diagnosis aside, it is clear that by the
turn of the century, when terms such as "allergy" and "anaphylaxis" were
being coined, those who began exploring such phenomena were not operat-
ing off of a blank slate. The prevalence of food allergy before allergy notwithstanding, both physicians and their patients, not to mention the general
public, had a whole host of opinions about the relationship between diet
and health and, particularly, chronic symptoms that resisted explanation or
effective treatment. The definitions, theories, politics, and economics of allergy during the twentieth century might well have completely transformed
the ways in which bizarre reactions to food were understood when compared with previous centuries, but many of the core issues that would shape
the debates remained.

TWO

Anaphylaxis, Allergy, and the Food Factor in Disease

DEFINITIONS CAN BE DANGEROUS. In 2013, the fifth edition of the *Diagnostic and Statistical Manual of Mental Disorders* (*DSM-5*) was published by the American Psychiatric Association (APA) amid a cloud of controversy. Although there are a number of debates surrounding *DSM-5* (nothing new in the history of this, the psychiatric bible), the one most often discussed involves the proliferation of psychiatric disorders included in the manual.[1] While a psychiatrist during the 1950s had only 128 diagnoses with which to contend, today's psychiatrists have more than 300 options, ranging from fairly standard and long-standing disorders, such as schizophrenia (and some have questioned its validity as well), to abstruse conditions, such as disruptive mood dysregulation disorder, which appears to give a psychiatric explanation for being moody.[2] Does this mean that we are all crazier, or should we start to think a bit more about how psychiatrists define mental disorder?

On the one hand, such an expansion simply reflects changes in psychiatry. During the past forty years, psychiatry went from being dominated by psychoanalysis, which grouped mental disorders into a smaller number of general categories, to biological psychiatry, which has been more eager to differentiate between what it regards as different psychiatric conditions, each reflecting specific neurological dysfunctions.[3] On the other hand, the propagation of mental disorders also hints strongly that many behavioral characteristics once seen as normal have now become pathologized. While the historian Edward Shorter has suggested that such proliferation might indicate that we are less resilient to psychosocial stresses of life, others have suggested that a wide range of political, economic, demographic, philosophical, and technological factors have played a predominant role in the emergence, if not the creation, of new mental disorders.[4] Either way, and overlooking the demise of certain historically important psychiatric conditions, such as hysteria, homosexuality, and multiple-personality disorder, it seems fair to say that the criteria for being mentally ill have been watered down during the past few decades. In fact, the World Health Organization (WHO) estimates that mental illness will be the most common disease worldwide within the next few decades.[5]

DEFINING FOOD ALLERGY

Could one say the same about food allergy? Epidemiological estimates certainly indicate that a growing number of people in a wide range of countries are allergic to food. Although the increase in other immune system disorders, such as multiple sclerosis and Crohn's disease, suggests that there might be underlying causes for the rising rates of immune dysfunction more generally, as with mental disorders, the way one defines food allergy has played a crucial role in indicating its pervasiveness.[6] But just as psychiatrists and the general public have disagreed about the definitions of various mental disorders, casting estimates about the rates of mental illness into doubt, allergists and other physicians have long debated about how to define food allergy. During the twentieth century, the disagreements that arose about defining allergy tended to revolve around two key themes.

First, and most important, was the degree to which a putative food allergy reaction could be proved to have an underlying immunological mechanism. Expressed differently, was there demonstrable evidence that the immune system had gone awry and was taking defensive action against a foreign food protein, as it might do if exposed to a harmful viral pathogen? For some physicians, though certainly not all, this criteria had to be met in order for a reaction to a food to be described as allergic. When such evidence was available, reactions of this sort were typically described as "true food allergy."[7] When it was lacking, the reaction was then dismissed as "food intolerance."[8] For those who resisted such narrow, immunologically focused definitions, preferring to employ a broader definition of food allergy, either the importance of such evidence was overestimated or the immunological mechanisms put forth as evidence for "true food allergy" were poorly understood. Immunity worked in mysterious ways, as it were, and an allergic response might denote more than simply a dysfunctional immune system.

Underlying such differences was a second theme: the tensions and incongruities between clinical experiences of food allergy and laboratory investigations of it. Clinicians, generally speaking, were less concerned about whether the symptoms presented by a patient were examples of "true food allergy" or "food intolerance," than they were in identifying the foods at fault and taking steps to eliminate them. Laboratory researchers, in contrast, were intimately involved in searching for the precise immunological mechanisms behind food allergy and, in turn, elucidating what they revealed about immunity and human physiology. Although there have been plenty of clinicians who have conducted research, and while many have argued that clinical practice could be improved by the knowledge generated in the lab, debates about how to define food allergy were and still are undoubtedly influenced by the gulf between theory and practice. In the preface of the second edition of *Food Allergy and Intolerance*, for example, the editors argued that better understanding of "the 'nuts and bolts' of the gut and its relationship to the immune system" would help improve the clinical treatment of food allergy. They also indicated that in some cases (the example provided was systemic candidiasis, a controversial type of yeast infection associated with irritable bowel syndrome), "the concept may be wrong but empirical dietary management can be successful."[9] The relationship between *Candida* and certain symptoms might never be experimentally proven, but for clinicians and patients who witnessed an improvement of symptoms following the prescription of diets designed to restrict the growth of such yeast, this lack of laboratory evidence mattered little.

Another example of this disparity between theory and practice can be found in the report of the joint committee of the Royal College of Physicians and the British Nutrition Foundation, "A Report on Food Intolerance and Food Aversion," published in 1984. The committee devised three definitions to describe untoward reactions to food:

- Food intolerance: "unpleasant, but reproducible, reaction to a specific food (or ingredient) which lacks either psychological or known physical basis"

- Food allergy: a form of food intolerance "in which an aberrant immune reaction to a food or component occurs"
- Food aversion: "psychological problem with ingesting particular foods, which would not occur if presented in disguised form"[10]

Although these definitions appear fairly straightforward, other allergists suggested that "diagnosis at clinical level is far more difficult to establish," leading to "claims that food allergic reactions are on the increase, whether supposedly due to agricultural or industrial food processes; the use of substances . . . that promote animal growth, preserve and stabilize raw foodstuffs and products for distribution."[11] In other words, official definitions may look definitive on paper, but they are often difficult to apply in practice, contributing not only to inflated rates of food allergy but also to "unproven hunches and speculations" about the underlying causes of such reactions, many of which have been rooted in concerns about the environment and emergent diseases of civilization.[12]

On the other side of such debates, clinicians inclined to narrow the definition of food allergy and, subsequently, downplay its epidemiological significance have also employed definitions selectively. During the early 1960s, for instance, attempts were also made to delineate different types of hypersensitivity,[13] partly out of concern with the "imprecise usage of the term allergy."[14] The British immunologists P. G. H. Gell (1914–2001) and R. R. A. Coombs (1921–2006) responded by describing four types of hypersensitivity reactions:

- Anaphylactic, involving the immediate release of pharmacologically active substances, such as histamine, which trigger an immune response
- Cytolytic, when an antigen present on the surface of a cell combines with an antibody to destroy the cell
- Inflammatory, caused by an excess of either antigens or antibodies
- Cellular, delayed reactions which are mediated not by antibodies but by white blood cells[15]

Although Gell and Coombs's classification was well received, and while all four reactions have been implicated in food allergy and intolerance, conservative allergists intent on restricting the definition of food allergy often ignored types two, three, and four, focusing solely on type one, that of anaphylactic reactions.[16] Definitions of food allergy, as these examples indicate, have historically been manipulated by allergists to suit their preconceived notions of what allergy is and what it is not.

In order to understand why the debates about defining food allergy have been so divisive and intractable, it is helpful to go back to the turn of the century when the terms "allergy" and "anaphylaxis" were coined. Throughout the twentieth century, as well as today, arguments about the frequency of food allergy have relied on definitions and conceptualizations of allergy that emerged during the first decade of the twentieth century, specifically those formulated by the French physician and physiologist Charles Richet, the Austrian pediatrician Clemons von Pirquet, and the lesser-known Irish physician Francis Hare (1858–1928).[17] In many ways, these researchers came from disparate personal and professional backgrounds, and enjoyed varying degrees of adulation and respect from their peers. While Richet was a laboratory physiologist who came from a privileged, scientific family and would win the Nobel Prize in 1913 for his work on anaphylaxis, von Pirquet was a pediatrician who also conducted academic research and whose novel term "allergy" took nearly two decades to become commonly used by physicians.[18] He committed suicide with his wife in 1929 for reasons that largely remain a mystery.[19] Least known of the three by far, Hare was a peripatetic clinician whose interests ranged from treating typhoid fever to treating alcoholism, yet he came to be cited by some food allergists and clinical ecologists as being the true founder of food allergy and clinical ecology, its unruly offspring. Despite these differences, the theories and speculations of Richet, von Pirquet, and Hare have served to frame the debates about food allergy ever since they emerged. Above all, they served to distinguish orthodox allergists, who saw food allergy in narrow terms, from more liberally minded food allergists, who saw it as a ubiquitous cause of chronic symptoms, and by the 1960s, clinical ecologists, who argued that it represented a profound disconnect between industrialized humanity and the natural environment.

In what follows, I describe how the ideas of Richet, von Pirquet, and Hare influenced how allergists would come to understand, diagnose, and treat food allergy from its infancy to throughout the twentieth century. Allergy—and food allergy—became clinically significant during a time of rapid transformation in Western medicine, a period of professionalization, specialization, expansion, international exchange of medical concepts and practices, and, importantly, improvements in many of the treatments and explanations physicians offered to patients. It was also a time of great division and uncertainty, as old ideas clashed with new, as clinicians struggled to transform revolutionary theories into therapeutic breakthroughs, and as national rivalries added intensity to many discussions. The rival notions of food allergy that emerged soon after the "birth of allergy" in 1906 were marinated in these underlying debates about germ theory, immunity, physiology, and even how best to generate useful medical knowledge. The disparate understandings of food allergy that developed, therefore, were enveloped in much deeper, often philosophical, issues about epistemology, the nature of individuality, the question of balance with respect to health, and the relationship between humans and the environment.

ANAPHYLAXIS AND THE "HUMORAL PERSONALITY"

In the early years of the twentieth century, two terms entered the medical lexicon that both clarified and muddied understandings of clinical phenomena, including asthma, hay fever, migraine headaches, and food idiosyncrasies, all of which had confronted and confounded physicians for centuries. Although "anaphylaxis" and "allergy" were often used interchangeably at the time to describe hypersensitive reactions to insect stings, pollen, food, and other foreign substances, they actually had quite different meanings in terms of their precise definitions and with respect to what they implied about immunity, immune dysfunction, and individuality. The differences inherent in these terms and how they would be applied by allergists, other physicians, and the general public played a considerable role in shaping the debates about food allergy that emerged.

In 1901, Charles Richet and his fellow Frenchman, zoologist Paul Portier (1866–1962), were invited by Prince Albert I of Monaco to join a cruise on his yacht, *La Princess Alice*, and investigate the sting of the Portuguese man-of-war (*Physalia physalis*) in an attempt to devise a protective antiserum for divers and bathers, including the good prince himself, who were often stung by the creatures.[20] While on board, they found that some laboratory dogs, having been injected with nonlethal amounts of *Physalia* toxin, died following a second dose.[21] This discovery was actually serendipitous; the dogs, whose individual reactions to various toxins were what interested Richet and Portier, had been reinjected in order to reduce the number of animals needed and, therefore, cut costs.[22] Following their return to Paris,

Richet and Portier continued investigating, now focusing on how the poison produced by a sea anemone (*Actinia sulcata*) affected dogs, mindful of what could happen after a second injection. The same phenomenon occurred. Moreover, they noted that whereas "death from the poison usually occurred slowly and gradually" over a period of up to three or four days, dogs that survived the first dose suffered "a dramatic, violent death a short time after the second injection," even if the second dose was extremely small, and even if a long time had elapsed since the first dose.[23] Richet coined the term "anaphylaxis" to describe this phenomenon: from the Greek *ana* (against) and *phylaxis* (protection).

Although Portier soon left the study of anaphylaxis to concentrate on marine biology, Richet continued to investigate the phenomenon. The historian Ilana Löwy and others have noted that the French physiologist François Magendie (1783–1855) had observed decades before the way some rabbits rapidly succumbed to shock after being injected a second time with albumin; Robert Koch (1843–1910) and the American experimental pathologist Simon Flexner (1863–1946) had also made similar observations.[24] Where Richet's work differed (though this point has often been overlooked) was his willingness to speculate about what anaphylaxis meant and how it might help answer difficult questions about human physiology and immunity.[25] At the heart of Richet's inquiries was the nature of human individuality, best modeled in a laboratory setting by man's best friend.

As Löwy persuasively contends, the fact that Richet used dogs for his laboratory experiments had implications for how anaphylaxis—and, eventually, allergy—would be understood by both physiologists and immunologists. Since dogs were more distinguishable, in terms of both physical appearance and personality than, say, guinea pigs, they appeared to have more individual differences. For physiologists like Richet, such "individual variations among laboratory animals (mainly dogs and cats) constituted important experimental data." Dogs, according to Richet, could undergo four separate stages of anaphylaxis, the respective symptoms ranging from mild itching and sneezing in stage one to fatal cardiovascular and respiratory trauma in the fourth stage.[26] Other dogs exhibited no symptoms whatsoever. Guinea pigs were less useful to Richet, since they were "extremely sensitive to anaphylaxis" and terminal heart failure often occurred only a few seconds after the injection.[27] For immunologists and bacteriologists, who typically used small rodents such as guinea pigs, "individual variations among the animals used in their studies . . . were 'noise' rather than 'signal,'" a distraction from developing a standardized, reproducible animal model that would help assess the effectiveness and safety of serum in serotherapy—the treatment of infectious disease by the injection of immune serum. As Löwy suggests, "Loyalty to these divergent experimental models did much to widen the gap between the immunological and physiological explanations of allergies," meaning that scientists would eventually "abandon earlier attempts to make 'biological individuality' (or in medical terms, 'idiosyncratic responses') into a legitimate study for basic scientific research."[28]

Richet intended his emphasis on individuality to connect meaningfully with classical medical theory and, specifically, humoralism. In "An Address on Ancient Humorism and Modern Humorism," his presidential speech to the International Congress of Physiology in 1910, Richet stressed the importance of each person's "humoral individuality" or "chemical constitution," which helped explain why different people reacted to different substances in the environment.[29] Food could be one of these substances. According to Löwy, Richet was particularly interested in "food-related anaphylaxis," since it "proved . . . that anaphylaxis was not just an artificial result found in laboratories or an iatrogenic side-effect of serotherapy, but an important physiopathological phenomenon."[30] According to Richet,

> It has long been known that some people are sensitive to cheese or to strawberries or to fish or to shellfish or to eggs or even to milk. Now the symptoms to be seen in such individuals on ingesting such and such foods are analogous to the effects of anaphylaxis: acute stomach pains, vomiting, diarrhoea, colic, erythema, urticaria, severe itching and sometimes cardiac troubles and fever. We know now that these are anaphylactic phenomena; this has become a pathological commonplace.[31]

Conditions such as food allergy, therefore, were not only interesting clinical phenomena in their own right but also potent indicators of the fundamental importance of individuality, which had profound implications for both medical researchers and clinicians.[32] As Richet explained in his 1913 Nobel Prize speech, his notion of humoral individuality was

> an entirely new idea. It was thought up to now . . . that with individuals of the same age, race and sex the humors would no doubt be chemically identical.

Well, it is not like that at all. Every living being, though presenting the strongest resemblances to others of his species, has his own characteristics so that he is himself and not somebody else. This means that henceforth study of the physiology of the species is no longer enough. Another physiology must be taken up, which is very difficult and barely broached, namely that of the individual.[33]

Later in his career, in the foreword to a book on alimentary anaphylaxis (Richet's preferred term for food allergy) co-written by his son, Richet stressed again the importance of individuality: "I am led to believe that there is no identity among the different alimentary anaphylaxes, and that each clinical case must be studied alone if one is to obtain a comprehensive idea of this difficult problem."[34]

While such an approach to allergy inspired many food allergists, Löwy has argued that Richet's call for a concerted investigation into biological individuality and its relation to physiology was never taken up by his successors in the laboratory. Richet's interest in the connection between body and mind with respect to immunity also had a mixed legacy. Perhaps understandably, given his interest in "metapsychical phenomena," Richet, as well as other contemporary researchers, including Ivan Pavlov (1849–1936), was deeply interested in the link between the mind and the body in physiological phenomena.[35] Although we may associate the fin-de-siècle period with the emergence of germ theory, disease specificity, and the subsequent need for pharmaceutical magic bullets, there continued to be a great deal of interest in the susceptibility of individual bodies with respect to foreign pathogens; every pathogenic seed, as it were, required fertile soil in order to thrive.[36] Individual susceptibility and emotional states could certainly be affected by environmental conditions, as the work of contemporary sanitary reformers and health organizations, such as the National Association for the Prevention of Consumption in Britain, would attest.[37] As the historian Otniel Dror has observed with respect to Anglo-American medicine, many scientists believed that the emotional experiences of test animals could affect the outcome of their experiments; they subsequently developed methods to record, manage, and control such emotions.[38] In the case of food allergy, the emotions of patients, including what would later be called "stress," played a considerable role in explaining why individuals' allergic reactions to the same amount of allergen might vary, even providing for some underlying explanation for food allergy altogether.[39]

ALLERGY: "ANY FORM OF ALTERED
BIOLOGICAL REACTIVITY"

With anaphylaxis, Richet had the ideal condition with which to emphasize how individuality—both psychological and chemical—was central to understanding human physiology. But despite Richet's confidence, his Nobel Prize, and his considerable influence, other conceptualizations of hypersensitivity materialized, challenging both Richet's concept and the use of the term "anaphylaxis." Löwy explains that this was partly because some of Richet's contemporaries, such as the Ukrainian-French immunologist Alexandre Besredka (1870–1940), came to the problem of hypersensitivity from different theoretical perspectives: bacteriology and immunology rather than physiology. Whereas Richet described himself as a "thoroughgoing humoralist," Besredka faithfully followed on from the cellular theory of the Russian zoologist Elie Metchnikoff (1845–1916), which "suggested that immunity was essentially a cellular phenomenon" and stressed the changes that occurred to cells and their structures during immune defense rather than the formation of antibodies.[40]

The attempt to apply theories of anaphylaxis to clinical practice, as well as clinical observations of hypersensitivity, also played a role in fomenting debate about Richet's conceptualization. Soon after Emil von Behring (1854–1917), a German physiologist and the first Nobel laureate for physiology in 1901, along with the Japanese bacteriologist Shibasaburo Kitasato (1853–1931), developed the first effective diphtheria antisera (serum containing antibodies) in the early 1890s, clinicians who employed serum therapy noticed that some patients developed severe reactions (serum sickness) upon repeated injections of antiserum.[41] The first case, which involved the fatal reaction of a two-year-old German child, was doubly tragic in that the diphtheria serum had not been administered in order to cure a case of the disease but, rather, prophylactically.[42] As Besredka suggested in *Anaphylaxis and Anti-Anaphylaxis*, serum sickness caused many mothers to doubt the treatment, "bringing the worst charges against serum therapy and raising the bogey of mishaps resulting from anaphylaxis."[43] In the first decade of the twentieth century, Besredka became interested in developing safer serum-therapy techniques by preventing anaphylaxis from occurring, something he described as anti-anaphylaxis. He realized that very low doses of sensitizing serum did not always elicit an anaphylactic reaction; in fact, some animals developed resistance to the serum following a series of low doses. While some investigators described this absence of reaction as "immunity to anaphylaxis," Besredka termed it "anti-anaphylaxis," which literally meant "anti-anti-protection."[44]

On the one hand, Besredka's notion of anti-anaphylaxis paralleled developments in clinical practice. At roughly the same time as Besredka's experiments, clinicians, such as Leonard Noon (1877–1913) and John Freeman (1876–1962) in the United Kingdom, and Karl Koessler (1880–1925) and Robert A. Cooke (1880–1960) in the United States, began to "desensitize" patients suffering from hay fever by giving them repeated doses of infinitesimal extracts of pollen, increasing the doses gradually and lowering patients' hypersensitivity over time.[45] The London physician Alfred Schofield (1846–1929) even reported desensitizing patients to egg in 1908.[46] This desensitization procedure would have enormous implications for the treatment of allergic conditions and would also be one of the factors that separated the practice of food allergy from the rest of clinical allergy (see chapter 3).[47] But, on the other hand, anti-anaphylaxis also represented a way to understand the relationship between immunity and anaphylaxis differently from that developed by Richet. For Besredka, "anaphylaxis and antianaphylaxis were essentially identical . . . anaphylactic shock was merely a sudden, uncontrolled desensitisation."[48] Whereas Richet stressed the way exposure to certain substances changed the chemical makeup of individuals by the creation of antibodies, Besredka believed that "anaphylactic or immune reactions were not primarily grounded in the chemistry of humoral antibodies" but instead reflected "the receptivity of target cells to pathogenic germs or their ability to react to toxins."[49]

Although Besredka left the direct study of anaphylaxis by the beginning of the First World War, his idea that anaphylaxis and anti-anaphylaxis were part of the same physiological process provides some context for the work of another investigator, Clemens von Pirquet, and how his novel term "allergy" would come to be used throughout the twentieth century.[50] Von Pirquet was an Austrian pediatrician who conducted experimental research and also held academic positions, including being appointed as the first professor of pediatrics at Johns Hopkins University, a position he held from 1909 to 1911 before returning to Europe.[51] Von Pirquet had employed serum therapy in his Vienna clinic and became interested in the mechanisms behind serum sickness, which afflicted some of his young patients. Working

with the Hungarian pediatrician Béla Schick (1877–1967), von Pirquet determined that the "clinical features of serum sickness were not the direct product of the antiserum but the outcome of a hypersensitivity reaction characterized by 'a collision of antigen and antibody.'"[52] Although von Pirquet
allowed that "the conception that the antibodies, which should protect
against disease, are also responsible for the disease, sounds at first absurd,"
he, like Besredka, determined that this was only the case if one downplayed
"the close parallels between immunity and hypersensitivity."[53] In order to
encapsulate both normal and pathological immune responses, and link the
two states, von Pirquet proposed the term "allergy" (from the Greek *allos*
[other] and *ergon* [reaction]) and defined it as "any form of altered biological
reactivity."[54] Underlying von Pirquet's idea that allergy included both functional and dysfunctional immunity was his definition of the resulting term
"allergen," which he explained as "a foreign substance which induces the organism to react in a changed manner to its single or repeated introduction
into the body."[55] The fact that von Pirquet highlighted "single or repeated"
exposures distinguished him from Richet, who stressed that anaphylaxis always required a second exposure.

Mark Jackson has suggested that von Pirquet's term "allergy" was coined
partly to "simplify understandings . . . of biological reactivity," and partly to
reflect idiosyncratic phenomena that clinicians had long recognized, including hypersensitive reactions to insect stings, pollen, and foods.[56] At first, von
Pirquet's term received a "scathing" reception, something the pediatrician
himself acknowledged.[57] Richet, for instance, thought the word was "unnecessary," and the American immunologists Robert A. Cooke and Arthur F.
Coca (1875–1959) argued that it was simply confusing, since it incorporated
both normal and pathological immune responses; the more generic term
"hypersensitivity" was preferable.[58] Most physicians and medical researchers appeared to concur with these critiques, at least to the extent that the use
of the term "anaphylaxis" far exceeded that of the word "allergy" between
1906 and 1926.[59] Due to these misgivings about terminology, lingering debates about humoral and cellular approaches to immunity, and, possibly, the
relative status of the assertive Nobel laureate Richet and the relatively cir-
cumspect pediatrician von Pirquet, physicians used the term "anaphylaxis"
to describe what would later be described as "allergy" until the 1920s.[60]

Eventually, however, such preferences shifted, partly because of the various ways the words were being employed in clinical practice as allergy rap-

idly emerged as a clinical specialty in its own right. By the mid-1920s, the term "allergy" was being used to describe a broad range of conditions, including reactions to food, insect stings, and mold, as well as a catchall for diseases such as asthma and hay fever. Perhaps the best evidence of the change in terminology occurred in 1929, the year of von Pirquet's death, when the *Journal of Allergy* was founded, replacing the *Journal of Immunology* as the publication of choice for allergists.[61] With respect to food hypersensitivity, the term "anaphylaxis" was increasingly, though not exclusively, associated with anaphylactic shock, an immediate, sometimes fatal, allergic reaction characterized by the rapid onset of swelling (particularly around the face, throat, and chest), nausea, skin eruption, and cardiovascular and respiratory difficulties.[62] An example of the refined way in which "anaphylaxis" was being used can be found in a case evocatively described in the *Canadian Medical Association Journal* (*CMAJ*) in 1926 under the title "Food Anaphylaxis." Immediately "after eating one-quarter of a peach," a thirty-five-year-old woman, "Mrs. P.," experienced the following symptoms, which were already becoming emblematic of food anaphylaxis:

> The fruit in her mouth immediately produced a sensation of formication [the feeling of small insects crawling on the skin] with nausea. A little latter there was a tight choking sensation in the throat and chest with crowing inspiration and "itching sensation" situated deeply beneath the sternum: the heart rate was markedly increased. Soon followed a distressing coryza [nasal congestion and mucous buildup] and conjunctivitis with swelling of the eyelids and lip. After two or three hours, the symptoms gradually subsided with a feeling of weakness and lassitude which lasted two or three days.[63]

Mrs. P.'s physician also mentioned that she had suffered similar reactions after eating bananas, apples, raspberries, walnuts, and, interestingly, aspirin, and made a connection between the onset of these reactions and her pregnancy three years before, when "she had a 'craving' for raw fruits which she satisfied to the limit." He added that she could eat cooked fruits and had no history of other allergic diseases, such as asthma or hay fever.[64]

For clinicians, the narrowing of the term "anaphylaxis" in cases of food hypersensitivity was relatively straightforward. As the use of the word was evermore restricted to cases of anaphylactic shock—fittingly, the sort of reaction induced by Richet in his experiments—what anaphylaxis was and was not became increasingly clear. Part of this clarity had to do with the recognizable symptoms associated with food anaphylaxis (especially the characteristic swelling) as well as their severity, but, more important, how quickly these symptoms appeared after eating a particular item of food. The immediacy of food anaphylaxis made it unmistakable, to the extent that many sufferers never bothered to consult a physician about the condition.[65]

The problem for both clinicians and their patients, however, was that not all cases of food hypersensitivity were anaphylactic. As discussed in chapter 1, there was a long history of associating more chronic complaints, such as migraine, asthma, and skin conditions, with idiosyncrasies to food. Not only were these reactions symptomatically different from anaphylaxis, but they were usually delayed rather than immediate, and therefore it was much more problematic to prove the link between them and a suspected food. For example, one case described a patient breaking out in urticaria (hives) and suffering gastrointestinal upset six hours after consuming buttermilk, the food ultimately deemed responsible.[66] Delays of more than twenty-four hours were also reported.[67] Moreover, the symptoms presented in such "subacute or chronic cases" often mimicked those associated with other conditions, meaning that patients could be given a number of inaccurate diagnoses before arriving at the true cause of their distress.[68] There were also technological issues, which made food allergy much more difficult to diagnose and treat than other allergies (see chapter 3). Underlying all such challenges were lingering questions about how to define food allergy, questions inextricably tied to the terms of Richet and von Pirquet and that remain contested to this day.

Richet's term "anaphylaxis" ceased to be a general word for hypersensitivity by the 1930s and became increasingly limited in cases of food hypersensitivity to anaphylactic shock, but this did not mean that the physiologist's original conceptualization of the term was forgotten. For Richet, anaphylaxis was a distinct, pathological state intimately connected to an individual's unique "humoral personality."[69] Moreover, it was an excellent example of immune dysfunction, the body reacting irrationally to foreign substances that should not have been perceived as any kind of threat or, even more disturbingly, to its own tissue, as in cases of multiple sclerosis, rheumatoid arthritis, and lupus erythematosus.[70] Anaphylaxis was a condition where the body simply got it wrong, mistaking ally from threat or self from non-self, to use Frank Macfarlane Barnett's immunological metaphor.[71] According to Richet, anaphylaxis was simply the humoral parallel of psychological individuality: "Since our humours contain an enormous number of imponderable substances . . . which most certainly exist in different proportions in different individuals, it follows that humoral differences can be no less than the psychological differences."[72] Richet's analogy inferred that there was no hidden logic behind such reactions, and, more to the point, in clinical encounters it was an individual's body—nothing else— that was at fault.[73]

Food anaphylaxis was in many ways the perfect clinical illustration of Richet's term, and not just because the immediate, intense, and highly dangerous symptoms of such reactions bore a marked similarity to those he induced in dogs. Such reactions were also characterized by their idiosyncratic, bizarre, and nonsensical nature. Why would a body react in such a way to a substance that, in healthy individuals, provided it nourishment?[74] If the body overreacted to a bee sting or serum, that might make some sense . . . but food? Whether it be Mrs. P.'s peach or peanuts today, anaphylactic food allergy was a confounding, disturbing phenomenon that defied explanation, suggesting that sufferers, or at least their immune systems, were profoundly dysfunctional. For clinicians influenced by Richet's notion of anaphylaxis, it was not only the patient's exceptionality and idiosyncrasy that mattered, but also his faulty immune system. Food anaphylaxis provided clear, indisputable proof of pathological immunity, and, for clinicians, it was this immediate, demonstrable evidence of immune dysfunction that had to be present if a purported reaction to a food was truly food allergy rather than simply a patient's intolerance or aversion to a particular food. Although symptoms other—and less severe—than anaphylactic shock (such as hives or an itchy mouth) could provide alternative evidence of immune dysfunction if they occurred soon after ingestion of the suspected food, and although certain clinical tests could also offer some (often disputable) proof of immune system involvement, food anaphylaxis came to symbolize food allergy for orthodox allergists. Since only a small number of foods tended to trigger such anaphylactic reactions, food allergy was subsequently perceived by such allergists as a fairly rare, albeit serious, problem represented by a limited range of symptoms.

Such was not the case for food allergists, who favored von Pirquet's definition of allergy as "any form of altered biological reactivity." For a start, von Pirquet's somewhat open-ended term almost automatically suggested a wide range of potential symptoms. Rather than perceiving food allergy as a condition limited to immediate, often anaphylactic, reactions, as did their orthodox colleagues, the more liberal-minded food allergists asserted that any number of chronic, otherwise unexplained symptoms could be manifestations of food allergy. As food allergy emerged—unofficially—as a distinct clinical specialty within allergy, the accumulation of anecdotal clinical evidence supporting such claims mounted. Although the wording of von Pirquet's definition might have had something to do with food allergists adopting such a catholic approach, the Austrian pediatrician's conceptualization of "allergy" as a term encapsulating both normal immunity and pathological hypersensitivity was also crucial. This flexible approach conveyed "an ecological and biological tenor" to allergy that captivated many food allergists, and following the postwar growth in food processing and food chemicals, a number of clinical ecologists, such as Theron Randolph, began emphasizing the environmental aspects of allergy.[75] In other words, allergy was not conceived by food allergists solely in terms of pathological immunity, as the orthodox allergists influenced by Richet envisioned, but as "an entirely appropriate protective response to dangers posed by widespread environmental and ecological damage."[76] Adding an additional dimension to such ideas about allergy as a "disease of civilization" or a "pathology of progress" were radical, yet popular, ideas about what constituted the ideal diet for human beings.[77] The theory behind the "Stone Age diet" advocated by the British psychiatrist Richard Mackarness (1916–1996) in *Not All in the Mind*, for example, contended that humans had not evolved to consume many of the foods associated with the rise of agriculture, such as wheat and milk, resulting in countless unexplained chronic health problems, including, as Mackarness's title hinted, mental illness.[78] Not everyone might react hypersensitively to the constituents of an industrialized diet based on grains, dairy products, refined sugars, and chemicals, but those who did signaled a warning to the rest about the potential dangers of a so-called civilized diet and, more broadly, the disconnect between humans and the environment.

THE FOOD FACTOR IN DISEASE

It could easily be argued that physicians such as Randolph and Mackarness stretched what von Pirquet meant by "allergy" all out of proportion, despite the pediatrician's all-inclusive definition. Given the long-standing and continued use of that term as metaphor for any form of profound dislike, this should not be altogether surprising.[79] But it is also important to note that von Pirquet, let alone Richet, was not the only fin-de-siècle theorist to which food allergists and, especially, clinical ecologists referred. Sandwiched in between Richet's description of anaphylaxis in 1902 and von Pirquet's coining of the word "allergy" in 1906 was the publication of Francis Hare's two-volume *The Food Factor in Disease* (1905), which would significantly influence food allergists and, later, clinical ecologists. Hare was a Dublin-born, Newcastle-educated physician whose varied career saw him serve as assistant-resident surgeon at the Brisbane General Hospital and medical superintendent of the Charters Towers Hospital in Australia, and later as the medical superintendent of the Norwood Sanatorium for Inebriates, in Beckenham, an asylum just south of London, which catered to wealthy alcoholics and drug addicts.[80] Hare's first claim to fame was "conquering" typhoid at the Brisbane General Hospital during the late 1880s, using a cold-bath treatment combined with "intense interest in the welfare of patients."[81]

Two aspects of Hare's approach to treating typhoid had a bearing on his investigations of the "food factor in disease." First, as his use of cold-bath therapy suggests, Hare emphasized the importance of simply reducing the temperature of those who were feverish from typhoid. Although his critics and many of his patients described Hare's cold-bath treatments as "burdensome," "barbarous," and "brutal," the Irish physician believed that "in the high temperature itself lay the main source of danger" in cases of typhoid, thus justifying the "harsh and unpleasant procedure."[82] On the one hand, Hare's focus on temperature reflected contemporary concerns about inflammation, first investigated by the German pathologists Julius Cohnheim (1839–1884) and Carl Weigert (1845–1904).[83] But on the other hand, it foreshadowed Hare's nutritional interest in "hyperpyraemia," a condition seemingly rooted in classical humoral theory and characterized by excess fuel (from the Greek *pureia* [fuel]). Hyperpyraemia was triggered by an imbalance between the intake of food and the expenditure of energy (in the course of vigorous exercise, for instance) and manifested in a wide range of chronic symptoms.[84] For Hare, an excess in fuel or food energy, much like excesses in heat, explained many chronic, unexplained health complaints, and "carbonaceous" foods—such as sugars, starches, alcohol, and other carbohydrates—were particularly problematic. Hare described patients as often having a hearty appetite for such carbonaceous foods and connected their attraction to them with the alcoholic's desire for alcohol, a topic to which he would turn while serving at the Norwood Sanatorium.[85] Food allergists influenced by Hare would later interpret the allergic individual's desire for the food that triggered his symptoms as a form of "food addiction," which resulted in a vicious cycle of excessive consumption of typically sugary, starchy food, followed by the onset of chronic symptoms, much like those witnessed by Hare.[86]

Hare also stressed that his endorsement of cold-bath therapy for typhoid was very much rooted in his clinical experience rather than in any underlying theory. Although Hare reported being indebted to the fever research of Sir William Osler (1849–1919), Carl von Liebermeister (1843–1901), and, especially, the German physician Ernst Brandt (1827–1897), he admitted that "the only qualification which I claim for the task is a sufficient personal experience of the disease, extending over upwards of 2000 cases."[87] Perhaps due to some of the criticisms of his cold-bath treatment for typhoid, Hare attempted to shift from this purely inductive approach when he turned to study the relationship between diet and disease in his next major work. Although Hare introduced *The Food Factor in Disease* by stating that a balance had to be struck between clinically based inductive knowledge and theoretically based deductive knowledge, he emphasized that his primary goal was to develop a theory, rooted in physiology, to explain his observations. This tension between inductive and deductive knowledge would be a recurring theme in the history of food allergy, symbolized above all in the respective outlooks of the two major American allergy associations: the American College of Allergists (ACA) and the American Academy of Allergy (AAA). While clinicians such as Hare and food allergists such as Arthur Coca were quite willing to theorize about the relationship between diet and disease, and while some allergists, such as John Freeman and Ben F. Feingold (1899–1982) would actively seek a balance between knowledge accumulated from clinical experience and that supported by laboratory experiment, just where to strike this balance remained debatable.[88]

Despite Hare's attempts to "take a deductive view," his magnum opus was in fact replete with case studies (including an appendix of eighty-six cases, stretching to more than one hundred pages), and it was these clinical encounters that influenced his admirers.[89] As with so many clinicians who would come to blame food for a host of otherwise unexplained chronic symptoms, Hare's interest in the "food factor in disease" began with an epiphany. In 1889, while in Australia, Hare treated an overweight man of about 215 pounds, prescribing him a diet that limited fats, carbohydrates, and alcohol and that encouraged the intake of protein.[90] He then lost touch for two years before bumping into him in northern Scotland. The patient

> informed me that he had ever since practically adhered to the plan of diet I had prescribed, not on account of the obesity, for he had fallen in weight to between eleven and twelve stone [154–168 pounds], but because he had quite ceased to suffer from periodic headaches. I then elicited for the first time that he had suffered from violent headaches since early boyhood: that the attacks had recurred at intervals of a month, three weeks, or a fortnight; and that, having tried many physicians and numerous drugs without relief, he had ceased to seek advice on their account.[91]

Although Hare initially regarded the alleviation of such "migrainous" headaches following the adoption of his diet as coincidental, he soon encountered another patient for which *"attacks of migraine ceased absolutely from the day on which he commenced dietetic treatment: they returned within a fortnight after the cessation of treatment, and they continued to recur thenceforward with their odd regularity.* No other alteration in his habits had been made."[92] Hare concluded that at least some instances of migraine constituted a "food disease," in which "something, derived from the ordinary food supply, remained unassimilated by the tissues and accumulated in the blood, inducing, at regular intervals, a kind of salutary explosion."[93] Once Hare "seriously entertained" the clinical implications of hyperpyraemia, he stated that "it was found to correlate and explain a large number of isolated clinical observations, otherwise inexplicable, or, at any rate, unexplained."[94] By the time Hare wrote *The Food Factor in Disease*, he had had six years' experience prescribing his fat- and carbohydrate-reduced diet, claiming that it gave him "results which for rapidity and decisiveness seems to me unsurpassed."[95]

Hare proceeded to describe how hyperpyraemia caused by inappropriate diet was related to a long list of chronic ailments, including asthma, gout, eczema, obesity, dyspepsia, catarrhs (colds), epilepsy, and a host of mental disturbances. For example, one of Hare's cases involved an "elderly gentleman" who complained of "intense mental depression." The gentleman

> had an excellent appetite, and, so far as could be judged by the absence of symptoms, a powerful digestion. His breakfast consisted of porridge and milk with

sugar, followed by eggs and bacon, or a chop or steak, also bread and butter and marmalade. The more depressed he became, the bigger the breakfast he ate ... as a result, his depression became intensified further. He was ordered a lighter—that is, a less carbonaceous—breakfast: porridge, sugar, and bread were interdicted, and he was allowed either a small chop or steak, or one egg with a little bacon, together with not more than half an ounce of toast. The depression ceased concurrently with the alteration of diet, and has not returned.[96]

As early as the mid-1910s, Hare's association of food and mental health problems would be reflected in the writings of other physicians, particularly those working with children, representing the start of a spirited debate about the link between food allergy and mental disorders.[97]

In order to supplement his own observations of hyperpyraemia, Hare referenced a large number of physicians who had also associated diet and chronic disease. In addition to discussing the dietary treatments of the neurologist Silas Weir Mitchell (1829–1914), who recommended fasting and a milk diet for neurasthenia, Hare cited the observations of John Fothergill and Edward Liveing on migraine and Henry Hyde Salter on asthma. It was Hare's ability to collate and link the dietary hypotheses of researchers specializing in a variety of conditions, compare them with his own clinical experiences, and synthesize an overarching theory to explain how food could cause so many disparate chronic health problems that explains why many food allergists cited him as the true founder (*pace* von Pirquet and Richet) of their discipline.[98] This was despite the fact that when Hare's explanations of hyperpyraemia are analyzed, few substantive similarities with how food allergy would come to be conceptualized (apart from blaming diet for a wide range of symptoms) can be found. Chiefly, Hare did not see hyperpyraemia in either immunological or even toxicological terms. Instead, he presented the condition very much as a classical humoral imbalance, often prescribing exercise in addition to diet, and noting that various forms of either therapeutic or unintentional bloodletting (bleeding a patient, menstruation, or simply having a nosebleed) sometimes resulted in spontaneous relief, particularly of migraine and psychiatric complaints.[99] Changes in climate and fasting could also elicit an improvement in symptoms.[100] Rather than focusing on such differences, however, subsequent food allergists simply concentrated on Hare's assertion that many of the chronic diseases that frustrated clinicians and their patients were caused by food. As Theron Randolph later enthused, Hare's "observations of virtually the full range of the localized and systemic manifestations of allergic/ecologic disturbances at this time is simply an amazing accomplishment."[101]

In the handful of times in which the dietary approach failed to work, Hare tended to blame the patient. Thirty-five-year-old "Mrs. B.," for instance, suffered from migraine but did not like to stay on the diet, even though it worked better than available pharmaceutical remedies. As Hare described: "She is, of course, well aware that she has it in her power to avoid them [headaches], but she prefers the intermittent punishment to the continuous dietetic restriction."[102] In another case, the patient, who also suffered from migraine, stopped taking the diet because she "was too readily satisfied with her improved condition, and constantly broke down in her observance of the dietetic rules."[103] Other patients found Hare's dietary advice easy to follow but struggled to get the required amount of exercise, with one asthma sufferer complaining that walking through Melbourne's "long uninteresting streets" was "anything but pleasant." Whenever this patient failed to complete his therapeutic evening walk, however, he immediately felt the effect.[104] Hare also blamed patients' impulsivity, impatience, and skepticism when the treatment failed.[105]

Such failures indicated that patients had to cooperate fully with their physicians in order for such dietary treatments to work. For Hare, this started with the patient providing an "accurate pathological life-history . . . since infancy." Although Hare believed such "life-histories," in addition to "an exhaustive physical examination," were "indispensable," he admitted that they did not "rank so high with the profession . . . for diagnosis—as formerly."[106] Hare's reliance on a patient's history would also be reflected in the clinical approach of food allergists, who were not able to use many of the new diagnostic tools used by allergists treating other allergies.

Hare's attempt to develop a theory to explain hyperpyraemia notwithstanding, *The Food Factor in Disease* demonstrated to subsequent food allergists and clinical ecologists the value of inductive knowledge; the accumulation of cases may not have provided much evidence individually but, cobbled together, they told a convincing story. Whether it was typhoid, asthma, or alcoholism, the patterns hidden in Hare's thousands of cases held the answer. In order for this inductive approach to be effective, the history, situation, and proclivities of each patient had to be investigated thoroughly, but eventually general explanations would emerge: cold baths cured typhoid;

low-carbohydrate diets combined with exercise ameliorated migraine; tapering alcohol consumption was preferable to immediate abstinence. Hare's explanations for why dietary errors triggered migraine, epilepsy, and depression may have harkened back to classical humoralism, but they nevertheless highlighted food as a key etiological factor. For food allergists and clinical ecologists, Hare provided conclusive evidence that diet was the starting point for any investigation of chronic health complaints.

● ● ●

INTERESTINGLY, Charles Richet, Clemens von Pirquet, and Francis Hare would all steer away from such inductive research by the beginning of the First World War, with Richet concentrating on spiritualism, von Pirquet turning to child nutrition, and Hare treating alcoholics and drug addicts. But that coincidence is one of the few similarities that can be drawn between these three very different researchers, who approached the topic of idiosyncrasy from such disparate perspectives. For Richet, recognition for his discovery was immediate and resulted in a Nobel Prize in 1913. A physiologist, he saw such reactions as evidence of how human beings (and dogs) all had unique humoral individualities, which, much like their psychological personalities, were shaped by their interactions with the environment. Anaphylaxis might have been a pathological immune reaction, but it was also a clear indicator that each human being was physiologically unique. In this way, the notion of anaphylaxis was a reaction against the nascent reductionism and determinism associated with germ theory and the era of magic bullets that accompanied it. But anaphylaxis, both as an all-encompassing term for hypersensitivity, as it was for the first two decades of the twentieth century, and as a specific clinical phenomenon outlined by Richet, also had its limits, especially when it came to food. For orthodox allergists who looked to Richet's notions of hypersensitivity and his novel term, the appellations "anaphylaxis" and, later, "allergy" were defined by only certain pathological responses to eating food. Reactions had to be sudden and severe, and, crucially, clearly indicate the involvement of the immune system if they were instances of "true food allergy." Although such conceptualizations of food allergy have been present ever since Richet's first publications on anaphylaxis, they have been reasserted during the past two decades with the rapid rise of peanut allergy, the archetypical anaphylactic food allergy.

Von Pirquet's notion of allergy as "any form of altered biological reactivity," in contrast, provided subsequent food allergists with much wider lens through which to view bizarre reactions to food.[107] Although von Pirquet's term, if not his precise definition, would eventually be embraced, it took two decades for this to happen. First becoming interested in hypersensitivity when the magic bullets promised by serotherapy proved dangerous to some of his child patients, von Pirquet's understanding of allergy was informed in part by Alexandre Besredka's view that immunity existed on a continuum from the protective to the pathological and in part by von Pirquet's own role as a clinician in Vienna. Von Pirquet's ability to connect serum sickness with idiosyncrasies to foods and other foreign substances has been described as an example of his "genius," his "brilliant ideas and lightning flashes of insight," but this was again due to his own clinical experience.[108] The "violent, itching, urticara-like skin rash" that signified serum sickness, as von Pirquet observed, was similar to those triggered by idiosyncrasies to "strawberries and crustaceans," reactions he would have encountered during his clinical practice.[109] Similarly, von Pirquet's liberal definition of allergy would eventually be the term that clinicians preferred to anaphylaxis, since it appeared to explain many of the chronic symptoms suffered by patients. As food allergists during the 1920s and 1930s began to build up a large body of clinical evidence, which appeared to demonstrate the clinical significance of food allergy, von Pirquet's definition appeared increasingly apt.

Although Hare's ideas about food and disease were not immunological, and while *The Food Factor in Disease* was not read by many food allergists until well after the Second World War (Theron Randolph found it difficult to even locate a copy), the eventual influence of his ideas demonstrates how many clinicians, particularly those drawn to clinical ecology, were willing to overlook the involvement of the immune system altogether in cases of food allergy.[110] Setting Hare's humoral theory of hyperpyraemia to one side, clinical ecologists such as Randolph and Richard Mackarness were instead drawn to the Irish clinician's ideas about food addiction, as well as his ability to attribute a plethora of intractable chronic disorders, including mental illness, to diet. Clinical ecologists were certainly eager to theorize about the origins of such food allergies and what they inferred about our relationship to the environment, but they were also drawn to Hare's clinical acumen, which they aimed to replicate. Ultimately, it was this, their ability to help patients overcome their debilitating symptoms, that mattered most for admirers of Hare, rather than the validity of any underlying explanatory theory.

Despite their disparate backgrounds and career paths, the ideas and terminologies of Richet, von Pirquet, and Hare set the stage for the debates about food allergy that divided the allergy community in the twentieth century. Although technological, economic, and political issues also contributed enormously to these disputes in the decades that followed, almost every argument about food allergy could be distilled to how one defined allergy and how one applied such definitions in clinical practice. Anaphylaxis denoted a restricted definition of food allergy, which was limited to certain reactions and, by extension, certain kinds of food. For orthodox allergist, who believed that the rates of food allergy were exaggerated, it was Richet's definition of anaphylaxis that mattered most. Allergy, as defined by von Pirquet, widened the spectrum, allowing for a greater array of symptoms, especially chronic complaints, to be included under its umbrella. Physicians who regarded food allergy as a widespread clinical phenomenon adhered to this definition, despite the opprobrium of their orthodox colleagues. But for some, including the clinical ecologists who defected from allergy in the 1960s, even von Pirquet's term did not go far enough. They, instead, turned away from the immune system and toward Hare, whose inductive process had convinced them that food played a key role in countless chronic health problems, including mental illness. Food allergy could mean very different things depending on one's definition of it.

THREE

Strangest of All Maladies

IN A 1939 PUBLICATION grudgingly described in the *Journal of the American Medical Association* (*JAMA*) as "another book on food allergy," the author Helen Morgan (1904–1989) proclaimed, "An age has dawned when medical science admits that simple foods may incite explosions that vary from a rash to a fatality."[1] Describing the furor, Morgan, a Pennsylvania home economist and poet, explained that

> the numbers who are saying "I can't eat that!" are reaching into the millions. They are sticking to it, defiantly. Backing them are the physicians, who were the first to scoff at "food fads" a decade ago. They know that victims of allergy are hypersensitive to certain foods, which means that they react differently from most people to ordinarily harmless food. If you're allergic, you may swell up like a balloon after eating a sprig of parsley or break out in a rash after a chocolate nut sundae.[2]

Morgan stated that many of the "cool, pontifical" doctors who had earlier eschewed food allergy now expressed a "perfectly schoolboyish enthusiasm" for it, believing that it might be a "cure-all" for "the orphans of medical science," such as "epilepsy, canker sores, indigestion, arthritis, colds, neuritis, sinus trouble, cold sores, conjunctivitis," and other health problems.[3] Although Morgan acknowledged that these symptoms were not always allergic, and that many people had taken to food allergy as they might have done to "mah-jongg and knitting," she insisted that even doctors who down-played the condition admitted that more than 7 percent of the American population suffered from such allergies.[4]

For what was essentially a recipe book, *You Can't Eat That!* did an impressive job of summing up the excitement and controversy generated by clinical and popular interest in food allergy during the first several decades of the twentieth century. Morgan accurately portrayed the "zest" with which the public had seized on the notion of food allergy and the sense that many physicians were uncomfortable with such zeal. She correctly asserted that physicians remained heavily reliant on their patients' insights in order to identify the offending foods in cases of food allergy: "The doctor will tell you frankly that without you he's lost. He needs your co-operation in allergy more than in any other disease. He is Sherlock, but you must be his Watson. It becomes a game, and it gets results."[5] Morgan recognized that food allergy was often perceived as a "disease of civilization," a disorder afflicting the "sensitive," those who were "more tender, more highly civilized, than the common herd," but she also revealed that this "strange and obscure" medical condition might have its origins in the murky depths of human history. Ironically, the hypersensitive had "never outgrown the instincts their ancestors had back in the jungle . . . the functions his Neanderthal cousin needed billions of years ago to smell the approach of a tiger."[6]

While Morgan's prehistoric timing might have been off, she nevertheless captured the contradictory, perplexing, and divisive nature of food allergy. She also, uniquely, provided a patient-centered view of the condition, outlining not only the frustration of dealing with undiagnosed food allergies but also the difficulty in finding "substitute foods" once the correct diagnosis had been made.[7] The foreword to Morgan's book, written by the Mayo Clinic gastroenterologist and medical columnist Walter Clement Alvarez (1884–1978), indicated that food labels tended to be incomplete, confusing, or inaccurate.[8] Food allergy sufferers might "get better," explained Morgan, but they also felt "awfully restricted. You become morbid about your fate. You sulk when your family dives into a strawberry shortcake or when your spouse rolls his eyes over a watermelon."[9] Moreover, patients also had to deal with the stigma associated with being on a special diet, because "the vast American public disapproves of people who diet," characterizing them as "sickly, neurotic, or vain." Worse still, many physicians believed that people claiming to suffer from food allergy were actually hypochondriacs and thus referred them to psychiatrists. *You Can't Eat That!* was written to help such people cope with the nutritional and emotional difficulties presented by an unsympathetic world full of dangerous foods.

In many ways, the decades immediately before and after *You Can't Eat That!* was published represented a zenith of sorts for the study of and, more important, the clinical appreciation of food allergy. Although the topic divided opinion, the debates surrounding food allergy had not yet generated the vitriol that would characterize them in later decades. Individuals claiming to suffer from food allergies might be viewed suspiciously by some physicians, as Morgan and Alvarez noted, but the idea that such symptoms were purely psychosomatic had not yet become commonplace among orthodox allergists. The fact that Alvarez was willing to support a book such as Morgan's hints that the topic of food allergy had attained a certain level of respectability in American medical circles during the 1930s and 1940s.

To a degree, Alvarez's interest in food allergy could be explained away by his own, self-diagnosed allergy to chicken and that William Mayo (1861–1939), one of the clinic's founders, was himself allergic to cottonseed oil. But both physicians' acceptance of such a diagnosis demonstrates that food allergy was viewed by many influential and powerful physicians as being a plausible explanation for otherwise unexplained complaints.[10] Although Alvarez was chided by some colleagues for studying the topic, Mayo, whose cottonseed allergy was severe enough to prevent him from dining in restaurants and other people's homes, encouraged him to keep researching and writing about it, which Alvarez and many others duly did.[11] In addition to hundreds of medical articles published during the 1930s and early 1940s, food allergy was the subject of numerous books, including recipe books like Morgan's; primers aimed at a popular audience, like *Allergy: Strangest of All Maladies* by Warren T. Vaughan (1893–1944); and textbooks, such as those written by Albert H. Rowe (1889–1970).[12] Health columnists in newspapers, ranging from the founder of the Battle Creek Sanitarium and breakfast cereal inventor John Harvey Kellogg (1852–1943) to the Johns Hopkins–educated physician, child expert, and mail fraudster Leonard Keene Hirshberg (b. 1877), also addressed the topic beginning in the 1910s, citing food allergy as a cause of respiratory, gastrointestinal, and skin ailments.[13]

Perhaps the strangest medical acknowledgment of food allergy is found in a 1933 article for the *Journal of the American Veterinary Medical Association* in which the health problems of "Marie," a young walrus calf captured in the Bering Sea and moved to the San Diego Zoo, were attributed to her cow's milk allergy. Not having a supply of walrus milk or knowing the composition of "sea mammal milk," her keepers instead fed her twenty-four 14.5-ounce cans of condensed milk daily, which appeared to trigger drooling, conjunctivitis, mucous discharge, "gastric distress," "papular eruptions," hair loss, and breathing irregularities. Once the milk was eliminated from the walrus's diet, facilitated by her emergent teeth and subsequent ability to eat fish and crustaceans, "immediate relief was experienced," and Marie quickly became a "popular performer" at the zoo, even making "appearances" on radio shows.[14]

Growing awareness of food allergy was also made evident by a nascent niche in the food industry that catered to those with allergies to staples, such as wheat, eggs, corn, and milk (though apparently not that produced by walruses).[15] Morgan outlined that

> in Oakland, California, there is a bakery where counters are filled with non-allergic delicacies. One of the largest cereal manufacturers in the country has recently put out an all-rye breakfast food. In Ohio, a special process has been invented in an effort to make cow's milk harmless; it is heated to remove traces of the grass or clover the cow ate, which causes troubles for some people. The potentialities of the soybean are being explored, not only for industrial uses, but to replace milk, butter, and meat in an allergic diet. Elaborate baby foods have been concocted that resemble the concentrated food pills the tabloids love to shriek about; they're a mixture of the minerals and vitamins a baby needs, without the foods that might start a rash.[16]

Specialty foods for food allergy sufferers were also advertised in the *Journal of Allergy* and other medical journals during the 1940s, including Ditex Oat Crisps (cookies free of eggs, milk, wheat, corn, and barley, and made of oatmeal, cottonseed oil, soda, salt, brown cane sugar, and artificial flavors), Ry-Krisps (a cracker free of eggs, milk, and wheat, and produced by Ralston Purina), Allerteen (a maple-flavored milk substitute), and Mull-Soy (a soy-based milk substitute).[17] Although Morgan cautioned that "apart from these ventures, the attention given the allergic's dietary needs has been woefully meager," she also recommended shopping in ethnic food stores—for instance, Chinese supermarkets for rice flour and Jewish shops for potato flour.[18] Alvarez also suggested that patients

explore also the foreign markets in large cities—the stores which carry the
foods of foreign origin which are sought by immigrants from other lands. Such
foods have the advantage that not only have they never been eaten by the sensitive person, but the plants from which they come are often so different botanically from those that supply the dietary needs of the average American that
there is only a small likelihood that the patient will be sensitive to them.[19]

Garbanzo beans from Spain; chestnut flour, lichi nuts, bamboo shoots,
mung bean sprouts, and citron from China; dates from the Middle East; pa-
paya from Florida; reindeer meat from Lapland; and taro flour from Hawaii
(where Alvarez was born) were listed as possible food substitutes. Although
the day "when the allergic people of America, over a million strong, get together to . . . secure in pure form in cans and cartons, properly labeled, all
sorts of new foods gathered from the ends of the earth" was still in the future, there were at least some alternatives for the food allergy sufferer.[20]

But despite popular, medical, and commercial interest in and, to a lesser
degree, acceptance of food allergy, it was also abundantly clear as early as the
1910s that the condition differed fundamentally from other allergic diseases.
Unlike allergies to pollen, animal dander, and dust, allergists soon learned,
food allergies could not be reliably diagnosed with the use of skin tests, nor
could they be treated effectively or safely with desensitization therapy. Instead, food allergists relied primarily on rigorous elimination diets to identify the foods that their patients should avoid. Whereas skin testing and desensitization required patients to be the passive recipients of diagnosis and
treatment, these elimination diets were reliant on both patient testimony
and participation if they were to be effective. Food allergists, therefore, developed symbiotic, cooperative relationships with their patients—or, in the
case of children, parents—which meant that they were sympathetic toward
patients' accounts of their symptoms, symptoms that other physicians
often dismissed as hypochondriacal or psychosomatic. In turn, patients
believed their clinicians' explanations for their problems and the solutions
they offered, particularly when the dietary advice they prescribed appeared
to work and because many food allergists themselves claimed to suffer from
food allergies, citing their own personal experiences. In part because of this
combination of diagnostic difficulties and the trusting relationship that existed between food allergists and their patients, many leading food allergists

produced startlingly high estimates of the prevalence of food allergy. While such estimates encouraged food allergists to increasingly suspect the condition as the hidden cause of chronic health problems during the interwar period, they also raised the ire of orthodox allergists.

NOT SKIN DEEP

In a relatively sympathetic review of a food allergy book by Herbert Rinkel (1896–1963), Theron Randolph, and Michael Zeller (1900–1977), the New York City allergist and former AAA president Will Spain explained the difficulties involved in diagnosing food allergy. Compared with all other "problems in clinical sensitization . . . food allergy was the most difficult to resolve," Spain declared, mainly because physicians were "shorn in at least half of his cases of the benefit of positive food reactions by skin test."[21] As such, they had to rely inordinately on the recollections of the patient, who lacked "objectivity in presenting his problem because of his whims, fancies, and aversions relating to various viands, ideas which are often construed by him as proofs of specific food allergy."[22] These factors, combined with the fact that food allergy symptoms tended to "mimic" those of other conditions, made it a problem that did "not lend itself to an easy solution."[23]

For most allergies, skin testing was a quick, accurate, and usually safe way to determine the substances to which patients were allergic.[24] The procedure, pioneered by Clemens von Pirquet in 1907 to test for reactions to tuberculin, an antigen used in inoculations for tuberculosis, involved introducing a small amount of the potential allergen, such as grass pollen or egg white, just below the skin and then waiting to see if the skin reacted by erupting in a wheal or welt. Further developed by the American allergist Isaac Chandler Walker (1883–1950), skin tests soon became the primary means by which allergists identified most allergens and assessed their severity: the more potent the allergen, the larger the wheal.[25] A number of different types of skin tests eventually emerged, including scratch tests, in which allergens were rubbed into an abrasion made by the allergist; prick-puncture tests, in which the allergen was injected into the skin via a puncture; and intradermal testing, in which a diluted food extract was simply injected just below the skin.[26] Following diagnosis of an allergy—for instance, to a specific pollen—the allergist would desensitize the patient to the allergen (a technique known as desensitization therapy or desensitization) by injecting microscopic amounts of the same pollen extract into the patient and then slowly increasing the dosage over time so that the patient developed a resistance to it. Eventually, the patient would be able to tolerate at least some exposure to the allergen in real-life conditions. Skin testing, therefore, was not simply a diagnostic procedure, but also the first step in treatment.

Up until the early 1930s, most physicians were comfortable employing skin tests to diagnose cases of food allergy, believing that the procedure was accurate with all allergens. As the New Jersey–born physician and cardiologist George Frederick Laidlaw (1871–1937) explained in a 1917 discussion about the relationship between hay fever and diet, "a patient who at any time has been poisoned or, as we now say, sensitized by any of these foods, still has circulating in his blood or fixed in his skin the reactive bodies to that food. These reaction bodies react to that food on the skin by redness and swelling."[27] In order to perform the test—often described as a "scratch test"—Laidlaw mixed "pure food protein" in a 5 percent solution and compared the reaction with a control injection of milk sugar. He assured that such tests were "simple and harmless if the scratch is not too deep and *if the protein is not injected beneath the skin*. If injected beneath the skin or rubbed into a deep scratch, the food proteins, like the pollen proteins, may be dangerous. If they are absorbed rapidly in to the circulation of a patient who happens to have been sensitized to any of them, there is serious danger of anaphylactic shock."[28]

Others concurred, believing that such dangers were worth risking. Writing in 1921, the British physician Arthur F. Hurst (1879–1944) depicted skin testing as being the routine approach to diagnosing food allergy–induced asthma.[29] In a 1922 article on the neurological manifestations of food allergy in children, a Minnesota pediatrician by the name of W. Ray Shannon also described using skin tests successfully, and three years later Shannon's fellow pediatricians George Piness (1891–1970) and Hyman Miller recommended them as well.[30] As the London physician Arthur Latham explained, although "a very careful history of an individual case and full inquiry into his habits and dietary will give considerable information," physicians could "only obtain accurate information by carrying out the skin test."[31] Skin tests, it appeared, offered the sort of evidence of immune response that signified a true food allergy.

But others were doubtful. According to one commentator, "the results of cutaneous sensitization tests are occasionally spectacular. On the other hand, they are much of the time indeterminate or highly confusing."[32] From a purely diagnostic point of view, the chief problem was that the tests often resulted in false positives and false negatives. Foods that provoked a wheal during a skin test in some cases did not appear to cause any clinical symptoms when tested in other ways—for example, using an oral challenge. Other times, the opposite occurred: a food that caused certain symptoms, as determined by an individual food challenge, did not provoke a reaction following a skin test. The risk of both false positives and false negatives meant that many food allergists believed that skin tests were completely without use. Why submit patients, many of whom were children, to a distressing and uncomfortable test if it led you in the wrong direction?[33]

Explanations for these false negatives and positives varied. Perhaps most obvious was the fact that before it entered the bloodstream, ingested food was digested and partially metabolized, thus consisting of a different chemical composition from that of pure food extracts prepared for skin tests. People who reacted allergically when they inhaled wheat dust, for instance, usually responded positively to wheat in a skin test; such tests in people who exhibited symptoms *after* they ingested wheat tended to be negative.[34] Food allergists also complained about the quality of food extracts, a criticism that persisted. The leading British allergist A. W. Frankland (b. 1912) grumbled as late as 1972, "Unfortunately, the testing solutions we use are grossly (immunologically) impure."[35] Thirty years later, Frankland was still dissatisfied, claiming that "a recent investigation demonstrated that only one out of five commercial walnut skin prick test solutions contained significant quantities of walnut protein."[36] There were also technical issues inherent in skin testing, which could lead to false negatives and positives. While the scratches themselves involved in the tests were difficult to standardize and often led to false positives, pricking too deeply in prick-puncture or intradermal testing led to false negatives.[37]

Fundamentally, however, food allergists' reservations about the accuracy of skin tests boiled down to debates about the definition of food allergy. If allergists restricted their definition of food allergy to cases in which there was clear evidence of immune system involvement, as orthodox allergists did, then a positive skin reaction was a necessary indicator of true food allergy. If they employed a wider definition of food allergy, as most food allergists did, then skin tests would capture only a limited number of cases. Or, as Frederic Speer (1909–1985) explained in 1975: "One school takes a restricted view. Its adherents insist on limiting the term to cases in which a skin test (or other objective method) demonstrates an antigen/antibody reaction. The other school takes a broad view, believing that whether objective tests are positive or not, any reaction that causes a typical, clear-cut allergic manifestation is allergy."[38] Speer, who preferred the second, broader view, argued that by insisting on the need for positive skin tests, allergists were depriving patients who suffered from "hidden food allergens," which often came in the form of ubiquitous foods, such as milk, corn, and eggs.[39] Allergies to these foods were especially difficult to identify not only because they were so commonly eaten but also because they were ingredients in baked goods, sauces, and processed foods.

Writing in the mid-1970s, Speer was reflecting on debates that had been under way for more than four decades and had ultimately riven the allergy community into rival, antagonistic factions. Although these divisions were rooted in the terms coined and definitions devised to describe hypersensitive reactions during the first decades of the twentieth century and, indeed, even earlier disagreements about idiosyncrasies, it was the issue of skin testing that caused the first momentous fissures. By the early 1940s, many food allergists—including Albert Rowe, Herbert Rinkel, Theron Randolph, and Arthur Coca—had independently determined that skin tests were an ineffective way in which to diagnose food allergy, and others concurred that the tests were not always accurate.[40] The Oakland-based Rowe, one of the earliest to critique the use of such tests in a 1931 textbook, also expressed his concerns about them in a 1944 letter to Randolph, stating that "I feel that this is so important that I have discussed the fallibility of skin tests on the very first page of my book on elimination diets as you have probably noticed."[41] The title of this book, *Elimination Diets and the Patient's Allergies*, made Rowe's diagnostic preferences explicit, and Rowe's specially designed elimination diets became quite popular and well regarded in food allergy circles, if not notorious in other quarters.[42]

For his part, Randolph, working as the chief of the Allergy Clinic at the University of Michigan Medical School during the early 1940s, began to question the accuracy of skin testing after he asked his patients to use elimination diets at home to confirm whether the findings from the skin tests he had conducted on them matched their own observations while on the diet. The patients reported many inconsistencies, prompting them to ask: "If the skin tests with foods are unreliable, why do you do them?"[43] Agreeing that this was a fair question, Randolph called a meeting of his staff, including medical residents from pediatrics, otolaryngology, and internal medicine, and asked them if they gained more reliable information from skin testing or from ingestion tests (simply asking a patient to consume a small amount of a suspected food allergen while in the clinic) and elimination diets. The consensus was that skin tests were less useful; Randolph, with the support of his staff, then decided to (apparently literally) "dump the skin test extracts for foods down the sink."[44] Reassessing this decision at a later date, Randolph recalled that "it was agreed that discarding the use of skin tests with food extracts—mechanically performed and literally interpreted—. . . had been beneficial."[45]

A review of Rinkel, Randolph, and Zeller's *Food Allergy* claimed that the three authors had "entirely abandoned" all types of skin testing because they were "insufficiently accurate in the diagnosis of food allergy."[46] Although this was not absolutely true—the authors did state that they could be used in combinations with other diagnostic methods and provided some recommendations on how to use skin tests more effectively—their accumulated clinical experience, including some trials, had convinced them that other techniques were preferable. A study of 659 patients indicated that skin tests for fourteen of what the authors believed to be the most frequent food allergens (including wheat, corn, egg, milk, coffee, and apple) were accurate in only 38 percent of asthma cases, 34 percent of eczema cases, 20 percent of gastrointestinal allergy cases, and less than 19 percent of urticaria cases.[47] Allergies to certain foods, including wheat, were even more difficult to identify with the use of skin tests. The "indisputable errors in skin testing with food extracts" notwithstanding, the authors bemoaned the fact that "they are used constantly and great emphasis is placed upon the occasional concomitant skin reaction and actual clinical sensitization."[48]

Despite these shortcomings, other food allergists, including the influential Warren T. Vaughan, were more equivocal about skin tests for food allergy, inferring that although they could not be judged as being as accurate as when used for inhalant allergies, the evidence they provided could be included along with that made available through other means, such as family history of allergy, patient testimony, and elimination diets. Between "the extremes of those who depend entirely on skin tests and those who consider them of no value," suggested Vaughan, were "the greater number of workers who recognize the shortcomings of food testing but who find it helpful enough to justify its use."[49] In other words, when dealing with a condition that was so difficult to diagnose, all testing techniques should be considered.

Despite Vaughan's cautious stance on skin tests, these tests remained a divisive topic in the nascent allergy community, partly because they represented more than just a diagnostic technique. To eschew skin testing was to take a provocative stance, one that could alienate oneself from many of one's colleagues.[50] For a start, it implied that one employed a broad, liberal definition of allergy, a view increasingly seen as unscientific at a time when attempts were being made in the United States to designate allergy as a distinct medical discipline. Although some allergists felt somewhat self-conscious about how skin testing was perceived in the broader medical community, the practice had the aura of a legitimate, quantifiable diagnostic procedure and, more important, provided a link between allergy, as a clinical practice, and the science of immunology.[51] To reject skin testing for food allergy was, in a sense, to sever the link between allergy and legitimate medical science.

Moreover, by dumping one's food allergy extracts down the sink, so to speak, one also cut oneself off from the "global economy of allergy," the pharmaceutical market involved in developing allergen extracts for both skin testing and, subsequently, desensitization.[52] Skin testing and desensitization not only meant the provision of a medical service, but also involved the development and sale of a pharmaceutical product: allergen extracts. In the case of hay fever, as Gregg Mitman explains, American pharmaceutical companies were quick to exploit the discoveries of the British allergists Leonard Noon and John Freeman regarding desensitization during the 1910s, undertaking extensive pollen surveys across the United States to identify the most problematic regional plant allergens.[53] Noon and Freeman then developed pollen extracts, which would be sold to allergists for use in their patients. In this way, skin testing, desensitization, and, later, other treatments for allergies, such as antihistamine products, corticosteroids, and bronchodilators, all of limited use to food allergists, linked the work of orthodox allergists with the research, marketing, and sales activities of pharmaceutical companies.[54] While this symbiotic relationship between allergists and pharmaceuticals would have major repercussions for how diseases such as asthma would come to be researched, conceptualized, and treated, it failed to materialize in the case of food allergy until the emergence of peanut allergy during the 1990s, meaning that food allergists lacked the financial support and inducements enjoyed by orthodox allergists.[55]

Finally, skin tests could be dangerous, especially in cases of suspected food allergy. One alarming example from 1921 involved two Cleveland pediatricians who used skin tests to determine what was causing a one-year-old infant's eczema and asthma. After an injection of egg extract, the boy developed a large wheal and experienced "severe and extreme" breathing difficulties and cyanosis (when the skin turns blue), to the extent that the physicians had to administer epinephrine to revive him. Despite this apparent evidence of an egg allergy, they re-inoculated the boy with egg a few days later, leaving him alone in the examination room for five minutes. When they returned, the child had stopped breathing. Epinephrine was employed once again and, fortunately, the child recovered. Strangely, the only lesson to be learned from this episode, according to the pediatricians, was to have epinephrine close to hand when performing skin tests.[56] Other patients were not so lucky, and, as early as 1929, compilations of fatalities were being recorded in medical journals.[57]

ELIMINATION DIETS AND OTHER DIAGNOSTIC ALTERNATIVES

Without skin tests, food allergists had to employ other methods in order to determine what foods were causing their patients' complaints. The most common alternative was the elimination diet, in which patients were prescribed a limited diet consisting of hypoallergenic foods. Although an elimination diet might appear on the surface to be a fairly intuitive and obvious way in which to diagnose an allergy, they were actually quite sophisticated, with different food allergists developing their own versions and adapting them to fit their patients' individual circumstances. The chief challenge was designing diets that provided the necessities of nutrition and simultaneously avoided all foods likely to trigger reactions, eventually establishing a baseline for testing suspected foods later. Once a patient had been on the diet long enough to be symptom-free, the food allergist would introduce common food allergens into the patient's diet, with the patient recording any reactions in a diet diary. More foods would be added until the culprits were identified. For this reason, at least one allergist favored the term "food addition diets," since foods were added over time.[58]

Among the elimination diets available to patients, the best known were the Rowe diets, developed by Albert Rowe at the Merritt Hospital in Oakland, California, in approximately 1927 and revised during subsequent decades.[59] Rowe, who had helped to found the Western Society for the Study of Hay Fever, Asthma, and Allergic Disease in 1923 with George Piness and Grant I. Selfridge (1864–1951), began suspecting in the 1920s that food allergies could be the hidden cause of many chronic conditions.[60] Since Rowe believed that nearly every food could trigger an allergic reaction and that "food allergens probably stay in the blood stream for days or even weeks after the elimination of the allergenic foods," his diets were long in duration and restrictive, more so than those devised by other physicians.[61] At the same time, though, it was crucial for elimination diets to provide at least basic nutritional requirements, especially when prescribed to children, given contemporary medical interest in the nutritional importance of vitamins and minerals, another new area of research.[62]

While Rowe argued that his diets were nutritionally sound, others questioned this claim and the effectiveness of his diets generally.[63] In an ardent article, "With What We Must Contend," an anonymous writer lambasted an allergist working in the northwest of the United States (most likely Rowe, given the contents of the diet and the fact that Rowe worked in Oakland) for restricting a three-year-old girl's diet to "whole rice krisps, rye, rice, arrowroot, leaf lettuce with oil and white vinegar, string beans, spinach, banana, pear, apple juice, grape juice, sugar, salt, butter and (small quantities) of lamb and beef" in an effort treat her asthma, even though skin tests revealed allergies to cat hair, feathers, silk, and dust. The author contended that not only did the patient's symptoms fail to improve with the diet, but infractions of the diet did not lead to additional symptoms. The frustration of the author was evident in the question that concluded the article: "Why was the child made to follow an unbalanced diet of approximately ten foods for almost two years during which her infections increased in number and intensity? Why?"[64]

Part of this anonymous physician's animosity toward Rowe and his diets may have been due to Rowe's sheer success in marketing his diets to both patients and other physicians. By the early 1930s, Rowe diets were being used in many allergy clinics and general practitioners' offices, and by the

1960s Rowe was reportedly earning nearly $200,000 from his clinic.[65] Such financial success might have had something to do with Rowe's contention that "criticism rolls of me like water off a duck."[66] Although opinions about Rowe diets were definitely divided, they were admired by some. One physician, writing in the *Dallas Medical Journal*, described how Rowe diets not only met all the criteria of an effective elimination diet but also were "well-rounded and palatable," intimating that they would be acceptable to patients.[67] Another writer, complaining that "the usual cutaneous food tests were of little or no value in the detection of the etiologic ingestant or ingestants," prescribed Rowe diets instead.[68]

Given their inherent restrictions and the time it took in employing them, however, Rowe diets and other elimination diets were difficult to implement. In a 1929 discussion of Rowe's approach to gastrointestinal allergy, for example, George Piness attested that although Rowe's cases were "really spectacular," they were dependent on a great deal of "hard work and constant observation," requiring patients to adhere to them for an inordinate amount of time, and, as such, were not ideal.[69] For Piness, who used skin tests at the Los Angeles Children's Hospital's Allergy Clinic, determining which of the foods responsible for a patient's reactions using elimination diets was simply too difficult. Alexander Sterling believed that Rowe deserved "a great deal of credit" for his diets but also questioned the time required for accurate diagnosis: "Personally, I find difficulty with this elimination diet. I should like to know how long a period it takes to determine, by elimination, whether a patient is really ill from the foods one suspects."[70] Such diets were also arduous for patients to carry out. As the Tennessee pediatric allergist William G. Crook (1917–2002), an enthusiastic proponent of food allergy, admitted: "My patients seem to have a lot of trouble carrying out elimination diets. Even though I give them my book and other instructional materials, they're often overwhelmed. And, too often, they don't carry out the diet properly. . . . Then no matter how carefully I tell them about taking foods away and adding them back, they still get confused."[71] Compared with a skin test, which would at least provide some evidence within minutes and was not reliant on patient cooperation, it was not surprising that many clinicians believed that the difficulties involved in the execution of an elimination diet outweighed the benefits.

Because of the problems inherent in both elimination diets and skin tests, other techniques were proposed. Some of these were simply variations of the elimination diet, modified to provide either enhanced accuracy or quicker diagnosis. In the former category, for example, was Randolph's diagnostic approach, which required a patient to fast for up to four days to make sure that all traces of food proteins were removed from her system As Randolph began to suspect the role of environmental chemicals as a cause of chronic symptoms, a condition he termed "multiple chemical sensitivity" (MCS), patients also had to be kept in a hermetically sealed environment where exposure to such chemicals would be eliminated.[72] In the latter category was the ingestion test, or individual food test, first suggested by the American pathologist William Waddell Duke (1883–1945) in *Allergy, Asthma, Hay Fever, Urticaria, and Allied Manifestations of Reaction.*[73] Although Duke failed to elaborate on exactly how to conduct such tests, the Kansas City food allergist Herbert Rinkel provided such details in his discussion of a case of gastrointestinal allergy that he treated periodically from 1927 to 1933.[74]

The patient, twenty-six years old when he first sought help from Rinkel, began suffering from upper abdominal distress in the summer of 1927. When the symptoms worsened in November of that year, he was diagnosed with acute appendicitis and his appendix was removed. Symptoms persisted for another year, when he was diagnosed as having a peptic ulcer and was given the Sippy treatment, a regimen devised by Bertram W. Sippy (1826–1924), which involved a five-day period of fasting, followed by hourly feedings of milk and cream and the administration of antacids.[75] Although the Sippy treatment provided temporary relief, the symptoms soon returned, and during the following four years the patient was diagnosed as having a ruptured ulcer and an acute intestinal obstruction, undergoing four subsequent surgeries. None of these procedures relieved his abdominal distress, and a number of the internists and surgeons involved in treatment speculated that the patient's problems were actually psychosomatic. Finally, in November 1932, Rinkel tested for wheat, egg, and milk allergies, using his individual food test. Each of the foods was found to cause not only the abdominal pains that were consistent with the symptoms presented earlier (and confused for other conditions) but also nausea, headache, nasal irritation, and itching in the mouth.[76] Skin tests for these foods, however, proved negative, confirming for Rinkel the usefulness of the ingestion tests.

Rinkel's case demonstrated the apparent effectiveness of individual food testing, but it also pinpointed the frustration and, indeed, iatrogenic dangers posed by undiagnosed food allergies and the willingness of surgeons to perform appendectomies and other procedures in the hopes of reducing symptoms. In 1949, the California pediatric allergist Ben Feingold—who gained both fame and notoriety during the 1970s as the promoter of the food additive–free Feingold diet for hyperactivity and also held a reputation as an orthodox allergist—similarly argued that many of the symptoms that resulted in children undergoing over a million "indiscriminate" tonsillectomies and adenoidectomies annually were actually caused by hidden allergies.[77] These allergic conditions often worsened following these surgeries. In other reported cases, cholecystectomies (removal of gall bladder) and hysterectomies (presumably to relieve suspected psychosomatic causes) were conducted without improvement in symptoms.[78] Rather than automatically referring their patients to the surgeon for invasive operations, Feingold argued that physicians should first eliminate the possibility of allergy.

Rinkel's individual food tests might be able to help patients avoid unnecessary surgeries and other treatments, but they, too, had their drawbacks. Primarily, they were most effective in cases in which the reaction occurred soon after ingestion of the suspected food, typically within an hour.[79] If reactions tended to be delayed, as many food allergists believed they could be, then such tests were less useful. They also, like skin tests, ran the risk of triggering severe reactions. Rinkel tests recommended that patients consume "an average portion" of the suspected food within a five-minute period, followed by feeding a half or quarter portion an hour later if no symptoms developed.[80] This could add up to quite a significant dose if the patient was truly allergic. In the case of Rinkel's gastrointestinal allergy patient, the milk test caused particularly serious symptoms, including those resembling anaphylaxis, and ephedrine and saline solutions were required for relief.[81] In another patient, who was given an ingestion test for corn, "violent symptoms," including an intense headache, chills, and neuroses, lasted for four days; in yet another case, an ingestion test for milk caused "effects so violent as to require intravenous aminophyllin [the agent found in bronchodilators used to treat asthma]."[82]

In order to supplement the evidence provided by the ingestion tests, some food allergists also performed leucocyte (white blood cell) counts as an additional proof of an allergic reaction, with abrupt changes to the number of leucocytes highlighting the likelihood of allergy. Using the so-called leucopenic index, which had been developed by Warren Vaughan in the early 1930s, was thought to identify two types of reaction not usually detected by

employing Rinkel's individual food test alone—delayed reactions and cu-
mulative reactions—whereas a single test would not induce a reaction, but
consuming the food four to five days in succession would.[83] Although leucopenic tests were often carried out, they also received "severe criticism"
from skeptics and had to be timed correctly in order to provide worthwhile
data.[84] As with skin tests, most food allergists viewed them as potentially
useful, but not a comprehensive or consistently reliable diagnostic tool.

Even more controversial than Vaughan's leucopenic index was the "pulse
test," developed by Arthur Coca, whose varied career included a professor-
ship at Cornell University Medical College (1910–1932), working as the medical director for Lederle Laboratories (1932–1948), founding the *Journal of
Immunology* in 1916, and serving as the president of the Society for the Study
of Asthma and Allied Conditions (SSAAC).[85] Coca, who believed that many
of his own health problems, including severe migraines, dizziness, and hypertension, were due to various allergies, began to investigate the diagnostic
value of the pulse test in allergy after his wife told him that her pulse raced
up to 160 beats per minute when she ate certain foods.[86] He first described
its use in *Familial Nonreaginic Food-Allergy*, the title of which hinted at not
only Coca's previous interest in the role of heredity in allergy (with Robert
Cooke, he had coined the term "atopy," a hereditary predisposition to allergic disease) but also his opinions about the definition of allergy and the diagnostic challenges this posed.[87] The term "nonreaginic" referred to reactions
that did not produce antibodies and, therefore, were not immunological in
nature.[88] As such, Coca's title demonstrated that he, along with most food
allergists, chose to define allergy broadly, embracing von Pirquet's notion of
"any form of altered biological reactivity."[89] Among those with whom Coca
debated about this broad interpretation of allergy was the Swiss allergist
Robert Doerr, who was nominated for a Nobel Prize in 1936 and who convinced many European allergists that a more restrictive, immunologically
based definition of allergy was preferable.[90]

Coca's pulse test was even more divisive than his liberal definition of
allergy. As described in a 1961 review in the *Journal of Allergy*, "Coca's initial reports were not accepted by most allergists who privately expressed
doubt and skepticism about the method. They questioned his findings as
to the normal pulse range, and the lack of control over such influences as
exercise, emotion, and complicating infections."[91] Although the authors of
this review expressed some sympathy toward the pulse test, stating that any

objective measure in the diagnosis of food allergy was helpful, most of Coca's contemporaries were "bitterly critical."[92] A review of *Familial Nonreagninic Food-Allergy*, for instance, outright rejected that the "diagnostic method described in this treatise as sufficiently accurate to determine sensitivity."[93] Even Coca's admirers, including Theron Randolph and Richard Mackarness, expressed reservations. Mackarness doubted the test's reliability but did allow that "it has the merit of great simplicity and patients can be taught to use it themselves in determining their own allergies."[94] For his part, Randolph believed that the test could be useful but admitted struggling to master the technique, adding that in cases of severe allergic reaction a drop in pulse might occur. He also feared that Coca's pulse test ran the risk of delegitimizing food allergy even more than it already was in the eyes of orthodox allergists, stating that "if we are going to sell the concept of food allergy we've got to sell it by means of objectively demonstrable evidence, which is going to be difficult enough to do; and that probably we'll never be able to sell it on the basis of pulse changes of the type Dr. Coca describes."[95] Aware of Randolph's reservations, Coca testily replied: "Not having mastered the time consuming art of interpretation of the objective pulse record your investigation of the disease is limited."[96] Such a sharp retort indicated not only the tenor of the personalities involved but also that food allergists were not always unified in their attempts "to sell the concept of food allergy."

Although Coca continued to employ, investigate, and promote his technique, publishing a popular handbook, *The Pulse Test for Allergy*, in 1959, it proved to be yet another controversial technique that both bemused and divided allergists. Or, as Will Spain lamented in his review of Rinkel, Randolph, and Zeller's *Food Allergy*, "The methods of diagnosis . . . are time-consuming, tedious, and complicated. But so is the condition of food allergy complicated. Anyone in search of a simple and easy diagnostic procedure for this clinical form of sensitization will not find it."[97] Expressed lyrically in the "Ballad of the Allergists," which dates from the early 1940s:

> Now that you know just what to use you sneak upon your victim, and scratch or
>   stick, or cut or prick, according to the dictum.
> Some say we nearly all react. Some say it's just the few. There's lacking unanim-
>   ity in just what wheals are true.
> Some even doubt that this reaction leads us ever right, and follow the sadistic
>   plan of sealing up air-tight their subjects in aseptic rooms on salt-free water
>   diet [Theron G. Randolph].

A purpura will quick subside, thus ran Pete Eyermann's theme, by leaving off all
   carbs and fats, but first of all protein.
And Albert [Rowe] cures his worsest ones by mere elimination. A spinach diet for
   six weeks will cure the constipation.
But Warren [Vaughan] got around all of this and figured out an index, whereby
   a thousand white blood counts might save a man's appendix.[98]

Given these difficulties and the lack of consensus, however expressed, it was
sensible that food allergists looked to another source of evidence in order to
diagnose food allergy: their patients.

INTELLIGENT AND COOPERATIVE PATIENTS

Despite attempts to develop food allergy tests that were more objective, most
food allergists remained reliant on elimination diets of one kind or another.
This being the case, food allergists were largely dependent on their patients
to provide accurate accounts of family history and symptomology, adhere
to the elimination diet religiously, and, ultimately, avoid the foods to which
they were allergic. As Albert Rowe, the prescriber of so many elimination
diets, declared, "The absolute determination of all the allergenic causes of
many allergic manifestations requires the intelligent and understanding cooperation and analysis of the patient."[99] Parents, typically mothers, also had
to be intelligent and cooperative in the case of allergic children, according to
the pediatric allergist Bret Ratner (1893–1957), of Bellevue Hospital Medical
College.[100] Rather than being the passive recipients of skin tests and desensitization, as were most allergy sufferers, food allergists' patients had to be active participants, being as central in the diagnostic process as the physician.
In turn, food allergists had to trust patients' ability to observe and describe
their own symptoms reliably. Far from branding their complaints as psychosomatic, as orthodox allergists did, food allergists were sympathetic to
the plights of their patients and took their health history accounts seriously.
In order to get the better of food allergy, food allergists and their patients
had to be partners.

A useful description of this partnership is found in Warren Vaughan's
Practice of Allergy, a lengthy textbook on clinical allergy that was first published in 1939 and went through three editions. Vaughan, who developed
the leucopenic index and was a cautious advocate of skin tests in cases of

suspected food allergy, was nevertheless convinced that the patient's testimony was crucial to an accurate diagnosis. The first step was the elucidation of the patient's own allergic history, including that of his family, all of which "must be painstakingly obtained."[101] As Vaughan explained, "One is often astonished at the wealth of information in the past and family allergic histories, if the patient is given an opportunity to describe his experiences and is helped along with pertinent questions. The comprehensive history is not always necessary for adequate therapy, but is essential for clearest understanding of the patient's illness and a clearer understanding of allergy."[102]

While a one-on-one interview was the best way for the patient to divulge such information, Vaughan also recommended using questionnaires, in order to get supplemental details. Here, too, the value placed on information provided by patients was explicit:

> Please record below any substances which you have found to cause symptoms mentioned below. . . . Describe in detail how they affect or affected you. Write down whether they no longer trouble you. If so, how long did they bother you? Please make your answers very explicit. Describe any other symptoms that you can attribute to some particular substance with which you come in contact. If you suspect certain things but cannot be sure, describe them and indicate that you just suspect them, and tell why you do.[103]

What is interesting about these instructions is not only the details requested, but more so the subtlety with which patients were expected to recount their experiences. Patients were asked to be "explicit," to provide details, to quantify, to qualify, and even to speculate. On another two-and-a-half-page form, which focused on patients' migraines, even more details were requested, highlighting yet again the premium placed on patient testimony.

And that was not all. Although Vaughan admitted that most physicians might "feel that with the preliminary anamnesis as comprehensive as it has been described there would be little left for the patient to tell in subsequent discussions," more evidence could be had following the initial diagnosis.[104] For instance, if a patient was diagnosed with an allergy to chocolate, she might then recall other instances in which chocolate likely caused a certain symptom. Moreover, Vaughan recommended arming the patient with more information about allergy so that he might be able to mine his allergic history further and "more intelligently to observe his response to contact with potentially allergic substances;" Vaughan's own *Primer of Allergy* served very nicely for such an education.[105] In order to take advantage of all this information, clinicians had to keep a comprehensive and current record of all their patients' experiences. Such records were useful partly because of the intractable nature of food allergy, meaning that a food allergist might treat a patient for a period of years, and partly also because, as Vaughan warned, "no two allergic cases are exactly alike in their symptom grouping, their sensitizations, and their response to treatment."[106] Patients, therefore, were treated quite seriously by food allergists; they were treated as individuals.

Given that many orthodox allergists believed their food allergy patients to be hypochondriacs, the emphasis food allergists placed on patient testimony, as well as the sense of partnership in the diagnostic process, is striking. It may have been than some of this trust boiled down to the simple fact that, ultimately, patients were on their own when it came to treatment of their food allergies. The diagnostic process might take up to a year to complete, but dealing with a food allergy once diagnosed was the responsibility of a lifetime and was largely left up to sufferers.[107] Although desensitization had some history in cases of food allergy, first being used in London by Alfred T. Schofield to treat urticaria and asthma caused by eggs, the practice had been largely abandoned on the grounds of safety, meaning that patients were left to their own devices to avoid problem foods.[108] As Helen Morgan ruefully observed, "Doctors consider their work done when they have played detective and uncovered your food enemies. They can't go into the kitchen and cook for you, too."[109] If food allergists were to experience any kind of clinical success, they had to empower their patients to take a leading role in both diagnosis and, especially, treatment.

The cooperative, sympathetic relationship food allergists enjoyed with their patients was further enhanced by the fact that many individuals came to food allergists as a last resort. Food allergists often relished their ability to help in such desperate cases. As a friend of Theron Randolph—and an allergy sufferer—remarked, "It is a grand life to be in allergy and get enthusiastic about curing the psychoneurotic, and the impossible."[110] Discussing how food allergies could cause fatigue and irritability in children, for example, Randolph acknowledged that "a common reaction is to assume that the child is a 'naughty brat' and to inflict various types of punishment to induce the child to 'snap out of it.'"[111] After effective allergy management, however, the improvement in the child's behavior demonstrated to all parties the importance of considering food allergy before demonizing the child or his parents.

In this way, the blame for symptoms shifted from resting solely with the patient (and her faulty immune system, parents, or mental state) to outside agents, specifically, food. By seeing their patients as not inherently damaged, and by perceiving them as intelligent, active partners in diagnosis and treatment, food allergists attracted many sufferers who had failed to find help elsewhere; this attitude also engendered a fierce loyalty in these patients. In the eyes of many patients, food allergists, unlike psychosomatically oriented allergists, were on the side of their patients, both empathizing with them and empowering them.[112] Relieved that their symptoms were "not all in the mind," patients and parents would play a key role in forming groups such as the Society for Clinical Ecology (SCE), founded by Theron Randolph in 1965 (renamed the American Academy of Environmental Medicine [AAEM] in 1984), and the Feingold Association of the United States, which stressed the link between food additives and hyperactivity in children. For these groups, clinicians such as Randolph and Feingold were granted near-hagiographic status, as opposed to the villains who downplayed such links.

Another crucial factor that played a substantial role in the sympathetic relationship that evolved between most food allergists and their patients, however, had more to do with the allergists themselves. Specifically, many, if not most, leading food allergists were patients themselves. Often, it was the clinicians' epiphany about their own food allergies that spurred them to consider the condition as a potent cause of mysterious chronic health problems. While such first-person success stories undoubtedly convinced many patients that they, too, might suffer from food allergies, they also raised the suspicions of orthodox allergists.

The case of Herbert Rinkel, for example, provides a fascinating, if disgusting, case of self-diagnosis. Rinkel was the son of a Kansas farmer who entered Northwestern University Medical School after serving in the First World War as a regimental photographer. Married and with a young son, Rinkel had very little money during his studies and subsisted on eggs that his father sent him from the farm. Throughout his studies, he developed a host of chronic symptoms, including a sore throat, inflamed ears, and a runny nose, which was especially problematic. As an avid photographer, his nose would run constantly while he developed film in his sink. Not being able to interrupt what he was doing, the "ropes of mucous" would run from his nostrils and onto the floor.[113]

Upon graduation, Rinkel opened a practice in Chicago and came across some of Albert Rowe's works on food allergy. Deciding to self-experiment to see if his nasal symptoms were allergic, he ate six eggs in rapid succession and waited for a reaction. Nothing happened, and, if anything, he felt better than normal. Determining that his problems must have a different cause— and not particularly inclined to give up eggs, which he continued (astonishingly) to like—Rinkel abandoned the hypothesis, but the symptoms, which now included headaches and fatigue, persisted. Four years later and in Oklahoma City studying allergy, Rinkel embarked on another self-experiment, this time eliminating eggs altogether from his diet. It would be the first time since he had started medical school that Rinkel would go through a day without eating an egg, and within a few days he began to feel better. Five days later, he ate a piece of birthday cake baked for him by his wife. Within ten minutes, he fainted and collapsed to the floor. After going through the list of ingredients with his wife, he discovered that the cake had included three eggs. Now highly suspicious of eggs, Rinkel avoided them for five more days and then ate one to see if the acute reaction would recur. It did and Rinkel subsequently began to check patients for similar "masked" allergies, eventually developing his individual food-testing technique.[114]

Rinkel's case bore similarities to those experienced by other food allergists. As with Rinkel, it often took many years for food allergists to diagnose their own food allergies, often because they were caused by foods eaten on a daily basis—like Rinkel's eggs—or because they were foods used as ingredients in baking or food processing, also like Rinkel's eggs. Despite having studied and written about food allergy for nearly a decade, Randolph, who knew that he himself was sensitive to peanuts and maple, was oblivious to his allergies to corn, wheat, and other cereal grains, the reactions to which caused headaches and "uncontrollable intermittent somnolence." After being alerted to the possibility by Rinkel, who was also allergic to corn, in 1944 Randolph "promptly diagnosed my own allergy to corn and with the avoidance of all cereal grains, dissipated my chronic fatigue and intermittent headaches as well as increasing my general level of competence."[115]

Similar epiphanies were also spurred by food allergists interacting or corresponding with one another about their allergies. After all, it was one thing to be convinced by one's patients that food allergies could trigger numerous symptoms; it was quite another if a colleague, especially a leading allergist, provided the evidence. In 1944, after Randolph published a paper on a case in which a patient's milk allergy triggered neurological symptoms, Rowe wrote to him, explaining that he thought himself to be "a neurotic individual only to find some 15 or 20 years ago that food allergy was entirely responsible for the difficulty."[116] Five years later, having been advised by Randolph to suspect corn allergy in a particularly recalcitrant patient, Rowe similarly discovered at the age of sixty that he was also sensitive to corn. As Rinkel reflected to Randolph about Rowe's corn allergy: "It stimulates lots of these fellows to think about it, you know. They go home and begin to check it and the first thing you know they find it is true."[117]

Although the allergies experienced by Rowe, Randolph, Rinkel, and others were extensive, the most allergic food allergist was possibly Arthur Coca, who suffered severe migraines, dizziness, and hypertension, which he blamed not only on food allergies but also on a number of other inhalant allergies. Randolph, who dated his interest in environmental allergy back to a speech Coca gave in 1933 to his senior medical school class, recalled meeting him for the first time in 1938 at Harvard, where Coca was speaking to the Sneeze, Wheeze, and Itch Club, subsequently and unimaginatively renamed the Boston Allergy Society. Coca arrived with a box, and Randolph, who happened to be on hand, offered to take it, along with his coat and hat. Coca demurred and kept the box under his arm. At the dinner that followed the speech, Coca refused his plate of food and, instead, requested an empty plate. When it arrived, he took food from the box, put it on the plate, and began to eat, clearly not trusting the kitchen staff with his allergies.[118]

Coca also suspected that he was allergic to numerous other substances, including dust, tobacco smoke, cooking gas, automotive exhaust, newsprint, cleaning chemicals, and perfume, stating that "fragrant females make me *miserable!*"[119] In order to avoid accidental exposure, he took extreme measures, including constructing a semidetached kitchen to prevent exposure to cooking gas, having his newspapers and magazines baked in the oven, installing air filters and dustproof covers to his bedding and upholstery, sleeping in a partially closed-off sunporch, and spraying all his rugs with Dust-Seal, an adsorptive mineral oil that reduced household dust.[120] Coca almost never ate out due to his fear of mistakenly eating foods to which he was allergic, and in his later years he avoided going out altogether. As Randolph remarked on the possibility of a rare Coca appearance, "I am delighted to hear that Dr. Coca is coming out to discuss this paper. This, really, is an unheard of honor. You may not know but he has rarely every ventured out during the past decade . . . he is fragile from the standpoint of reacting to tobacco smoke and to odors."[121] It is possible that Coca never made it to the discussion mentioned by Randolph, as he died the following month, having lived to his mid-eighties in spite of all his allergies.

THE SCALE OF THE PROBLEM

Perhaps due in large part to their own personal experiences, as well as their willingness to trust their patients' testimony, food allergists were inclined to suspect food allergy as the cause of potentially every chronic health problem encountered in the clinic, with precious few foods exempt from the list of culprits. From the gastrointestinal tract and the skin to respiration and the brain, virtually every system of the body was susceptible. Among the long list of complaints thought to be caused by food allergy included alcoholism, arthritis, asthma, colic, depression, diarrhea, dizziness, eczema, epilepsy, fatigue, flatulence, gastroenteritis, giddiness, hay fever, hyperactivity, incoordination, indigestion, insomnia, irritability, migraine, nervousness, rhinitis, stuttering, ulcers, urticaria, violent behavior, and vomiting.[122] According to Coca, ever the most enthusiastic of food allergists, allergy was also at the heart of even more conditions, including cancer, glaucoma, hypertension, male-pattern baldness, multiple sclerosis, and even the common cold; in fact, one of Coca's chapters in *The Pulse Test for Allergy* was "You Don't Catch Your Colds—You Eat Them." Coca also argued that many of the tribulations associated with old age were particularly allergenic: "The problem of old age will surely change when the new knowledge of food-allergy is put to universal use. Instead of planning for the care of the 'aged,' we shall have to find the work for them which they will certainly demand in their emancipation from the allergic handicap."[123]

Due to the astonishing array of conditions perceived as potentially allergic in nature, it followed that many food allergists estimated that a large percentage of the population were sufferers, whether they knew it or not. Warren Vaughan, for instance, calculated that more than 60 percent of the American population was allergic to one food or another, a figure that Coca judged as "essentially correct if it is not possibly somewhat conservative."[124] In making his approximation, which was based on a survey of the town of

Clover, Virginia, Vaughan included what he described as both "frank" and "fortunate" food allergy sufferers.[125] Fortunate sufferers, those who had so-called minor allergy, reacted to foods that were eaten relatively rarely, such as "cucumber, watermelon, strawberry, tomato, onion, and cabbage."[126] Such sufferers were fortunate since allergies to these foods were fairly easy to identify; indeed, Vaughan acknowledged that many such individuals were able to diagnose them without medical assistance. They were also fortunate because of the possibility that if they avoided the food for long enough, they might eventually lose their sensitivity to it.

Frank sufferers, however, reacted to common foods, such as wheat, milk, eggs, beans, and potatoes, which also tended to be hidden in baked goods, sauces, and pre-prepared foods, such as canned soups and stews. These sufferers were much less likely to identify the cause or causes of their ailments. Moreover, since such foods were consumed on a daily basis, the frank allergic were unlikely to become naturally desensitized, meaning that their chronic symptoms, many of which might have been incorrectly diagnosed by physicians as having different origins, were unremitting.

Most other food allergists did not adopt Vaughan's terminology of fortunate and frank sufferers, but they did recognize the scale of hidden or "masked" food allergy, as Rinkel termed it, urging other clinicians to consider it as an explanation for undiagnosed chronic health problems.[127] Such pleas fell on deaf ears, leading Albert Rowe to lament that "failure of the majority of physicians and specialists, including most allergists, to recognize, study, and control such allergies is . . . one of the main deficiencies in medical practice today," accounting "for much unnecessary morbidity, invalidism, and even mortality."[128] The concerns of Rowe, who endeavored to emphasize the ubiquity of food allergy at medical meetings and in the media throughout his career, were echoed and even inflated by other food allergists in the years that followed, as environmental theories of allergy began to flourish.[129] The British psychiatrist-cum-food allergist Richard Mackarness, for instance, argued that allergy "was the greatest cause of illness in Western civilization," blaming "the industrial production of food" for its rise.[130] While such claims did little to convince orthodox allergists that rates of food allergy were anywhere near that projected by food allergists, they struck a chord with the general public, whose suspicions about the food supply and the chemicals found in it increased during the postwar period.

Although the controversies that surrounded food allergy would be magnified by the postwar environmental movement, they were rooted in long-standing debates within the allergy community about the scope and significance of the condition. An editorial in the *Journal of Allergy* declared: "Controversy rages around the clinical importance and frequency of food allergy in a more lively manner than around any other subject in the field of allergy. The reason for this undoubtedly lies in the difficulties which beset the clinician when he sets out by clinical experiment or observation to investigate it."[131]

Partly because of earlier debates about how to define allergy, partly because of the difficulties in diagnosing food allergy and the resulting reliance on patient testimony, and partly because of food allergy enthusiasm, orthodox allergists had long expressed grave doubts about the impact that food allergy and food allergists had on the reputation of allergy as a legitimate medical discipline. Allergy, much like psychiatry, was a marginalized field within medicine that struggled to attract "high-grade men" into the discipline, let alone funding for research.[132] Ben Z. Rappaport (1897–1981), president of the AAA in 1953, for example, contrasted the $27 million allocated for cancer research by the National Research Council during the period 1947 to 1951 with the $800,000 provided for allergy research during the same period.[133] Rappaport warned that allergists would have to "tell the story of allergy over and over for a long time to produce the necessary impact on public attention and opinion" and reduce such 'disparity.'"[134]

To orthodox allergists, however, that story would not include a chapter on food allergy. Although many leaders within the allergy community lamented that medical schools underestimated the significance of allergy, the apparently extravagant claims of food allergists made matters worse, hampering their efforts to improve the standing of allergy. As Leslie N. Gay (1891–1978), president of the SSAAC in 1927, charged in 1948: "We have directed our efforts constantly toward the improvement of the standard of men who are interested in Allergy. Unfortunately, allergists have a rather low rating among internists in this country. This is due primarily to the fact that they have not 'lived down' the reputation acquired many years ago—that the majority practiced quackery."[135] Coming from Gay, who had attacked the books of food allergists, such as Rowe, Vaughan, and Coca, it is clear whom he thought were quacks.[136] He stated in a review of Rowe's *Elimination Diets and the Patients' Allergies*:

To any physician who is a disciple of Rowe, I am sure that this publication will be very helpful in the preparation of menus for patients suspected of having some food sensitivity. As the reviewer does not agree with the opinion that food plays such a major role in allergic diseases, expecting in infants, young children, and a small proportion of adults, it is natural that the opinion expressed is critical. The manual is written with such didactic positiveness that one who is inexperienced might accept "food sensitivities." Unfortunately, the tendency toward a broad interpretation of the definition of allergy, accompanied by reports of cases inadequately studied and not followed for a sufficient period of time, has frequently led to undue emphasis upon the prevalence of food allergy.[137]

For Gay and many other orthodox allergists, food allergists such as Rowe, whose "positiveness" attracted "disciples," did little to establish the legitimacy of allergy as a whole.

The gulf that existed between orthodox allergists, such as Gay, and food allergists, such as Rowe, was also reflected in the United States by the outlook of the societies that emerged to represent American allergists. Representing orthodox allergists, many of whom were situated in universities, was the AAA, which was formed by the merger of the SSAAC, based on the East Coast, and the American Association for the Study of Allergy, based on the West Coast, in 1943, and now known as the American Academy of Allergy, Asthma and Immunology (AAAAI). Clinicians found their home in the ACA, founded the previous year, and now known as the American College of Allergy, Asthma and Immunology (ACAAI). Each association also had its own journal, the *Journal of Allergy* and the *Annals of Allergy*, respectively. Whereas the AAA valued academic research, supported the development of immunological theory, and generally downplayed the significance of food allergy, the ACA put greater stock in the knowledge derived from clinical encounters, gave a forum for the discussion of food allergy (and, to a lesser extent, clinical ecology) at its meetings and in its publications, and, as a result, was less likely to minimize the prevalence of the condition.[138] Representing the interests of academic allergists eager to establish allergy as legitimate medical science and the desires of clinical allergists to raise awareness among other physicians about the prominence of allergy as a major cause of ill health, respectively, the AAA and the ACA were often at cross-purposes when it came to understanding allergy and its prevalence, and food allergy, ever contentious, was at the heart of these divisions.

• • •

DESPITE THE MISGIVINGS OF ORTHODOX ALLERGISTS, it was impossible to amputate food allergy from allergy, much like a gangrenous limb. Food allergy was too integral to the ways most clinicians as well as the general public understood allergy, something that early allergy researchers accepted. When early investigators, such as Charles Richet, Clemens von Pirquet, Milton J. Rosenau (1869–1946), and John Anderson (1873–1958), listed the clinical manifestations of allergy, they mentioned allergies to various foods just as readily as hay fever and asthma, emphasizing the long-standing acknowledgment of such reactions. Perhaps more so than any other allergic disease, food allergy symbolized allergy during these years. But it did not take long to realize that despite being part of the family, food allergy, like an unruly child, did not follow the same rules.

Neither did food allergists. Stripped of the tools employed by other allergists, food allergists had to discover other ways to diagnose and treat patients. In the process, they distanced themselves from orthodox allergists not only in terms of their diagnostic and therapeutic techniques and the economies associated with them but also with respect to how to understand allergy. To learn about food allergy, one had to be a detective, unconventionally investigating each case on its own merits with the full cooperation of the patient, yet also gradually building up a body of inductive, anecdotal evidence that would provide insights for the next case, and the one after that. In order to gather enough clues to make the correct diagnosis, food allergists also had to be much more holistic in their approach than their orthodox colleagues, who reduced the practice of allergy to skin testing and desensitization therapy.[139] Over time, and often through their own personal experiences, food allergists came to believe that food allergy was responsible for much of the undiagnosed, chronic illnesses suffered by patients. And while critics might scoff at their self-proclaimed accomplishments, arguing that even faith healers could elicit a placebo effect, food allergists did manage to run successful clinics, which thrived for decades, indicating that if they failed to convince some of their colleagues of the importance of food allergy, they did convince their patients.

Despite dabbling in a dubious area of medicine, part of this success was also due to the fact that many of the most notorious food allergists were well-respected physicians, leaders within their incipient field. Albert Rowe, Arthur Coca, and Warren Vaughan took turns as presidents of allergy associations. While Coca had held high-level positions in both academia and industry, Vaughan came from medical royalty. His father, Victor C. Vaughan (1851–1929), as well as being one of the earliest allergy investigators, "was a leading figure in US medicine during the late nineteenth century and throughout the Progressive Era," serving as dean of the University of Michigan Medical School (1891–1920) and as president of the American Medical Association (AMA) from 1914 to 1915.[140] Many other food allergists held leadership positions in other associations and were cited regularly as pioneers in their field. Perhaps most important, food allergists were regularly invited to present papers at medical meetings and published voluminously in leading medical journals. During the first half of the twentieth century, food allergy—and food allergists—enjoyed a certain amount of respectability.

This soon changed, as the claims of food allergists and clinical ecologists became enmeshed with the environmental movement, and orthodox allergists strove even harder to safeguard the legitimacy of their field. Food allergy would not return to a position of priority for three decades, when mushrooming rates of peanut allergy thrust it—or at least one version of it—back onto the agenda. But although peanut allergy and other anaphylactic food allergies are treated seriously today, the notion that chronic conditions, such as migraine, asthma, and mental disorders, could be caused by what one eats is still ridiculed in many quarters. It is true that, just as in the 1930s and 1940s, much of the evidence to support such claims remains anecdotal, inductive, patient-driven, and, to many skeptics, unconvincing. Nevertheless, such "orphans of medical science" often remain undiagnosed and untreated. Perhaps in dismissing the innovative, creative, patient-focused, and time-intensive methods food allergists employed and adopted out of desperation in order to help their patients, medicine lost something it has struggled since to recover.

FOUR

Panic?
Or the Pantry?

IN 1957, Ethan Allan Brown (1906–1979), then president of the ACA, declared:

> In this age of chemicals and synthetics there is truly no limit as to what sub-
> stances may be discovered as causes of allergy. . . . It is not too much to expect
> that one or several new ubiquitous allergens may be discovered at any time.
> This would, of course, change overnight the present practice of allergy. Among
> these might be the more than 1,000 "additives" now ingested with foods and
> now certified for safety but not to allergenicity.[1]

If this was not alarming enough, added to it was allergists' struggle to answer basic questions about the root causes of allergy, including: "Why do
mammals become allergic? Why do they become allergic when they do?
Why do they become allergic to one substance and not another?"[2] For many
food allergists after the Second World War, the answers to Brown's questions about what caused allergy had much to do with his previous comments about food additives. What made people allergic? During the postwar
period, many people suspected that changes in the environment and the increasing number of chemicals in the food supply were responsible.

To a degree, the 1950s, 1960s, and 1970s represented the environmental turn in food allergy, the decades in which food additives and processed
foods, such as corn derivatives and refined sugar, were highlighted by food
allergists as being particularly disruptive allergens. Such thinking reflected

heightened concerns about the environment which had emerged in the United Kingdom during the 1930s and 1940s, with the rise of the organic food movement and the foundation of the Soil Association (1946), and had taken hold in the United States during the 1950s.[3] Although the modern environmental movement is often believed to have been launched with the publication of Rachel Carson's *Silent Spring* in 1962, her exposé of the ecological and health impacts of agricultural chemicals, however momentous and influential, could be alternatively interpreted as the articulation of fears that had been percolating for more than a decade but had not yet been expressed so eloquently, or so persuasively.[4]

For a start, Carson (1907–1964) was prompted by others already campaigning against the use of pesticides. A series of letters between Beatrice Trum Hunter (b. 1918), a New Hampshire writer and lay nutritionist, and Carson reveal how the latter was influenced by the former's campaign to stop the United States Department of Agriculture (USDA) from spraying New England with DDT to control a gypsy moth infestation.[5] Hunter had been liaising with a group of wealthy Long Islanders, including Marjorie Spock (1904–2008), sister of the pediatrician Benjamin Spock (1903–1998), who had begun legal action (which was ultimately unsuccessful) to stop spraying DDT in their region. She wrote a letter to the *Boston Herald* about their cause on January 12, 1958, which moved Carson to ask the New Hampshire author for her references. Hunter, who had reviewed Carson's *The Edge of the Sea* for her local newspaper, responded within days with an eight-page litany of evidence, which not only spurred Carson to investigate further but also formed the foundation for Carson's *Silent Spring* research.[6] Hunter went on to play a major role in the clinical ecology movement.

Another example of nascent concern about food chemicals during the 1950s was the passage of the Delaney Clause, or Food Additive Amendment, in 1958, which amended the Food, Drugs, and Cosmetics Act of 1938 to ban all food additives that were found to cause cancer in laboratory animals.[7] The Delaney Clause, named after the New York congressman James Delaney (1901–1987), had its origins in the Chemicals in Food Products hearings, which began in 1950. It took nearly a decade for the amendment to be passed, partly because of the lack of governmental or scientific interest in investigating food chemicals, and partly due to the "extensive and intensive" nature of the hearings themselves and the political maneuvering that followed, thus highlighting the contentious nature of the topic.[8]

While the passage of the clause provides some evidence of American concern about the use of food chemicals, the controversy it engendered also acted to unify food manufacturers, chemical companies, agricultural interests, and sympathetic scientists against such ideas. Documentation of such a backlash, which certainly included attacks on Rachel Carson and *Silent Spring*, can be found in a variety of contemporary newspapers, journals, and broadcasts, but perhaps the most illustrative example is *Panic in the Pantry* (1975), a reactionary polemic that ridiculed the connection between food chemicals and ill health of any sort.[9] Written by the New York City epidemiologist and author Elizabeth A. Whalen and the Harvard nutrition scientist Frederick J. Stare (1910-2002), *Panic in the Pantry* sarcastically branded those who questioned food additives as faddists. While Stare established Harvard's Department of Nutrition largely on the back of food industry funding in 1942, Whalen continues to serve as president of the industry-friendly lobby group, the American Council on Science and Health (ACSH), which she helped found in 1978.[10] Dedicated to "those of us who look forward to meals," and festooned with cartoons and letters to the Food and Drug Administration (FDA) from panicked consumers, the book's chief objective was to undermine the organic food movement, the health food and vitamin industry, and the Delaney Clause, but many of its barbs could have easily been leveled at food allergists as well.[11] The one allergist mentioned in the book was Ben Feingold, whose food additive–free diet for hyperactivity had recently gained international attention. Given that Feingold himself had previously been a fairly orthodox allergist, sparring in particular with his Bay Area rival Albert Rowe, there were certainly easier targets available.[12] As early as 1950, twenty-five years before the publication of *Panic in the Pantry*, Theron Randolph had voiced concern about retaliation from the "corn people" after he had identified corn as being an especially problematic and ubiquitous allergen found in innumerable processed foods.[13] As Randolph's concerns spread from corn to chemicals in the environment, he and his allies felt even more marginalized by orthodox allergists and under fire from the food, chemical, and pharmaceutical industries.

But the environmental movement was not the only external factor influencing allergy during the postwar period. One section of Brown's editorial discussed another potent theory for allergy, which had recently emerged, as well as his opinion of it: "In present-day journals (the editors of which should know better) there are papers (by physicians who should also know better) stating that not only asthma, but all allergy as such is 'psychoso-matic.' . . . The less one knows of any aspect of medicine, the more likely one is to believe that it is all psychosomatic. . . . Much of this literature is excellent fiction."[14] As Brown despairingly indicated, allergy had also taken a psychosomatic turn.[15] To a degree, examining the psychological compo-nent of an allergic reaction was nothing new. Many physicians who studied asthma prior to the twentieth century, including Jan van Helmont (1577–1644), Thomas Willis (1621–1675), John Floyer, and Henry Hyde Salter, had acknowledged that a patient's emotional state could cause or exacerbate an attack, with Salter listing both "remote nervous irritation" and "psychical irritants" as two of the four primary triggers of an attack.[16] Shortly after Cle-mens von Pirquet's coining of the term "allergy" in 1906, other physicians, including the influential Canadian Sir William Osler, also expressed the belief that asthma contained a "strong neurotic element."[17] But during the 1940s and 1950s, the stress on such "irritants," now deemed to be psycho-somatic factors, became predominant in allergy. Due to the influence of the German psychiatrist Erich Wittkower (1899–1983) and his concept of the "al-lergy personality," Helen Flanders Dunbar (1902–1959), an American psycho-analyst who co-founded *Psychosomatic Medicine* in 1939 with the Hungarian psychoanalyst Franz Alexander (1891–1964), and the general psychoanalyti-cal zeitgeist of the period, the psychological state of the patient would soon be foremost in the thoughts of many allergists.[18]

It should be no surprise, particularly given the symbiotic relationship food allergists had with their patients, that orthodox allergists stressing the psychosomatic clashed concussively with those who emphasized food, environmental pollutants, and dietary chemicals. After all, the last thing a food allergist was wont to do was to dismiss a patient's chronic symptoms as psychosomatic and possibly refer them for psychotherapy or some other form of treatment. On the contrary, food allergists expressed a great deal of pride in determining that a patient's problems were not psychological but due, instead, to food. Widening the divide between the two models of al-lergy even farther was the belief that some food reactions manifested them-selves in mental disorders. In other words, the patients seen by orthodox, psychosomatically oriented allergists might well come across as mentally disturbed, but the root cause of their disorder was not to be found in the Oe-dipus complex or some other psychoanalytical explanation: their problem was an allergy to food. Putting an artificially colored cherry on top of such debates was that during the 1960s and 1970s, food chemicals were specifically implicated in the unresolved mental disorders of many patients, including children.

In this way, disputes about food allergy during the postwar period were framed on competing ideologies, one rooted in the emerging environmental movement and concerns about processed foods and food chemicals, and the other centered on the mid-twentieth-century fascination with psychosomatic medicine and Freudian psychoanalysis. In order to understand the impact of both of these models of allergic disease, this chapter concentrates on how the relationship between mental illness and food allergy was variously depicted by food allergists and psychoanalytically oriented allergists. The resulting divisions split the allergy community and, indeed, led many food allergists to abandon both the field—and the concept—of allergy itself.

PUZZLING NERVOUS STORMS

In 1950, the New York allergist T. Wood Clarke surveyed 171 Canadian and American allergists about the relationship between allergy and "character problems" in children.[19] Clarke, a consulting allergist at Utica's Marcy State Hospital, explained his motivation by describing the case of a fifteen-year-old boy, who had been referred to him in 1945 by his late colleague Richard H. Hutchings (1867–1947), a past president of the American Psychiatric Association and editor of *Psychiatric Quarterly*. The boy, who had been "happy and amenable" as a child, had been suffering for three years "from attacks of acute excitement during which he would rage around the house smashing china and furniture."[20] Seemingly destined for institutionalization, the boy was examined by Hutchings, who had been interested in Clarke's work on allergy and epilepsy. Discovering that the boy was also afflicted with eczema, hay fever, and asthma, Hutchings referred him to Clarke. Skin testing indicated that the boy was allergic to oat, wheat, feathers, pollen, cat dander, and house dust, and Clarke promptly prescribed the removal of the offending foods from the boy's diet and desensitization for the inhalant allergies. According to Clarke, "The results of removing the oat and wheat from his diet were dramatic in the extreme. Almost overnight the boy's entire character changed. From being unhappy and apprehensive he became, in a very few days, happy and co-operative. He has had no outbreaks of temper for five years. He is friendly and full of fun. He is now doing well in college."[21]

The case, along with the similarly successful treatment of a woman admitted to Marcy State Hospital a dozen times for "episodic mental disorder," and that of a "morose boy, who had been expelled from four schools as incorrigible," made Clarke curious.[22] Perhaps, he speculated, many "problem children" were in fact simply victims of allergy or, to be more specific, "cerebral allergy" or "neuroallergy."[23] Eager to determine if other allergists had experienced similar cases, Clarke discussed the issue at the 1949 ACA meeting, where it was agreed that he continue to investigate.

The results of Clarke's survey were published in the *Annals of Allergy* and *Psychiatric Quarterly*, and read at the 1950 ACA meeting. Of the 171 respondents, 95 of them, or 56 percent, assured Clarke "that they had noticed personality changes due to allergy which corrected themselves when the allergic element was eliminated." In terms of the remaining 76 respondents, 58 did not tend to treat children or had not noticed such a phenomenon, 9 believed that allergy had nothing to do with personality, and 7 believed that allergy was psychosomatic. In sum, the survey revealed to Clarke that he "was on the right track" and that both allergists and child psychiatrists ought to be alerted to the problem of neuroallergy.[24] Psychosomatic factors, it appeared, "could travel in reverse gear."[25]

The bulk of the rest of Clarke's article consisted of case studies and opinions provided by his respondents about the issue. While the Boston physician Abraham Colmes affirmed that there was "no doubt in the mind of any physician who is practicing allergy that food sensitivities do bring about definite changes in children's behavior," Fannie Lou Leney (1902–1994), an Oklahoma pediatric allergist, attested that "practically every day since I have been practicing allergy, mothers come in with the statement that 'Johnny is so irritable,' or 'his disposition is so much better since he is on his diet,' or that 'he is as mean as the devil when he eats a certain food.'"[26] Other contributors added that controlling a child's allergies could have a marked effect on her school performance. William A. Thornhill remarked that "when a child is sent to us for allergy . . . I find the grades . . . may be low. After a semester or a year of allergy control, these youngsters make a distinct rise in their class standing."[27]

While many of the examples provided echoed Thornhill's observation about scholastic improvement, others stressed that the successful treatment of schoolchildren with neuroallergy also helped with psychosocial development. An eleven-year-old boy whose allergies to "celery, cauliflower,

PANIC? OR THE PANTRY?

peas, citrus fruit, oatmeal, and chocolate," made him "irritable, stubborn, rowdy, and introverted," was able to "regain" his friends once these foods were removed from his diet.[28] Preschool-aged children were also subject to such miraculous transformations. One "extremely irritable, 'spoiled'" three-year-old had struggled "exceedingly" with toilet training and was difficult to control, but when a number of offending foods, including, interestingly, peanuts, were removed from her diet, she became "a happy child, easily controlled."[29] Nonetheless, some parents remained unconvinced. The Michigan allergist Gerald C. Grout recounted the case of a ten-year-old boy who was found to be sensitive to "several of the more common foods, principally corn, wheat, chocolate, and orange," and whose irritability and personality changes had gradually improved following avoidance of these foods. The boy's "mother stated that it was difficult for her to believe, but she had finally been convinced that the complete reversal in the child's attitude and loss of irritability had accompanied improvement in the allergic symptoms. She further stated that prior to allergic management the child had never smiled and that now he is a very happy child."[30]

For Clarke, such anecdotes provided convincing evidence that many a child's undiagnosed allergies marked one out unfairly as a "problem child," a troubled soul who

> rarely has a pleasant life. He is punished for being naughty and disobedient. He has a difficult time in school, is disliked by his teachers and hated and tormented by his schoolmates. If his characteristics are due simply to a mean and selfish nature, he may get his just deserts: if they are due to faulty home training, his parents certainly get theirs. If, on the other hand, they are the result of a mental illness, he deserves great sympathy and every possible effort to correct the underlying physical or mental cause. If the cause is an allergic reaction . . . he deserves a thorough allergy study. A little time spent on this may change the whole course of a child's life. Allergy tests and appropriate treatment may be far more effective than either beatings or other forms of punishment.[31]

Even more worryingly:

> The "problem child" frequently grows up to be a normal, although often an erratic, adult. He may, however, end up as a true psychotic. . . . If every child who has to be sent to a state hospital, or every "problem child" seen our offices, or child guidance clinics, could be given a thorough allergy study, it is not too

much to hope that some, perhaps many, would be found to be allergic, could
have their allergy treated and could be returned to their homes normal emotionally as well as physically.[32]

The proper diagnosis of allergies, therefore, was central to stemming the
tide of mental disorder that alarmed many American physicians in the postwar period.[33] In the minds of allergists like Clarke and his respondents, the
field of allergy should no longer content itself with performing scratch tests
and desensitization; it could indeed play a role in treating and preventing
mental illness.

But how did an allergic reaction cause such psychiatric symptoms? When
some of the statements provided by Clarke's contributors are analyzed, it becomes clear that many allergists believed that mental health problems were
a secondary effect caused by the stress and strain of dealing with chronic
allergies, rather than a direct manifestation. As Louis Tuft (1898–1989), past
president of the SSAAC, declared, "I have seen a number of children in whom
the correction or improvement of the allergy has been followed by definite
lessening of the emotional instability and by better behavior."[34] The allergist
Frank F. A. Rawling (b. 1910), who had co-authored articles with Theron Randolph on drug sensitivity, concurred:

> So often during the first visit no mention is made of the child's behavior, and
> the only concern with the parents is the presenting allergic symptoms. How-
> ever, when the allergic situation has been brought under control, it is amazing
> how much emphasis is placed by the parents upon the altered behavior of the
> child. The stock phrase that is heard frequently is, "He is a different child to live
> with."[35]

Others similarly noted that successful treatment of allergy could improve
anything from a child's sleeping and eating habits to schoolwork and general disposition.

Clarke himself acknowledged that improvements in behavior could well
be simply a "pleasing and notable" by-product caused by the reduction of
physical symptoms. He even admitted that allergists should "pay more attention to the psyche of their child patients," hinting that psychosomatic
factors should also be considered.[36] But in countless other cases, the problem was purely neurological, an allergic reaction that caused swelling in
brain tissue, just as an allergy to strawberries might cause a rash on the skin

or a seafood allergy could trigger a facial edema. Such reactions were not so different from allergic migraine headaches. Citing the research of Victor Vaughan, the father of Warren Vaughan, who had "proved conclusively that one of the most common causes of migraine headaches was the ingestion of food against which the patient had an allergic sensitivity," Clarke argued that an intracranial edema or impaired vascular function in the brain could cause a variety of "bizarre neurologic symptoms," including those associated with mental illness and epilepsy.[37]

Although Clarke claimed that neuroallergies of this sort were the least appreciated of allergic manifestations, they had been observed by clinicians for decades. Eighteenth- and nineteenth-century physicians had already associated migraine headaches with food idiosyncrasies; within a decade of the birth of allergy, others were hypothesizing about its relationship to behavioral problems. One early description can be found in an article by a Detroit pediatrician, B. Raymond Hoobler, which discussed the symptoms associated with food sensitivities in infants. Along with intestinal, dermatological, respiratory, and anaphylactic reactions, Hoobler listed neurological symptoms, including irritability, restlessness, fretfulness, and insomnia.[38] In another journal article that would be cited repeatedly, the Minnesota pediatrician W. Ray Shannon similarly claimed that "food proteins to which the patient has become sensitized" could cause "extremely restless," "introspective," "nervous," "high-strung," "cruel," and "out-of-sorts" behavior as well as poor school performance.[39] Such children "could not sit still" and "were very hard to manage."[40] Other physicians, such as Alfred T. Schofield, Oscar M. Schloss, William Waddell Duke, George Piness, Albert Rowe (who described such symptoms as "food toxemia"), Wilmot F. Schneider, Theron Randolph, and Hal M. Davison (1898–1958), also observed how food allergies could trigger mental disorder in both children and adults, with Walter Alvarez describing such reactions as "puzzling nervous storms."[41]

In retrospect, it striking how similar many of the symptoms depicted by such physicians resembled what in 1957 would be termed "hyperkinetic impulse disorder," what is today known as attention deficit hyperactivity disorder (ADHD).[42] Schneider's article, "Psychiatric Evaluation of the Hyperkinetic Child," for example, began by describing the way teachers of the 1920s might have thought that the hyperkinetic child "had either St. Vitus Dance or pinworms, or, if a boy, needed a circumcision." Unfortunately, "too little attention is given by the general physician and pediatrician to the role of allergy."[43] Citing similar references, an article by Randolph in 1947 implicated food allergy even more specifically in the behavioral problems of childhood.[44] One of Randolph's cases involved an eight-year-old boy who, in addition to nasal obstruction and hearing difficulties, presented a range of behavioral problems, including "progressive fatigue, listlessness, irritability, crankiness . . . restlessness, jitteriness, inattentiveness, and apparent difficulty in concentration," all of which hampered his schoolwork.[45] In order to treat the somatic symptoms, the boy underwent a tonsillectomy and two adenoidectomies, all of which were ineffective. Once Randolph had determined that the boy was allergic to a range of foods and removed them from his diet, all the symptoms disappeared.

In 1954, three years prior to the coining of the term "hyperkinetic impulse disorder," many of the behavioral symptoms described by Rowe, Randolph, Clarke, Schneider, and others were encapsulated by the Kansas City pediatric allergist Frederic Speer in his term "allergic tension-fatigue syndrome."[46] Speer began his discussion of the syndrome by juxtaposing it with psychosomatic approaches to allergy, stating how

> the psychosomatic approach is now used in a wide field of medicine, with so much enthusiasm, in fact, that it is often forgotten that this relationship may operate in the opposite direction, and that somatic disease may often be the cause of disorders of feeling and behavior rather than the effect. This especially applies in pediatric practice, in which the patient's ability to express his complaints is limited and an organic basis for nervous manifestations may easily be overlooked.[47]

Speer's call to look beyond psychic explanations for behavioral problems in children mirrored similar efforts by psychiatrists who also turned to the nervous system for explanations. While some believed that many hyperactive children were the victims of brain damage, suffered either perinatally or during early childhood (giving rise to the use of the term "minimal brain damage"), others suspected underlying neurological disorder (resulting in the subtle switch to "minimal brain dysfunction").[48]

The symptoms delineated by Speer's allergic tension-fatigue syndrome could be grouped into two broad categories. The first category, representing the "tension" aspect of the syndrome, was characterized by hyperkinesis and irritability; the second, representing "fatigue," was characterized by sluggishness and torpor.[49] Such children were "torn between two extremes of feeling."[50] The hyperactive behavior Speer observed in such children attending his clinic was often marked and bore a striking resemblance to the descriptions of hyperkinetic children found in psychiatric journals:

> At school he is said to be the prime disturbing influence in his class. His actions when he visits the doctor clearly indicate that this must be so. When he bounces into the office he immediately announces, "Hurry up, I have to leave." In the reception room he is continually on the move, flitting from one activity to another, spending little time on anything. One minute he is hanging on his mother, the next exploring a desk and fingering and upsetting its contents . . . he is a study in impatience, talkativeness, and squirminess. He keeps up a constant babble of comments, jokes, and questions. He twists from one side to the other, attempts to lift himself by his hands, and in various other ways demonstrates his inability to restrain himself from virtually uninhibited activity.[51]

In addition to these behavioral symptoms, such children presented other signs of allergy, such as nasal congestion; sneezing; and dark rings, wrinkles, or bags under their eyes. Once physicians became aware of these signs, Speer argued, it became easier for them to recognize that such behavioral problems were not the result of underlying psychic problems, brain damage, poor parenting, or simply the actions of a "naughty brat," but were actually allergic. Why had the medical community failed to recognize neuroallergy? According to Speer, who traced the connection between food and mental health problems back to Robert Burton's *Anatomy of Melancholy* (1621), three factors, which had often undermined the theories of food allergists, were at fault: overenthusiasm; the rise of psychogenic theories; and, finally, the failure of skin tests to provide additional evidence.[52] As a result, he argued, many children were being diagnosed with mental disorders and prescribed psychiatric drugs when they should be treated for allergies.

HUMAN ECOLOGY AND THE CHEMICAL ENVIRONMENT

Up until the Second World War, the foods implicated in neurological reactions were identical to those that would cause gastrointestinal, dermatological, and even anaphylactic reactions, with milk, eggs, and grains being the most frequently cited culprits. Beginning in the 1950s, however, food chemicals became the prime suspects for many allergists.[53] To an extent, food allergists' increased focus on food chemicals simply reflected the fact that, following the war and the rapid development of food-production technologies, the number of additives found in the food supply increased, with the corollary that some people reacted to them. But to others, food additives represented something more sinister, an unwelcome intrusion of chemicals into people's diets that not only resulted in a host of bizarre symptoms but caused society itself to degenerate, becoming more violent and detached. Rising concern about the allergenicity of food additives also prompted some to contemplate whether foodstuffs associated with the emergence of agriculture millennia before, including milk, wheat, and corn, were similarly unhealthy, calling into question what was really "natural" for humans to consume. In this way, worries about food additives fomented alarm about the modern diet more generally and, increasingly, its role in mental illness.

All this does not mean that food additives were not consumed in the first half of the century. As the historian Harvey Levenstein has described, the use of food chemicals in American food production was highlighted as problematic as early as the 1880s and was indicted, along with other food-production practices, in Upton Sinclair's influential novel *The Jungle* (1906), which helped to inspire the Pure Food and Drug Act of 1906.[54] According to the historian Derek Oddy, similar developments occurred in the United Kingdom at roughly the same time, with "chemical preservatives, such as borax or formalin . . . used extensively in foodstuffs to extend shelf life."[55] That country's Adulteration of Food Act (1860) and Sale of Foods and Drugs Act (1875) were also early indications of concern about the chemicals used in food production for both legitimate and suspect purposes. Moreover, agitation about such additives persisted throughout the first half of the twentieth century. In the United States in 1933, for example, Arthur Kallet (1902–1972) and F. J. Schlink (1891–1995), both of whom worked as industrial engineers before becoming consumer advocates, co-authored *100,000,000 Guinea Pigs: Dangers in Everyday Foods, Drugs, and Cosmetics*, a scathing indictment of the food and chemical industry, as well as the "feeble and ineffective" Pure Food and Drug Act.[56] They claimed that many of the foods consumed by Americans were not only "worthless" but actually "dangerous" because of the chemicals used in their processing or preservation.[57]

There was a key difference, however, between the prewar perception of chemicals highlighted by muckrakers and whistle blowers, such as Sinclair, Kallet, and Schlink, and those views that would cause controversy in the postwar years. Most of the chemicals used in food production and identified as being problematic during the first half of the twentieth century were well known to be hazardous to human health and were recognized as such. Their use by food producers was perceived as either illicit or at least highly dubious, seen as a blatant attempt to stretch out food using hidden chemicals or inedible substances, preserve it with toxic substances beyond the point of when it should be consumed, or disguise it when it did spoil using coloring agents. When informed by Kallet and Schlink that lead arsenate was being sprayed on fruits and vegetables to prevent damage from insects, most consumers were justifiably alarmed, being at least somewhat aware of the toxic properties of arsenic and lead.[58] Earlier use of other chemical preservatives, such as boric acid and formaldehyde, was similarly recognized as suspect, if not outright illegal, given their toxic effects on human health.

After 1945, however, the situation became more complicated. The new food chemicals as well as food products that had been developed as part of the war effort were not regarded primarily as ways in which food producers could scurrilously increase their profit margin, though they often were just that, but rather as signifiers of scientific progress. As the DuPont slogan testified, food additives were simply an example of "Better Things for Better Living . . . Through Chemistry." Chemicals were no longer added to foods illicitly or even surreptitiously but very much on purpose and in the open. Consumers were well aware of such substances and eager to embrace them. The chemicals that made TV dinners and instant cake mixes possible were thought to liberate homemakers, freeing them—at least to an extent—from the kitchen's drudgery. As Levenstein explains with respect to the development and use of such food additives: "[M]ost American consumers were impressed by these achievements, and until well into the 1960s they showed little concern for the methods and ingredients which food processors employed to turn out a host of new products. . . . There was little inclination to question the products of the food business, which seemed to make life easier for the housewife with each new chemical breakthrough."[59]

Now meals were easier to prepare, and chemicals enhanced them with flashier colors, novel flavors, fewer imperfections, and increased shelf life. As a spokesman for the USDA retorted in response to *Silent Spring*'s warnings about DDT, "the balance of nature is a wonderful thing for people who sit back and write books or want to go out to Walden Pond and live as Thoreau did. But I don't know of a housewife today who will buy the type of wormy apples we had before pesticides."[60] William S. Gaud, the administrator of the USDA, even claimed that agricultural chemicals, such as pesticides and fertilizers, had contributed to a "Green Revolution," not only in the industrialized world but across the globe, allowing for more intensive, more productive agriculture, and amounting to a revolution "as significant and beneficial to mankind as the industrial revolution."[61]

But at what cost? For many food allergists, food additives were more than simply another allergen to which people could react; they were also a sign of the dangers that chemicals could pose to human health. As early as 1948, a Pennsylvania allergist, Stephen D. Lockey (1904–1985), speculated to the Pennsylvania Allergy Society that food dyes, especially the yellow azo dye tartrazine, could elicit untoward reactions, including urticaria and asthma.[62] Linking the chemical structure of such dyes to salicylates—low-molecule chemicals that are found naturally in aspirin and many fruits—Lockey began prescribing a diet that restricted such substances. He later wrote extensively about the hidden dangers of these and other chemical agents.[63] Ironically, some of the coal-tar dyes that Lockey identified as problematic were being used to flavor and identify corticosteroids, which allergists had begun to prescribe widely to mitigate against allergic reactions. By that time, other allergists, most notably Theron Randolph, had also begun writing about the dangers of synthetic food dyes as well as other chemicals.[64] Although Herbert Rinkel, Randolph, and Michael Zeller did not discuss food additives at length in *Food Allergy*, Randolph claimed to have first become concerned about them in the mid-1940s. He did not publish his observations about them, as well as pesticides, industrial solvents, liquid fuels, mosquito abatement sprays, and petrochemicals, until 1954.[65]

In the years leading up to that year, Randolph had experienced a series of profound professional and personal tribulations, which, though distressing, had in other ways freed him to begin his crusade against "the chemical environment." Randolph separated from his first wife in 1949, after eight years of marriage, and divorced soon after; his former wife moved to another part of the country with their three sons. While Randolph found being separated from his sons "hard to take," he remarried in 1954, this time to a woman who had been hyperactive as a child and subject to rhinitis, migraine, asthma, depression, and cardiac irregularities when exposed to gas fumes. Tudy

Randolph's health problems spurred Randolph to further investigate the role of chemicals in allergy, and she also became a key ally and confidante, working tirelessly in his clinics.[66]

Professionally, Randolph had also been divorced from Northwestern University, at which he had taught since setting up his private practice in Chicago in 1944. Soon after his arrival at Northwestern University Medical School and its subsidiary, Wesley Memorial Hospital, Randolph announced his interest in food allergy, which immediately set him apart from his colleagues, and by 1947 began writing *Food Allergy* with Rinkel and Zeller. During the course of research, writing, and ongoing clinical work, Randolph became increasingly convinced that refined sugars, especially those derived from corn and beet, caused many of his patients' chronic health problems, including "brain fag" or "brain fog," a self-described constellation of neurological symptoms.[67] Prior to the book's publication, Randolph began making his views about the role of sugar in allergy more public. In 1949, he testified before the FDA's Bread Hearings, requesting that the sources of sugars be made clear on food labels.[68] Other participating allergists, sponsored by the Corn Products Research Foundation, downplayed the need for such labeling. The following year, Randolph presented his views at a medical staff meeting at Wesley Memorial, along with a motion picture of a woman who fell into "an acute psychotic episode" after a blind test of beets and beet sugar. Although many of the medical students were intrigued, Randolph's chairman was not, retorting that the woman was clearly hysterical.[69] Soon, though not before the publication of *Food Allergy*, Wesley Memorial prohibited Randolph from listing his Northwestern affiliation in his publications, leaving him to cite his private office instead. This was to be the beginning of the end and, in the early summer of 1951, "the ax finally swung"; Randolph was dismissed from Northwestern Medical School, which branded him as "a pernicious influence on medical students."[70]

Randolph was understandably dismayed by his dismissal, which he believed had been orchestrated in part by the "corn people" and in part by his immediate superior at Northwestern, Samuel M. Feinberg (1895–1973). Feinberg, in whose name there is now a chair of medicine at Northwestern, was a formidable force within American allergy, due to his position at Northwestern, his ties to the AMA, and his impressive publication record, having written, among other works, one of the first allergy handbooks (1934) for general practitioners.[71] Although this handbook stressed the allergenicity of all foods, including corn, by the 1950s Feinberg was well established as an orthodox allergist who bemoaned the way "the label of 'food allergy' has been grossly misused."[72] Prior to his role in firing Randolph, Feinberg had attacked Randolph's views on sugar in *JAMA*, claiming that "the experience of the vast majority of experienced and well-trained allergists and immunologists has been diametrically opposed" to such ideas; had written a scathing review of *Food Allergy*; and even had tried to undermine Randolph's position as president of the Chicago Allergy Society.[73] According to Randolph's friend Harry Clark, Feinberg's animosity to Randolph had to go beyond a difference in opinion about food allergy: "I suppose most of it must be jealousy because in Feinberg's first book he admits allergies to all foods even corn, I believe. I shouldn't be a bit surprised if he's being paid and told what to do by the corn people. His attack was too direct. Surely he can't be as self confident as all that." Adding his support for Randolph's cause, Clark continued: "I can't tell you how much I admire you for fighting back at such injustice. But please do be careful, and if there is anything I can do, even if it's just to give you moral support. . . . It seems incredible to me that anyone working as hard as you have should still have to protect himself against little people."[74]

Despite the support of Clark and other friends, as well as his initial intention to take his case to the courts and the Chicago press, Randolph eventually decided to abandon any hopes of returning to Northwestern and spent the rest of the 1950s rebuilding his career. He remained president of the Chicago Allergy Society (1951–1953), set up the Rockwell M. Kempton Medical Research Fund (which changed its name in 1960 to the Human Ecology Research Foundation), and established the first "comprehensive environmental control unit" (CECU) at St. Francis Hospital in Evanston, Illinois, in 1954, eventually transferring the unit to the Lutheran General Hospital in Park Ridge, Illinois, in 1959.[75] By 1960, which for Randolph represented a "dividing line" in his career, the Illinois physician had helped to launch a subsection of the ACA called Allergy of the Nervous System, and founded a support group for chemically sensitive patients called Chemical Victims, which later changed its name to the Human Ecology Study Group. A year later, one year before the publication of *Silent Spring*, Randolph finally published a comprehensive account of how he believed human health was being jeopardized by the increasingly chemical environment.

Human Ecology and Susceptibility to the Chemical Environment, first published in four successive issues of *Annals of Allergy*, dealt with chemicals that came in contact with humans through the air, common objects (such as newspapers, cars, toiletries, or furniture), water, and the modern diet.[76] Allergists, Randolph claimed, had confused reactions to certain types of foods with hypersensitivity to the chemicals used in their cultivation or production. One of Randolph's patients, for example, discovered that he routinely developed a headache after eating commercially available apples and peaches, "but was able to eat . . . *unsprayed* fruits with impunity."[77] Unfortunately, warned Randolph, such residues were difficult to eliminate, even with rubbing, washing, or cooking. In addition, many so-called organic farmers were not trustworthy, succumbing to economic pressure to ensure improved appearance, increased yield, and against loss.[78]

Headaches were not the only neurological symptoms that typified such reactions. Randolph estimated that "about a third of my present practice is devoted to the problems of mental illness and related behavioral abnormalities. The way that this aspect of the work is increasing, it is not unlikely that this type of work may come to dominate my time."[79] One of these patients, a surgeon, suffered from chronic fatigue, insomnia, "sexual maladjustment," hyperactivity, and depression, none of which were alleviated by psychiatric treatment.[80] After adopting "a chemically uncontaminated diet," as well as "avoiding eggs and potato," his "sexual adjustment is now satisfactory. He is apparently a happier and more pleasant person, insofar as his family and associates are concerned, and he is *far more productive* in his work."[81] Reflecting on such psychiatric symptoms, Randolph speculated "that susceptibility to and maladaptation to the chemical environment and illnesses associated therewith are early manifestations of degeneration," an assumption on which others would soon expand.

Human Ecology and Susceptibility to the Chemical Environment received mixed reviews, as did virtually all of Randolph's publications. Fellow travelers, such as Beatrice Trum Hunter, equated his efforts with that of Rachel Carson in launching the modern environmental movement and described *Human Ecology* as a book "with profound implications for all."[82] Randolph also received letters of support from public-health workers, including a pair of high-ranking staff from the California Department of Public Health, who praised it as "extremely interesting and enlightening," illuminating "a subject that seems to have received far too little attention in the past."[83] An article in *Archives of Otolaryngology*, "Ahead of Their Time," even likened the work of Randolph, as with that of Rinkel, to the Hungarian physician Ignaz Semmelweis (1818–1865), whose theory of puerperal sepsis was ridiculed by his co-workers at the Vienna General Hospital, resulting, just like Randolph, in his dismissal.[84]

Others, however, scoffed at Randolph's efforts or decried them as scare-mongering: "In a time of war, it may be an indictable offence to spread information the nature of which is likely to cause dismay and depression among one's fellow citizens. This text will certainly cause uneasiness among the susceptible."[85] Perhaps worst of all, many journals chose not to commission it for review.[86] This was despite the fact that the publisher Charles C. Thomas, which produced most of the leading allergy volumes, printed two thousand copies of it, all of which sold. The book would be reprinted several times, though Randolph complained that it was difficult to find it in Chicago book stores.[87]

Although Randolph's efforts received some recognition—he was asked by Senator Hubert Humphrey (D-Minn.) to testify before Congress about pesticides in the early 1960s and was later called before the FDA's Peanut Butter Hearings in 1966—he increasingly felt ostracized from the mainstream medical community. He struggled to get published in major journals, and his paper proposals were often rejected at leading medical conferences, including both the ACA and APA meetings; Ethan Allan Brown, the editor of *Annals of Allergy*, remained one of his few allies.[88] Fed up, Randolph decided to abandon the field of allergy altogether and, on April 7, 1965, formed his own association, the Society for Clinical Ecology (SCE), in the unlikely location of Las Vegas. Describing his disenchantment and the need for the new medical specialty, Randolph explained that

allergists have been handicapped by self-imposed limitations of their field. Despite allergy having been originally defined as altered reactivity, the allergic concept of disease has since lost much of its usefulness by being restricted largely to hyper-reactivity, interpreted principally in terms of antigens and antibodies and limited essentially to localized clinical manifestations. A more clinically oriented and useful view is needed as a basis for understanding the long-term effects of a person's surroundings on his health and behavior.[89]

For Randolph, this split from allergy represented the culmination of nearly twenty years of struggle against what he saw as obstinate forces who were simply not willing to listen for ideological, political, or financial reasons. Ten years earlier, in a letter to Harry Clark, he had threatened to abandon the term "allergy" altogether, preferring to describe his patients using the terminology of sensitization and adaptation, which he had recently adopted from the Hungarian-Canadian physiologist Hans Selye (1907–1982).[90] Although Clark had convinced him to stick with "allergy" at that time, now this divorce was complete as well. SCE's foundation represented a clear break with an allergy community that was itself moving on. The SCE and Theron Randolph would certainly participate in the debates about food allergy that escalated during the next two decades, but would do so from the position of a rival discipline with different, ecologically based aims and little concern for orthodox allergy.

THE POLLUTANTS WE INGEST

In the same issue of *Annals of Allergy* in which the final chapter of *Human Ecology and Susceptibility to the Chemical Environment* was published, a much less emphatic article appeared. Written by the San Francisco pediatric allergist Ben Feingold, the piece frankly described the failure of the author's five-year mission to develop a technique to desensitize patients to flea bite allergy, something of a local problem.[91] As Feingold explained glumly: "In no case did the response to the challenging bites show an improvement over the original challenge before treatment was started. In every instance the reaction was either the same as before the course of treatment or . . . the degree of reactivity was actually increased."[92] Initially, there was no connection between the ill-fated flea experiments and Randolph's essays on clinical ecology, but this soon changed and the San Francisco allergist was thrust headlong into the debates about food additives and mental disorder.

Bemused by his inability to develop a desensitization extract, Feingold hypothesized that the reason might lay in the possibility that the reaction was haptenic, or a toxicological reaction caused by low-molecular-weight chemicals (haptens), in this case found in the saliva of fleas. Haptens were too small to induce an allergic reaction on their own; they had to combine with proteins of larger molecular weight in order to induce an allergic response.

Intrigued by such mechanisms, Feingold decided to investigate further during the late 1960s and early 1970s, and soon discovered that many of the chemicals used as food additives were also haptens.[93] After a series of serendipitous clinical encounters, he became convinced that such food chemicals, particularly synthetic food-coloring agents, were indeed responsible for the apparent escalation in the rates of hyperactivity in children. He began prescribing a food additive–free diet, dubbed the Feingold diet, in the early 1970s. Despite Feingold's previous position as chief of allergy for Kaiser Permanente, his attempts to convince his colleagues fell flat. Stung by rejection, the normally self-confident Feingold abandoned his efforts to win over his peers and in 1974 wrote the best seller *Why Your Child Is Hyperactive*, a book aimed, at least superficially, at parents.[94]

The story of the Feingold diet is described elsewhere, but a few aspects of it should be emphasized to understand just how divisive and widely popular the topic of food additives and mental health became during the 1970s.[95] Unlike many of the debates between food allergists and their orthodox colleagues, which were restricted to the medical community, the controversy surrounding the Feingold diet became a decidedly public affair, attracting international media attention and government inquiries. Although Feingold threw himself headlong into the furor, his position as a leader in the allergy community and, more important, as an orthodox allergist who had precious little time for Randolph or Oakland rival Albert Rowe, made him an unusual proponent of the link between food additives and mental disorder.

Certainly, many of Feingold's contemporaries, including the Tennessee food allergist William Crook, the New York pediatric allergist Doris Rapp, and the British psychiatrist Richard Mackarness, all of whom were heavily influenced by Randolph, would have been much more likely to have become the most infamous critics of food additives of the 1970s.[96] Crook, who called food allergy the "Great Masquerader," often describing how it could cause behavioral problems in children, went on to write a best-selling book, *The Yeast Connection*, about the relationship between candida yeast and chronic disease, a topic that continues to divide opinion.[97] Rapp helped to popularize Frederic Speer's allergic tension-fatigue syndrome, highlighting the facial signs of it in children. Although she was originally skeptical of the relationship between food allergy and mental health, she was eventually won over by Speer, Randolph, Crook, and others, and appeared on *The Phil Donahue Show* to raise awareness about the issue in 1988.[98] She continues to be active. Mackarness, who founded the first British National Health Service clinical ecology clinic in Basingstoke, pioneered the so-called Stone Age diet, in the belief that humans had not evolved to consume foods, including wheat and milk, developed since Paleolithic times (in fact, today's weight-reduction version of Mackarness's Stone Age diet is called the "Paleo diet").[99] Although Mackarness also thought that the Stone Age diet could aid in weight loss, the title of his book, *Not All in the Mind*, and his role as a psychiatrist indicate that he was also deeply interested in its positive effects on mental health.[100] But, instead, it was Feingold who came out of retirement after a series of personal health scares during the late 1960s to become the spokesperson for parents who sought an alternative explanation—and solution—for hyperactivity, by then the most common childhood psychiatric disorder.[101]

The Feingold diet sparked a dispute about hyperactivity, which has yet to be resolved, with recent studies in the United Kingdom reigniting the issue.[102] To a degree, the Feingold debates have had a somewhat narrow focus, concentrating primarily on artificial colors, in addition to flavors and preservatives to a lesser extent, as the chemicals in question, and with hyperactivity the behavior of concern. It was Feingold himself who restricted the parameters of the debate. Fearing even more reprisals from the food industry, he had to be convinced to add the preservatives BHA and BHT (butylated hydroxyanisole and butylated hydroxytoluene) to his list of banned foods, but he refused to add refined sugars, despite acknowledging in private that they were problematic. For this reason, Feingold's theory was seen by many clinical ecologists, including Randolph, as being too limited.[103] But this did not mean that Feingold did not speculate about the broader and long-lasting effects of food additives. In a chapter called "The Pollutants We Ingest," in *Why Your Child Is Hyperactive*, as well as in some of his academic publications, Feingold went further than almost anyone in warning his readers about their potential impact.[104]

For Feingold, the chief danger posed by such chemicals was not to physical health in the form of cancer or immune dysfunction but to social disorder. Citing the ethological theories of Nobel Prize laureate and animal behaviorist Konrad Lorenz (1903–1989), Feingold claimed that "overrapid" environmental change, best typified by food additives, helped to explain "the sharp upward curve of aggression and violence during the past twenty-five years."[105] No longer restricted to American slums, the "attack by fist, knife and gun has spread to the stamping grounds of the middle class and into wealthy suburbia; the snarl of frustration and rage spills out universally and from unlikely mouths."[106] The time was nigh, according to Feingold, "to look at these chemicals . . . in regard to the human species as a whole . . . to coldly question whether or not some of them have the possibility of disrupting the normal neurological pathways."[107] The threat posed by food additives, therefore, transcended the struggles faced by hyperactive children and their families: it had the potential to disrupt all of society.

ALL IN THE MIND

Despite Feingold's initial hopes to devise a theory that would attain scientific legitimacy, he was constantly faced with skepticism. Among the most repeated detractions was the one commonly rehearsed in discussions of food allergy: that psychosomatic factors were overlooked. Specifically, the Feingold diet's effectiveness was nothing more than a powerful placebo; it was the charismatic, grandfatherly allergist's power of suggestion, in addition to changes in the domestic routine, that were responsible for improved behavior, not the diet itself. Although Feingold would retort that there "may be an element of placebo, but the whole practice of medicine is placebo," there was irony in his outrage. During the 1960s, Feingold himself, as did many other orthodox allergists, had investigated the psychosomatic aspects of allergy, concluding that it did indeed play a role.

The research Feingold had undertaken focused on two groups of women: one whose members had "true allergic disease" verified by skin tests; the other being "nonreactive allergic" patients whose skin test reactions were weak or nonexistent but still reported allergic symptoms.[108] Subjecting both groups to psychological testing, Feingold found that

weaker reactors tend to be more deviant on the personality inventory. Stronger reactors are able to claim an attitude of closer affiliation with society and more adequate and satisfying interactions with others. The less sensitive tend to be dissatisfied with things as they are, more complaining, and more active in their attempts to do something about their complaints than the strong reactors. These are differences related to the dimension of sensitivity to allergens and suggest that clear psychological differences may be found between those with allergies and those with nonreactive allergies.[109]

These observations highlight Feingold's orthodoxy as an allergist and also imply that he believed that many "nonreactive allergies" might be psychosomatic and, more specifically, hypochondriacal. Although Feingold argued elsewhere that such effects could also be "contributory rather than primary," and although he had reversed his position by the time he began his hyperactivity crusade, Feingold's initial views about psychosomatic allergy were echoed by many orthodox allergists during the postwar period.[110] For some patients, allergies were all in the mind.

Although the psychological state of patients was long believed to be a factor in allergy, by the 1940s and 1950s, many allergists and the general public believed that "psychological events are primary factors as a cause of allergic disease." [111] As the New York allergist Harold Abramson (1899–1990) declared in a historical overview of the subject: "Even in their relatively primitive therapy, our medical ancestors not only seem to have recognized syndromes of hypersensitivity but have also stressed a relationship between the psyche and allergic diseases."[112] For example, whereas "nervous tension" aroused by a carriage failing to turn up might trigger an asthma attack in one late-nineteenth-century patient, other physicians noted that hay fever was most common in highly nervous people.[113] While many of these early accounts indicate that psychosomatic factors were of secondary, rather than primary, importance, by the 1940s the psychological state of patients was paramount in the minds of many allergists and, not surprisingly, psychiatrists.

One of the first such examples of the psychosomatic trend appeared in 1941, a treatise on psychogenic factors in bronchial asthma, co-authored by Thomas Morton French and the psychoanalyst Franz Alexander.[114] Five years later, a special issue of the journal *Nervous Child* was published, which also discussed how bronchial asthma, as well as other allergic diseases, could be rooted in psychosomatic factors. Asthma, according to one of the authors, could often be triggered when none of the suspected allergens were present. How was this so? The answer involved psychological factors, including "fear, anger, and anxious doubt," as well as "emotional conflict."[115] In the cases presented, maternal rejection loomed large.[116] Asthmatic attacks "occurred as a reaction to the danger of separation from the mother or loss of her love," acknowledgment of which remained "deeply repressed and continuous throughout the patient's life."[117] Since desensitization and avoidance of the suspected allergens were ineffectual in such cases, psychotherapy was required.[118] These observations contrasted wildly to Albert Rowe's arguments that most cases of bronchial asthma were caused by reactions to food.[119]

Other allergic diseases were similarly subject to psychogenic factors. Another article in the *Nervous Child* blamed a girl's eczema on the fact that her mother "neglected her," returning to work soon after giving birth and leaving the infant in her grandmother's care. Whenever the girl visited her grandmother in later childhood, her eczema would disappear, only to break out even worse when she returned home.[120] The relationship between such dermatological reactions and hereditary predisposition to allergy were explained elsewhere in the issue:

> Now let us suppose that an infant endowed with these biological heredities has his first skin manifestations. . . . The child experiences stimulation in an organ system which has all the properties to be used for an adequate discharge of libidinal energies. . . . The child may then turn from curiosity to voyeurism; from pride and childish boasting to exhibitionism; from hostility, rage, and guilt feelings to sadomasochism; from love to self-love. All these can be acted out on the skin.[121]

If such "psychosomatic interplay"—for example, scratching an itch—was prohibited by the child's parents, not only would this increase the pleasure derived from it, but scratching would also serve as an outlet for subsequent conflicts between parent and child.[122] In the case of a fourteen-year-old girl with chronic atopic dermatitis, the mother prevented her daughter from sucking her thumb by putting her arms in braces and sprinkling pepper over her thumb. The treatment lasted until the girl was eighteen years old, and because of it, "she hated her mother fiercely. Her hatred found the best outlet in scratching."[123]

Although psychotherapy and hypnosis were commonly cited as the required treatments in such cases, more drastic measures were often required. "Parentectomies," which involved removing children from asthma- or allergy-producing homes, could be warranted in intractable circumstances.[124] Despite the sensational terminology, a parentectomy could be accomplished simply by sending a child away to school. In one case, a ten-year-old girl with severe asthma attended a school where the allergens to which she reacted were known to be present. The fact that her symptoms soon abated indicated that psychosomatic factors, rooted in the domestic environment, were of fundamental importance. According to the study's author: "The allergist

must begin now to consciously utilize all of these basic data of psychodynamics so that he may incorporate within his practice not only the information obtained from the basic sciences from physics and chemistry but
also from the basic science of psychodynamics."[125] Of course, the opposite
argument was often made by food allergists: that psychiatrists should learn
more about allergy.

Given their completely different approaches, food allergists and their
psychosomatically oriented counterparts routinely accused one another
of misunderstanding what was at the root of allergy and, by extension,
misleading their patients. As former president of the SSAAC, Leslie N. Gay,
lamented in a review of Albert Rowe's *Elimination Diets and Patients' Allergies*: "It is unfortunate that allergists rarely consider the psychosomatic
side of human behavior . . . permanent relief is obtained when a thorough
study of his home environment and of his many mental problems is made,
and when these all-important factors are adjusted."[126] In a review of Warren
Vaughan's *Strange Malady*, Gay similarly claimed that many an "inexperienced or over-enthusiastic allergist confuses the digestive symptoms of a
patient, who is nervous and harassed by financial or domestic problems,"
again emphasizing the role of the patient's psychological state.[127] In response, food allergists believed that allergists who were psychosomatically
inclined not only were misguided but also failed to act in the best interests
of their patients. In 1950, a letter from Harry Clark to Theron Randolph asserted: "Psychosomatic medicine is going to be hard to fight. It is like Christian Science in that the onus is entirely on the patient to get himself better.
Too bad someone cannot keep such stuff out of the *Annals* [*of Allergy*]."[128]

What both approaches did share was frustration with the traditional
methods of skin testing and desensitization therapy.[129] Whereas food allergists blamed the ineffectiveness of skin tests on a limited conceptualization
of allergy, psychosomatically oriented allergists attributed it to their belief
that the underlying problem was not immunological but psychological. How
could two groups of allergists come up with such different explanations?
Apart from underlying philosophical differences and motivations—both
psychoanalysis and ecology were powerful postwar ideologies—the answer was largely epistemological. Allergists influenced by psychosomatic
approaches to allergy seem to have been swayed by its theoretical heft
rather than its therapeutic effectiveness. This was an approach to allergies
where deduction was paramount. The articles written about psychosomatic

allergy in *Nervous Child,* for instance, delved deeply into psychoanalytical theory, applying it to patients' backgrounds and discussing how underlying psychic tension might resolve itself in allergy, but the writings failed to describe much about therapy. In these cases, knowledge of allergy and its psychosomatic aspects was not driven by clinical experience as much as by preexisting theoretical maxims, which were rooted in psychoanalysis and could be applied to allergy.

While environmental ideology motivated many food allergists by the 1960s along with the emergence of clinical ecology as an alternative to allergy, food allergy, in contrast, remained primarily an inductive enterprise. The gradual accumulation of clinical experience was the evidence that mattered for food allergists; certain accepted immunological theories about allergy were often ignored, since food allergy did not appear to follow many of its rules anyway. If taking food additives away from the diet of hyperactive children seemed to ease their symptoms and help them do better at school, then so be it. If a Stone Age diet allowed psychiatric patients to return to their families and regain employment, it did not really matter why this was the case.[130] Hypotheses were often offered to explain such phenomena, but they were not fundamentally important to many food allergists and clinical ecologists. Results, however, were. As Randolph described, highlighting the influence of his predecessors, ranging from Francis Hare to Hans Selye:

> The point to emphasize here is that the original observations of these pioneers which led to the present concepts and techniques of clinical ecology were all made inductively, in that they were based on thousands of detailed clinical observations of chronically ill patients in the course of their responses to given environmental exposures. This accumulated knowledge led to hypotheses which were then confirmed and extended as they were applied more widely in the practice of medicine.[131]

For Randolph, the accumulation of evidence eventually convinced him that foods and food chemicals could and did cause somatic symptoms; they could also trigger a wide range of mental disturbances. As such, it was not patients' flawed psyches or dysfunctional upbringings that should be blamed; it was the inhospitable environment in which they lived, made no safer by ineffective government regulators. Such patients were not neurotic, hysterical, or hypochondriacal, but they were, as Mackarness put it, "chemical victims."

What might the typical patient have made of all of this? Suffering from chronic health problems that often went undiagnosed or untreated for long periods of time, many patients turned to allergists out of desperation, having failed to gain succor from other physicians. Depending on which allergist he saw, a patient's problem might have been interpreted as either psychosomatic, inferring an internal, psychological problem that required psychiatric treatment, or allergic, possibly triggered by substances in the increasingly chemicalized food supply. The patient might then have ended up in therapy or fasting in a Randolph-style CECU. Although many patients might have balked at either fate, it is clear from the eventual success of clinical ecology as at least an alternative to conventional medicine, as well as the eventual demise of psychosomatic allergy, that the latter alternative was deemed to be more attractive. There are many possible explanations for this (including the possible efficacy of the approach), but chief among them is the fact that food allergists saw patients not as damaged or dysfunctional but as casualties of a hostile environment. They were like canaries in a coal mine, overreacting to chemicals in the environment that would ultimately be harmful to all. And it was this—the chemical environment, not the patient—that had to be changed.

● ● ●

THE MENTAL HEALTH of food allergy sufferers is once again occupying the minds of allergists. A number of studies emerged recently that have hypothesized that the strain of dealing with severe, anaphylactic food allergies can lead to mental health problems in patients and their families.[132] Seeing mental stress as a consequence of allergy rather than a cause is nothing new, but it does distract somewhat from our understanding of the subtler ways in which psychological factors can have an impact on the functioning of the immune system. Often lost among the debates about food allergy and mental illness has been the idea, long familiar to many allergists, that stress can play a secondary, rather than a primary, role in both normal and pathological immune response.[133] Just as emotional turmoil might make one more vulnerable to an infection, psychic stress could exacerbate immune dysfunction, transforming a mild reaction into one that would require medical attention.[134]

In a way, it is strange that more was not made of this simpler, less contentious connection between stress and immune response during the postwar period, when Hans Selye's notion of general adaptation syndrome was achieving recognition.[135] But instead of regarding stress as a broader concept that might pacify or even unify food allergists and their psychosomatically oriented rivals, each group adapted it for its own purposes. While emotional stress was paramount for psychosomatic allergists, clinical ecologists saw stress in physical terms, "the struggle to adapt to a noxious agent."[136] Theron Randolph even claimed that his conception of "specific adaptation syndrome," the adaptive process by which susceptible people succumbed to the "long-term inurement of environmental excitants" was a "clinical counterpart of Selye's general adaptation syndrome."[137] Much like allergy, stress was a term that could be mutated to fit the needs of those who employed it.

It is possible that if allergists had instead interpreted the relationship between allergy and mental illness in a more pluralistic way, a more sophisticated, holistic, and complex understanding of food allergy and its causes would have developed. But to project such hopes into the past also belies that American medicine during the postwar period was not inclined toward heterogeneity. One only has to look as far as the field of psychiatry to see parallel examples of dogmatism and factionalism. In both cases, compromise was eschewed not only on the basis of ideology but equally in the name of scientific respectability, as both allergy and psychiatry were perceived as being less legitimate and scientifically sound than other fields of medicine. Just as allergy was split into environmental, psychosomatic, and orthodox camps, psychiatry was represented by psychoanalysts, social psychiatrists (who emphasized the social determinants of mental health), and biological psychiatrists (who stressed neurological explanations and pharmaceutical solutions), along with so-called anti-psychiatrists, who questioned the legitimacy of mental illness altogether. And as with allergy, there were few attempts to compromise; ultimately biological psychiatrists won the debates, and the other disciplines slowly faded away.[138] A similar process occurred in allergy. In both allergy and psychiatry, there was little willingness for conciliation or developing more complicated, multifaceted explanations for immunological or psychological phenomena, a situation that continues to this day, much to the detriment of the disciplines themselves and the patients they serve.

FIVE

An Immunological Explosion?

A STRANGE STORY APPEARED on the ABC News Web site in the spring of 2013. Graced by the headline "Weird Food Allergy Stresses Mom, Baffles Doctors," the article described the difficulties faced by seven-year-old Tyler Trovato, a food allergy sufferer.[1] An astonishingly wide range of foods—including chicken, turkey, rice, sweet potatoes, bananas, and even his mother's breast milk—caused Tyler severe gastrointestinal distress and shock-like symptoms, so he subsisted on a tiny list of items, including, oddly, peanut butter sandwiches and milk. This was not, however, the bizarre aspect of the story. What bewildered physicians was that Tyler's allergy did not appear to involve the immune system; it did not seem to be mediated by immunoglobulin E (IgE), what has become known as the marker for "true" food allergy reactions. Because of this, it could not be detected by skin or blood tests. Adding to the confusion was the fact that Tyler's symptoms tended to occur two hours after he ate an allergy-inducing food and did not include the dermatological symptoms often associated with anaphylaxis. Not fitting the conventional definition of an allergy, Tyler's rare condition was instead described as food protein–induced enterocolitis syndrome (FPIES).

The portrayal of Tyler's allergy as a "weird" and "baffling" condition requiring a novel name neatly demonstrates just how far removed the conceptualization of food allergy had become in 2013 from the way it had been understood for most of the twentieth century. Most food allergists, in opposition to their orthodox colleagues, believed that foods can indeed cause all sorts of strange reactions, the underlying mechanisms of which remain fairly mysterious. As such, Tyler's symptoms, though worrying, would not have been seen as particularly unusual. Certainly all the foods to which he reacted would have appeared somewhere on Warren Vaughan's tables of common food allergens; there were precious few that were not.[2] In addition, many food allergists, led by Arthur Coca and Theron Randolph, were also loath to restrict allergy to examples in which clear evidence of immune system involvement was present, largely because this excluded many patients, including themselves, who suffered from chronic ill health.

Instead, food allergists thought that allergy itself should be defined broadly, in line with Clemens von Pirquet's original meaning of the term. As Frederic Speer wrote in a 1967 editorial: "The term of von Pirquet and Schick is our term. No word better describes the problem with which we are concerned. And no word is a better symbol of the plain fact that the diseases of allergy belong to us."[3] "Any form of altered biological reactivity" would certainly encompass the symptoms presented by Tyler Trovato. Moreover, the beliefs of Speer and other food allergists about the use of the term "allergy" were rooted in their roles as clinical allergists, rather than in underlying immunological theory. How to determine what was a food allergy was shaped in part by the difficulty in diagnosing food allergy, and in part by the high value placed on the clinical encounter and the accumulation of inductive evidence that such cases provided over time. Clinicians such as Albert Rowe, Herbert Rinkel, Warren Vaughan, and even some orthodox allergists, such as Ben Feingold, trusted the results their methods garnered, instead of definitions that did not seem to match their observations. Food allergists' faith in elimination diets and food avoidance was no doubt compounded when they treated their own self-diagnosed allergies, when their own headaches, fatigue, asthma, or depression were relieved by dietary changes.

These approaches to food allergy, widely regarded as the most intractable of the allergic diseases, were understandably contested and increasingly so during the postwar period when concerns about the environment and food additives leached into the practice of allergy. Disputes about food allergy, its definition, diagnosis, prognosis, and treatment also caused schisms between the clinically minded ACA and the academically oriented AAA, with both associations attempting to balance the interests of their members against the galling task of asserting allergy's legitimacy as a clinical practice and as a medical science.[4] For those on the extreme end of the food allergy spectrum, such as Randolph, these tensions reached the breaking point by the 1960s, leading to the creation of clinical ecology as a distinct discipline. But for a considerable percentage of clinicians, food allergy continued to be understood much as it always had been: a perplexing clinical condition that did not play by the same rules as other allergic diseases and, accordingly, had to be diagnosed and treated differently.

Chapters 5 and 6 describe the process by which this all changed, when food allergy, long portrayed as the ugly duckling of immunology, finally came of age as a legitimate, serious medical condition and topic of inquiry to even the most orthodox of allergists, a topic worthy of patient advocacy, public-health campaigns, legislation, and voluntary industry action. While chapter 6 outlines the role of the peanut in this process, this chapter focuses on an earlier and prerequisite step: the discovery of IgE and its impact on not only understandings of food allergy but also the discipline of allergy itself. Described by Gregg Mitman as "the holy grail of allergy," IgE was discovered in 1966 by two Japanese immunologists, Kimishige Ishizaka (b. 1925) and Teruko Ishizaka (b. 1926), a husband-and-wife team working at the Children's Asthma Research Institute and Hospital in Denver, Colorado, a fitting place for such a discovery, as Mitman's work on the history of asthma would attest.[5] At roughly the same time, Swedish researchers, led by Gunnar Johansson (b. 1938) and Hans Bennich (b. 1930), had independently discovered the same antibody (temporarily named IgND, after the initials of the patient involved in the research), and subsequently organized a WHO-funded workshop in 1968 that established the identity of IgE as a new immunoglobulin class.[6] With IgE, orthodox allergists finally had a biomedical marker that proved unequivocally when a reaction was allergic and immunological. For allergists of a conservative persuasion, "true" food allergy, in which the presence of IgE could be proved, could now be distinguished from food intolerance, in which it was absent. The former was the business of allergists; the latter was not. As such, it is highly appropriate that allergists cite 1967, the year after the discovery of IgE, as when the first description of FPIES, the "weird" and "baffling" food reaction typified by no evidence of IgE, appeared.[7]

In addition to defining allergy itself, varying levels of IgE in patients were also thought to help determine the severity of an allergy. Johansson and Bennich soon developed radioallergosorbent tests (RAST) to detect the presence of IgE in human serum, an innovation that hinted at the replacement of "the more primitive skin test in clinical practice," which some allergists feared were perceived by most physicians as "a strange way to cure disease."[8] The phrase "IgE-mediated food allergy" entered the immunological lexicon as a way to describe such reactions, the "true" allergic nature of which there could be absolutely no doubt.[9] Such allergies were also described as fitting the description of "Type 1 hypersensitivity" made by P. G. H. Gell and R. R. A. Coombs in their 1963 classification system, a schema designed to add clarity to the definition of allergy.[10] Finally, research into the wider role of IgE in the body hinted that the antibody might play a diagnostic role in other immune dysfunction diseases as well as a role in the physiology of cancer, all of which helped put allergy research in the medical spotlight.[11]

Historian Mark Jackson acknowledges that many allergists regard the discovery of IgE as "a seminal moment in the transformation of allergy from a 'cinderella subject' into a legitimate science."[12] The discovery was also hailed as a "milestone in modern medical research" in the New York Times, providing proof to orthodox allergists that they had been correct all along, thus representing a clean break with a less enlightened past.[13] Furthermore, IgE promised to open "up a vast new area of research into allergic diseases," which could feedback into improved clinical allergy practice.[14] But, despite this sense of optimism, tensions remained. While IgE was treated as a godsend by orthodox allergists, many food allergists and clinical ecologists were nonplussed. IgE might help to explicate the mechanism behind some allergies, but this did not encapsulate the delayed, chronic, and lingering reactions to foods that posed the greatest challenge to clinicians. More worryingly for those who had heralded the arrival of IgE was emerging evidence that its use as a marker for allergy was more complicated than first thought. Similar problems emerged with RAST, much to the dismay of allergists eager to abandon skin testing.

But, whereas such chinks in the new paradigm promised by IgE might have provoked a demand for more pluralistic thinking, the opposite occurred. Just as orthodox allergists increasingly entrenched their position with respect to what constituted a "true" food allergy, food allergists and especially clinical ecologists similarly became more dogmatic and, according to some, more radical. Furthermore, as the new field of clinical ecology diverged from allergy, its boundaries became more unclear, especially with the emergence of even more questionable practitioners who began selling new diagnostic tests and therapeutic regimens directly to patients. The accuracy and ethics of these blood tests, which promised to identify even the most recalcitrant of allergens, were challenged vociferously by orthodox allergists, often through the auspices of the AAA. Ironically, such tests were inspired by IgE's very discovery and the development of RAST, their legitimate cousin. Fueled by these bones of contention and many others, the tensions between clinical ecology and organized allergy were eventually played out in the courts. IgE, potentially a unifying and decisive force for the discipline of allergy, instead further divided a field of medicine already riven by disagreement.

FROM BENCH TO BEDSIDE

The difficulty in fusing the link between laboratory immunology and clinical allergy—or between "bench and bedside"—is a theme familiar to historians who have investigated the history of immunity and its disorders.[15] Early allergists, including Clemens von Pirquet himself and John Freeman, were eager to retain and build on the connection between laboratory investigations of immunity and the treatment of allergy.[16] With the activities of allergists even compensating for the science of immunology before the immunological breakthroughs of the 1960s, some immunologists, most notably the Danish Nobel laureate Nils Jerne, argued that these bonds were maintained throughout the twentieth century. However, research on the history of allergy by Jackson and others, as well as the history of food allergy, suggest otherwise. Despite the intentions of many leading allergists, particularly those with university positions, to establish their discipline as merely the clinical arm of immunology, the relationship was more of a "marriage of convenience"—at least for orthodox allergists—than a "wedding of love."[17] Even Freeman, who believed that immunological theory was useful for allergists and engaged in research himself, remained a "self-confessed empiricist," trusting clinical evidence above all.[18] As a result, allergy remained "relatively untouched by the tyranny of immunochemistry or by the laboratory revolution," content "to be shaped largely by the pragmatic concerns of clinical practice rather than the need to elucidate theoretical issues in the laboratory."[19]

Not surprisingly, many allergists believed that this state of affairs was not in the best interests of their discipline. In the United States, in particular, attempts to associate allergy with the science of immunology during the mid-twentieth century were influenced by the assumption, held by many allergists, that their field was situated on one of the lower rungs of the medical ladder, somewhere alongside psychiatry and far below cardiology or oncology. Although allergists could see themselves as fairly successful in clinical terms, some believed that allergy was not much more than a glorified craft practice rather than a medical science. As a result, the discipline struggled to attract the best medical students, to become board certified by the American Board of Medical Specialties (this eventually occurred in 1971), to attain funding for research, and to gain a representative allocation of time and resources in the medical school curriculum.[20] Or, as the former AAA and ACA vice president Jerome Glaser (1898–1985) bemoaned in 1956: "Allergy is sadly neglected in the medical schools of this country. Some department heads look upon it as scarcely more scientific than witchcraft. . . . There is no question that allergy has been a sort of 'stepchild' of medicine either ridiculed or ignored."[21] Leading allergists produced a number of troubling statistics, which mirrored such concerns. Ben Z. Rappaport, the AAA president in 1953, complained that allergy ranked twenty-sixth of the twenty-nine diseases listed for National Research Council support between 1946 and 1951.[22] The ACA president, Orvil Withers, similarly grumbled that based on the amount of allergy content in a typical internal medicine textbook, medical students might assume "that less than 0.05 percent of internal medicine dealt with allergic patients . . . 10 to 20 percent of all the persons who visit physicians' offices are allergic, even though allergy may not be the presenting complaint."[23]

According to some, one way to help overcome such indignities was to embrace immunology more explicitly. As Max Samter (1909–1999), president of the AAA in 1958, contended: "The art of allergy which we practice is based on tradition—the joint experience of generations of allergists. Experience, however, is only the beginning; the art of allergy must now be persuaded to adopt and perhaps to be altered by its own unruly offspring, the science of allergy."[24] The "science of allergy" to which Samter referred meant immunology, implying that allergists should pay attention to laboratory investigations and that reactions, which were nonimmunological, were not bona fide allergy.[25] Since the immunological basis for many reactions to food was often difficult to prove, the specter of food allergy loomed large. Speaking about the overdiagnosis of food allergy, the New York pediatric allergist

Walter R. Kessler argued: "In the majority of instances . . . it has not been possible to produce objective evidence for the existence of an antigen-antibody reaction and such a mechanism has been assumed rather than demonstrated. . . . Even when the diagnosis is based on good clinical observation, it may not be possible to demonstrate an immunologic mechanism."[26]

Kessler, as with many other orthodox allergists during the heyday of psychosomatic allergy, stressed that "parental attitudes and a variety of other psychologic factors" contributed enormously to the unfounded idea that food allergies could cause a wide range of symptoms, particularly behavioral problems in children.[27] Similarly, in an article that warned of the psychological dangers of the indiscriminate use elimination diets, Edward L. Pratt, a Dallas pediatrician and chief of staff of the Children's Medical Center, advised that it was

> highly important to discriminate untoward reactions from eating a food, a complex mixture with its variable emotional connotations, from reactions following the ingestion of a rigidly defined, specific substance. In everyday practice this difference may sometimes be irrelevant, but to those interested in the role of allergy in Medicine, the distinction is vital. . . . Continuation of noncritical attitudes towards food allergy can only further debase this subject and may well lead to neglect of its true value, to the detriment of the patient.[28]

In order to avoid such debasement, allergists were encouraged to embrace immunology and the resultant insights and respectability it would bring. And, with the discovery of IgE, it was thought that the scientific foundation for the practice of allergy could finally be established.[29]

Such thinking reflected long-standing attempts to establish firmly the link between the clinical practice of allergy and the science of immunology, an aspiration that took some time to achieve, particularly with food allergy.[30] Although laboratory investigations of serum sickness provided good evidence of this association in some allergic diseases, it was unclear, for at least the first two decades of the twentieth century, whether allergic or, more precisely, anaphylactic reactions to food were immunological at all.[31] During those years, according to the immunologist and historian Arthur Silverstein, anaphylaxis was often thought to be caused by a potent toxin or poison, an understandable assumption considering that Charles Richet's initial experiments were on the venoms excreted by sea creatures. An early challenge faced by allergy researchers who believed, like von Pirquet, that allergy was simply an exaggerated version of a normal immune response, was therefore to demonstrate the mechanism involved in such phenomena.[32] Although most of the research that emerged, including that of Milton Rosenau and John Anderson, provided support for von Pirquet's claims, other investigators, including Victor Vaughan, remained convinced that anaphylaxis was toxicological in nature.[33]

One of the first steps in resolving these debates occurred in 1921, when two researchers, Otto Carl W. Prausnitz (1876–1963) and Heinz Küstner (1897–1963), undertook a daring self-experiment that not only would show that such reactions were immunological but also would pave the way for identifying the antibodies involved.[34] Küstner happened to have an unusual allergy to fish, but while he could eat raw fish with impunity, he was "exquisitely sensitive" to it when cooked.[35] Although responding to only a cooked food was rare—heating food proteins was thought to reduce their potency as allergens—it was not completely unknown, and would later be noted by both William Duke and Albert Rowe in the case of roasted peanuts and cooked fruits, respectively.[36] Prausnitz, who did not have fish allergies of any sort but suffered from hay fever, regarded this as an opportunity to determine whether the reaction was immunological or toxicological, as many of his contemporaries thought. After convincing his colleague to participate, Prausnitz injected Küstner's blood serum into his arm and, a day later, tested to see if he reacted by injecting a fish solution. Sure enough, a wheal developed immediately, demonstrating that Küstner's sensitivity had been passively transferred and strongly suggesting that immunological antibodies had been involved. This passive-transfer reaction became known as the Prausnitz-Küstner, or P-K, reaction. These tests were developed as alternatives to skin testing for allergies when, for example, a patient had skin problems or recurrent asthma, or when the direct tests were thought to be too distressing for certain patients, such as children and infants.[37]

Prausnitz and Küstner's self-experimenting did not end there. Prausnitz asked Küstner if he would be willing to reverse the experiment, this time testing to see if his hay fever could be transferred to Küstner. Although Küstner initially hesitated, he eventually agreed and was injected with Prausnitz's sera. Surprisingly, when Küstner was injected with the appropriate solution of rye-grass pollen, his skin did not erupt in a wheal. While Prausnitz was left to puzzle over why this was the case, Küstner abandoned the study of allergy for a career in obstetrics. The solution to the riddle would not materialize for forty years, when Prausnitz, who had fled Nazi Germany for England in 1935, returned to his homeland and visited his former colleague. Küstner admitted that he had "not been keen on the passive transfer experiments" and had suspected that Prausnitz was unwell and feared the possible health hazards inherent in receiving his serum. As a precaution, therefore, he surreptitiously boiled the pollen solution for ten minutes before injecting it into his arm, thus attenuating the potency of the allergen.[38]

Despite this act of sabotage, the pair's earlier experiment provided an impetus for researchers to identify and describe the antibodies believed to be involved in allergic reactions. Strangely, given his later focus on nonreaginic allergy, it was Arthur Coca who termed the substance involved the "atopic reagin."[39] Technological limitations hampered these efforts until the late 1930s, when developments in ultracentrifugation and electrophoresis (which allowed molecules to be separated by weight and electrical charge respectively) permitted the molecular structure of various proteins to be explored in more depth.[40] A series of structural studies emerged, which began the process of characterizing the different proteins found in sera, including antibodies, or what would also become known as immunoglobulin molecules. Different immunoglobulin classes were soon identified, including IgM (the first antibody that responds to invading pathogens), IgG (which also protects the body from infection), IgD (the purpose of which is not entirely clear but likely involves the activating of B cells, which make antibodies against antigens), IgA (found in numerous bodily fluids, including mucus, saliva, and breast milk), and, finally, IgE.[41]

When IgA was first isolated in serum by the Belgian researcher Joseph F. Heremans (1927–1975) in 1958, and its function was explained by immunologist Thomas Tomasi Jr. (b. 1927) in 1965, many suspected that it might be one of the "elusive 'reaginic' antibodies responsible for human atopic allergies."[42] Given its presence in mucus, a fluid associated with many allergic reactions, it did have some role to play, but a report by the influential allergist Mary Hewitt Loveless (1899–1991) concerning an allergic patient with low levels of IgA, as well as the failure of researchers to demonstrate that it could trigger skin reactions, undermined this theory. Only a few years later, however, the Ishizakas—along with Johansson and Bennich in Sweden—discovered a different antibody in the sera of a person extremely allergic to ragweed.[43] This became known as IgE, the secretive antibody believed to be the key to both understanding and identifying allergic reactions.[44]

Although most of the excitement generated by the discovery of IgE was in relation to its role in allergy, some researchers wondered about its broader function in human immune defense. The immunologist and artist Debra Jan Bibel noted that immunity has often been described using the metaphor of combat, with the various immunoglobulins taking on various military roles, including "shock trooper" (IgM), "principal infantry soldier" (IgG), "adjutant or training liaison" (IgD), and "specialized perimeter defender or sentry" (IgA).[45] Although Bibel described IgE as "the engineer" of the defense forces, "initiating the release of inflammatory agents to slow the progress of pathogens and to attract and aid the access of phagocytic cells, the tanks," its role in immune dysfunction suggests that it might more accurately resemble a Dr. Strangelove figure, providing robust, yet ultimately self-destructive, defenses.[46] Likewise, an early editorial in the *Lancet* observed that IgE was mainly understood with respect to the pathological reactions it could trigger.[47] While allergy might be an example of "too much of a good thing," the good thing being IgE, questions remained about why IgE was present in human bodies in the first place.[48]

TUMORS AND TAPEWORMS

Two separate possibilities soon emerged, both of which were investigated separately by the Ishizakas and the Swedish team.[49] First, building on earlier speculations about the relationship between allergy and cancer, it was suggested that rates of IgE were inversely linked to rates of certain types of cancer; in other words, people who suffered from allergic diseases were less likely to develop tumors.[50] Although some postulated that since allergy and cancer were also associated with young and old patients, respectively, the connection might just be coincidental, others hypothesized that the inverse relationship centered on IgE's possible role in checking the growth of cancerous cells.[51] Indicating that research in this field is accelerating, in 2006 the term "AllergoOncology" was coined to describe the study of the potential link between IgE and cancer.[52]

Second, roughly concurrent with the discovery of IgE was the revelation that it also helped protect the body from parasitic worms, or helminths.[53] As researchers acknowledged, it was only in the twentieth century that humans living in places with clean water and effective sewage systems became free from endemic helminthic infections. Where such parasitic infections were still commonplace, as in much of the developing world, allergies were far less common. Given the ubiquity of such infections, so much so that some researchers have suggested that to be afflicted with helminths is a "normal" state for all mammals, it followed that for the vast majority of human history IgE served a functional purpose.[54] With humans living in the developed world no longer coming in contact with such parasites, however, IgE was thought to have redirected itself to otherwise harmless environmental antigens.[55]

Recent investigations have extended this intriguing hypothesis, positing that even the structures of helminth and allergen molecules are quite similar, and even recommending helminthic treatment of immune disorders.[56] Notwithstanding the potential of this research to answer fundamental questions about the nature of allergy, the helminth hypothesis did not generate nearly as much excitement in the allergy community as the simple fact that IgE had been discovered, although some studies did emerge. One of these compared IgE levels in white and Métis (mixed aboriginal and European) populations in Saskatchewan, determining that the higher levels of the antibody in Métis people were due to their higher rates of helminthic infections.[57] Another study examined the epidemiology of allergy in the tropics, concluding that the difficulty in determining such rates was the omnipresence of endemic parasites, resulting in elevated IgE rates, which thus skewed results.[58] But despite these limited forays, allergists remained unimpressed. As a result, most of the research that investigated the connection between IgE and parasites was conducted either by researchers focusing on developing countries or by researchers concentrating on animal experiments, with the findings being published in journals aimed at laboratory researchers rather than clinicians.[59]

This apparent disinterest is all the more surprising since the links between IgE and both cancer and helminthic infections would have provided additional evidence for orthodox allergists and their contention that for a reaction to be allergic, proof of the underlying immunological mechanisms involved had to be demonstrated.[60] Both hypotheses hinted that allergies mediated by IgE were fundamentally different from those where immunological involvement could not be ascertained. If IgE did have a more fundamental role in human immune defense—in either curtailing cancerous cells or fighting off parasites—then that would suggest that the pathological effects of such antibodies when they overenthusiastically responded to food and other harmless foreign substances (meaning allergies) had deep immunological meanings, however poorly understood. Seen in this way, allergies and allergists had a significant role to play in answering basic immunological questions about how the body distinguishes friend from foe, and self from non-self. With respect to the intractable debates about how to define allergy, more insights into IgE's normal function might also have provided more ammunition to fight presumptions made by clinical ecologists that allergy was not an immune dysfunction so much as a hypersensitive response to a hostile environment. While the environmental hypothesis might have the ring of truth, at least with respect to helminthic infections, the fact that IgE could not be detected in the patients apparently suffering reactions from foods and chemicals indicated that such responses were essentially different. Such an assessment would not have mattered much to clinical ecologists, who remained blasé about IgE, but would have strengthened the position of orthodox allergists, further refining the definition of allergy.

IgE IN THE CLINIC

Most orthodox allergists, however, did not think of IgE in this way. Instead, it was seen partly in ideological terms but also as a godsend to clinical practice. An article on the impact of IgE on the practice of allergy by two Mayo Clinic consultants, John W. Yunginger and Gerald G. Gleich, for example, listed two main benefits. The first was RAST, which the authors believed to offer several advantages over skin tests. RAST was a spinoff of the work of Bennich, Johansson, and Leif Wide (b. 1934) on what would become IgE.[61] The test, which was an in vitro rather than an in vivo procedure, was first produced by the Swedish pharmaceutical company Pharmacia Diagnostics, which trademarked the name RAST.[62] Since elevated IgE levels were associated with a number of nonallergic conditions, a test that checked for antibodies to specific allergens was required.[63] RAST essentially involved taking serum from a patient and combining it with the suspected allergen. If the serum contained antibodies to the allergen, it would bind to the allergen, providing evidence of an allergy. The addition of a radio-labeled anti-IgE antibody would then determine the level of radioactivity, which was proportional to the level of serum IgE for the allergen, thus indicating the severity of the allergy. According to Yunginger and Gleich, RAST provided more quantitative results, was not affected by drugs in the patient's system, correlated closer with the severity of the disease, and was safer and more convenient for patients, particularly infants and those with skin problems, than skin testing.[64] Second, RAST could be modified to measure the potency of commercial allergy extracts, permitting the standardization of such allergens and more consistency in their use.[65] The authors mentioned the possibility that basic research into the "biologic function, genetic control, and metabolism of IgE" might provide improved desensitization and other therapies, but no further detail about how this might occur was provided.[66]

The tone of Yunginger and Gleich's article was optimistic and enthusiastic, not only hinting that IgE could pave the way for improvements in the clinic but also implying that the pharmaceutical industry and commercial laboratories might also benefit enormously from the sale of RASTs and standardized allergen extracts as well as laboratory services.[67] Although the authors warned that some challenges remained—purchasing the automatic gamma scintillation counters required for the test was expensive ($8,000) and the availability of radioimmunoassay materials was limited—they reassured their readers that these problems would be overcome.[68] Moreover, the initial RAST studies that emerged in the early 1970s, albeit many of them conducted by members of the Swedish team that helped invent the procedure, emphasized its accuracy in diagnosing a wide range of allergic disease, including some food allergies. The new procedure was seen to be as effective as skin testing but without its negative connotations. RAST appeared to provide good initial evidence that IgE might indeed herald an immunological revolution in allergy.

Before long, though, questions began to emerge about RAST and IgE, along with their importance in clinical allergy more generally. With respect to RAST, clinicians soon complained about its lack of sensitivity when compared with skin tests. As the Texas pediatric allergist William T. Knicker explained, "Enthusiasm for *in vitro* testing quickly dampened when it became apparent that the initial commercial RAST was relatively insensitive, being negative in too many patients."[69] This was the opposite problem of skin tests, which could often produce too many false positives. As more comparison studies were published pitting RASTs against skin tests, the results tended to be equivocal.[70] Although modifications of RAST were developed, all promising more sensitivity, an official position paper from the

American Academy of Allergy and Immunology (AAAI) indicated that the test had not, in fact, allowed allergists to abandon skin tests.[71] The position paper compared the merits of each test, finding that although both tests were relatively accurate when "optimally performed," RASTs were said to be less sensitive, slower to produce results (two to three days versus forty-five minutes for a skin test), and more expensive.[72] Whereas RAST was preferred in patients suffering from serious dermatological complaints and was considered to be safer overall, more convenient, more reproducible, and easier for nonallergists to conduct, the superior sensitivity of skin tests remained paramount. Knicker advised using both tests for best results, but he hinted that reimbursement for conducting both from medical insurers was unlikely. According to Knicker, insurers were already getting parsimonious about paying allergists to do either test, particularly since it was thought that less-expensive nonallergists (laboratory workers) could perform and interpret the in vitro RAST. Rather than debate endlessly about which test was better, Knicker urged his colleagues to concentrate on making sure that all allergy testing remained their responsibility and something for which they were adequately reimbursed.[73] If anything, RAST was making the practice of allergy more, rather than less, complicated.[74]

Other hopes for IgE proved to be short lived. One early objective had been to establish standards for IgE levels in allergic and nonallergic patients. Such measures would provide more objective criteria by which to diagnose allergies and determine their severity. In 1970, the British Medical Research Council began this process by establishing its own standards, and WHO followed suit in 1973, revising its preparations in 1980 and 2013.[75] But, as Mark Jackson notes, it became clear that these levels varied markedly, with genetics, sex, age, and the environment all affecting results.[76] Smoking, for instance, was shown in a number of studies to elevate IgE levels, as did excessive drinking.[77] Other underlying health conditions, including cancer, helminthic infections, celiac disease, and cirrhosis, could also raise levels.[78] In one study, depressive patients were seen to have particularly high IgE counts when compared with alcoholics, schizophrenics, and test controls, raising yet again the complicated relationship between allergy and mental health.[79] Most of these reports urged that more research be required in order to determine basal rates of IgE to establish standards and thus understand more comprehensively the role of IgE in human physiology.[80]

The immunological revolution was seen to be fleeting for allergists in other ways, with some admitting that while IgE had helped to clarify a few aspects of allergy, it had not made an enormous difference to clinical practice. A. W. Frankland put it bluntly in 1972, stating that "immunologists have characterized for us the unique immunoglobulin IgE, but so far this has not benefited our atopic patient."[81] According to Frankland, this was because IgE-mediated allergies were not particularly difficult to diagnose; it was allergies to which there were no associated IgE antibodies that were problematic. Food allergies, as usual, were the most confounding, demonstrating to Frankland that dysfunctional immunity was not about only IgE: "[A] boy recently under investigation for purpura produced by chocolate, bananas or milk, could reproduce the syndrome by a provocation test with the offending foods, but we have no immunological test to demonstrate why such a patient reacts in such a peculiarly specific manner. Immunity has certainly gone wrong when a child becomes allergic to chocolate."[82]

Likewise, Frankland declared that RAST "was not assisting me, as yet, to give greater help to my patients. There still remains a large gap between the advances made by the research laboratory and the clinical application of their studies."[83] Finally, Frankland considered that he and his fellow allergists "may think that we understand more about our allergic patients now, but perhaps we are only beginning to understand what a complicated sequence of events occurs in any allergic reaction."[84] Such thinking made sense for allergists who believed, like Frankland, that many allergies were not IgE-mediated, as well as those who emphasized the psychosomatic aspects of allergy. Was there a relationship between levels of IgE and stress? If so, many of the allergists who had previously claimed that allergy was primarily psychosomatic were not investigating it.

Other allergists concurred. In a letter written to Leonard Bernstein, chairman of the AAA's Research Council in 1972, John C. Selner (1936–2006) asserted, "In spite of the immunological advancements making possible new insights into many of the phenomena of allergy, innumerable patients present with clinical pictures that defy definition and treatment."[85] Selner, a Denver pediatric allergist who became the president of the ACAAI in 1992/1993 and who set up the short-lived Environmental Care Unit at Presbyterian Hospital in Denver, added that allergists dealing with food and chemical allergies, in particular, were shunted aside by the new

immunological focus: "Some practitioners have reported phenomena related to food ingestients and chemical exposure which can't be explained
by our present insight into immunologic mechanisms. When investigating
these reports, I believe there is a tendency to dismiss them out-of-hand."[86]

For food allergists, such studies might have been interesting, but they
lacked clinical relevance. IgE mattered in only some allergic responses, as
Frankland indicated, and those that were easiest to diagnose in particular. In an article, "Food Allergy: The Great Masquerader," William Crook
suggested that one of the reasons for this was that IgE-mediated allergies
tended to cause reactions in the respiratory tract. Non-IgE-mediated allergies, the validity of which orthodox allergists questioned, could cause symptoms elsewhere, including the nervous system, gastrointestinal tract, and
skin.[87] Anaphylactic reactions to foods, which certainly affected the respiratory tract, were in the former category (IgE-mediated allergies), but most
food allergies were in the latter (non-IgE-mediated allergies). As such, IgE
effectively divided physicians into two camps, the first being "Group A," who
reserved the term "allergy" for "reactions in which the immunologic mechanisms are known to be operative."[88] These cases amounted to IgE-mediated
or Type-1 allergies, which were immediate and diagnosable by the use of
skin tests, even in cases of food allergy. "Group B" physicians (Crook being
one of them) also recognized non-IgE-mediated allergies, which neither skin
tests nor RAST picked up, and were typically due to masked food allergies.
Recognizing that IgE had entered the lingua franca of allergists, but simultaneously undermining it, Crook proceeded to iterate his belief "that non-IgE
mediated food allergy plays a crucial role in causing behavior and learning
problems in children," as well as a wide range of other conditions.[89]

An example of a "Group A" physician was Charles D. May (1908–1992), who
edited *Pediatrics* between 1954 and 1961 and who wrote a commentary on
food allergy in the same issue of *Pediatric Clinics of North America* as Crook's
article.[90] May, an ardent opponent of food allergists, lampooned Crook's description of food allergy as the "Great Masquerader," arguing that it was better described as the "Current Crutch" and insinuating that the approach of
Crook and other "preachers of dubious beliefs" was not only intuitive, imaginative (in a bad way), and unscientific, but little more than "quackery," based
only on "flimsy testimonials."[91] For May, the only scientific approach to food
allergies was to see them "on immunologic grounds," determining the "char-
acterization of the antigens and antibodies involved in the pathogenesis of

symptoms through their interactions with the tissues." Because such immunological elucidation was difficult, given the

> complexity of the antigenic constituents in foods and the enormous variety of specific antibodies induced in the characteristic heterogeneous response to each antigen, along with the variable responses of tissues . . . uncritical claims of relations of foods to symptoms can be expected, and unsupported "systems" of diagnosis and treatment will flourish. . . . The afflicted and the uncritical will join in creating another quackery by resorting to some "system" as a crutch to hobble along with until better means of relief can be found.[92]

Although orthodox allergists had never been particularly shy to use strong language in their criticisms of food allergy, inferring that practitioners such as Crook were essentially quacks lowered the debate to another level. IgE may not have brought orthodox allergists the diagnostic and therapeutic breakthroughs that some had envisioned, but it did give them renewed confidence in the ideological battles that continued to rage about the definition, extent, and meaning of allergy.

BEYOND IgE, BEYOND ALLERGY

May was not, of course, the only "Group A" physician to savage food allergy and clinical ecology. A review by Wayne Lake of Lawrence D. Dickey's *Clinical Ecology* in *Annals of Allergy* opined that the evidence supporting the discipline was "vague," "anecdotal," and often provided by "remote researchers as [Arthur] Coca and [Albert] Rowe"; in short, the book amounted to "intellectual pollution" or "drivel."[93] Writing a letter to the journal in response, Crook attempted to take claim the moral high ground, stating that

> I fully realize that many "orthodox" allergists and immunologists still do not accept delayed onset, non-IgE mediated food allergy, even though it has been repeatedly described by clinicians during the past 50 years, beginning with [W. Ray] Shannon and Rowe in the 1920s. . . . [I]n the complex, complicated field of allergy today, there are bound to be differences of opinion and Dr. Lake certainly has a right to express his opinions. Yet I feel those who describe alternate methods for studying and treating allergic and ecologically induced diseases deserve to present their philosophies and methods without being ridiculed and slandered for their efforts.[94]

Although Crook added that the review was "biased, superficial and unfair," his tone hinted that if the protagonists in the debates were more civilized, if not actually open-minded, more patients could be helped.

Similarly, Theron Randolph's editorial in the following issue of *Annals of Allergy* suggested that compromise was possible. Randolph also suspected that much of the divisiveness had been triggered by the so-called revolution in clinical immunology: "Progressive disinterest of most allergists in the human environment came to be expressed in certain quarters as assertions that alleged clinical responses to foods, and especially environmental chemicals, were not allergic because known immunologic mechanisms were not apparently known."[95] Elsewhere, Randolph admitted that the discovery of IgE supported the "immunologically restricted interpretation of allergy," but he still maintained that "great gaps remain between allergy as defined immunologically and allergy as practiced empirically and pragmatically by clinical ecologists."[96] Much of this boiled down to basic differences between laboratory and clinical medicine. As Randolph explained: "It is unreasonable to demand that clinical practitioners behave as if they were laboratory scientists. They cannot do so. To dismiss the careful and honest observations of such doctors, however, is to negate one of the most fruitful sources of scientific knowledge."[97] Summing up, Randolph insinuated that either orthodox allergists could accept the validity of clinical ecology or the two fields could agree to disagree and continue to move in opposite directions.

By the 1980s, it became less likely that orthodox allergy and clinical ecology could in fact coexist, even in isolation. Both factions increasingly entrenched their positions, with the AAA taking the lead for conservative allergists, and SCE, which changed its name to the American Academy for Environmental Medicine (AAEM) in 1984, doing the same for food allergists and clinical ecologists. For its part, the ACA remained slightly more conciliatory, considering the establishment of an Environmental Ecology Committee in 1976, on the suggestion of Randolph, and regularly holding symposia on food allergy, which the AAA had by then refused to do.[98] But even the clinically oriented ACA had its limits, urging that "rigid control" should be maintained over the content of such symposia, with the presentation of "controversial methods" being kept to a minimum and accompanied by plenty of time for rebuttal.[99] While the definition of allergy remained central to the festering debates, issues relating to such "controversial methods," which affected the economics of allergy practice, served to transform what was essentially an scientific dispute into a legal one.

Two practical issues involving the politics and economics of allergy also factored into the deteriorating relationship between clinical ecology and mainstream allergy. The first was medical certification. The American Board of Allergy and Immunology (ABAI) had formed in 1971 as a conjoint of the American Board of Internal Medicine and the American Board of Pediatrics. Prior to 1971, allergy had existed as a subspecialty of internal medicine (from 1936) and pediatrics (from 1941). Under the auspices of the American Board of Medical Specialties (ABMS), established in 1933, member boards set standards of practice and professionalism, certifying physicians as qualified specialists in their particular area of medicine. Although board certification was—and is—voluntary, it carried a degree of prestige, which benefitted physicians financially in terms of attracting patients and referrals, and helped with their career progression for allergists with academic or hospital appointments. It also demonstrated the viability and respectability of a particular area of medicine, which mattered enormously to those concerned about the status of allergy.

Notwithstanding these benefits, board certification of allergy had long been a matter for debate. Some allergists, such as Leslie Gay, believed that subspecialization in pediatrics and internal medicine was preferable, since it required allergists to demonstrate their proficiency in these "basic fields"; others disagreed, including George Piness, who petitioned the ABMS for independent certification repeatedly during the late 1940s and the 1950s.[100] Apart from concern about the legitimacy of allergy, Piness argued that the discipline's status as a subspecialty resulted in the "injustice" that otolaryngologists and dermatologists could not specialize in allergy unless they were also certified in internal medicine or pediatrics.[101] Regardless, the Los Angeles allergist's overtures were continually rebuffed, much to his consternation and that of his supporters. When allergy finally achieved board status in 1971, the discipline gained more control over what constituted allergy and who could be called an allergist. Not surprisingly, it became difficult for not only clinical ecologists but also otolaryngologists, who often followed the tenets of clinical ecology, to attain certification.[102]

While physicians practicing clinical ecology could practice without certification as long as they had a medical license, getting medical insurers to pay for such procedures was another issue. Randolph had set up an ecology unit in Zion, Illinois, in 1975, and established another "comprehensive environmental control unit" at Henrotin Hospital in Chicago in 1983.[103] Such units were not prohibitively expensive to set up (Henrotin Hospital spent $130,000 on the facility, including adequate air-conditioning and ventilation), but given that up to 15 percent of Randolph's patients were too ill to be diagnosed as outpatients and had to stay in the unit for days at a time, these units were costly to run.[104] Unfortunately for patients and Randolph, health insurance companies were increasingly reluctant to pay for such procedures. Legal action taken by one patient spurred Blue Cross to reimburse Randolph's clinic in the late 1970s, but in 1982, Blue Cross refused once again, and the federal Medicare program and private providers followed suit. By early 1986, Randolph was forced to shut down his units due to the lack of insured patients.[105]

The AAA also attempted to influence the course of the debates surrounding the issues of both certification and insurance coverage, with the conundrum of diagnosing and treating food allergies looming large. Asserting their control over what counted as legitimate diagnosis and therapy, both the ACA and the AAA conducted double-blind trials to test the efficacy of controversial diagnostic and therapeutic techniques used by food allergists. In 1974, the ACA's Food Allergy Committee published its study on sublingual testing for food allergies. (Sublingual testing, as the name indicates, simply involves placing a drop of food allergen extract under the tongue of a patient.) The ACA's trial demonstrated that the method was not reliable, with "patient anticipation" of a positive finding resulting in too many false positives. Such tests, according to one of the committee's members, provided "an attractive means for the patient to express his conscious or subconscious belief that the food being tested caused untoward reactions in the past." Therefore, sublingual testing did not "provide maximal value for the fees the patients pay" and had to be regarded as merely "experimental."[106] Shortly after the ACA trial, the AAA conducted its own trial of the "Rinkel method of immunotherapy," a sublingual technique of desensitization. Although Herbert Rinkel had used his method to treat all types of allergies, the AAA opted to test its use only on hay fever caused by ragweed. Ultimately spending $20,000 on the clinical trial, the AAA determined that the Rinkel method was no more effective than a placebo.[107]

As soon as these tests were discredited, though, even more controversial tests sprang up to take their place. Just as the discovery of IgE spurred new diagnostic technologies, such as RAST, growing public interest in and awareness of food and chemical allergies during the 1970s and 1980s fostered a controversial health industry revolving around alternative testing methods and therapeutic approaches to food, chemical, and other allergies.[108] Most of these tests involved patients providing blood samples, which would be tested for either the presence of immunoglobulins, elevated levels of white blood cells, or "cytotoxicity" (cell toxicity). While some providers, such as the Immuno-Nutritional Clinical Laboratory (the "Leading Food Allergy Lab in the US"), marketed to physicians and listed assays to treat both immediate (IgE-mediated or Type 1) allergies and "food immune complex assays" for delayed reactions, others promoted their wares directly to consumers, advertising in numerous newspapers and magazines. Under such brazen headings as "Allergy Testing Breakthrough" and "Disaster Linked to the Food You Eat!" such tests promised to diagnose the root cause of a whole host of problems, including headaches, fatigue, skin problems, gastrointestinal troubles, asthma, arthritis, and depression.

Reminiscent of the hawkers of patent-medicine cures of times gone by, the manufacturers of such products capitalized on growing food fears, the inability of modern medicine to treat many chronic complaints effectively, and the notion—ironically fueled by the discovery of IgE and the development of RAST—that an individual could determine his food allergies simply by posting a sample of his blood to a laboratory. One such lab, the New York Metabolic Group ("Specialists in modern allergy testing and treatment"), placed a full-page advertisement in the *New York Times*, headlined "The Foods You Love May Not Love You." It included the cartoon of a man being strangled by a rather poor rendition of a lobster. The text below the heading reads "Oranges could drive you bananas. Sweets could make you sour. Poultry could make you feel fowl. In fact, you could be allergic to anything from soup to nuts. And not even know it. . . . And in most cases it's the foods that you crave that are doing the most harm."[109] Claiming that the lab's "state-of-the-art" cytotoxic test rendered "the time-consuming scratch test obsolete" by testing for 175 different foods, the advertisement promised that patients would not only be placed on a rotary-diversified diet and vitamin program designed just for them, but also receive advice from a "culinary expert" about how to prepare appropriate meals.[110] Within weeks, or perhaps even days, patients could expect to "experience more restful sleep, increased energy, easier digestion, less irritability, and an overall heightened sense of well being"; they would probably even lose weight.[111]

The AAAAI's archival collection of such advertisements indicates its concern about such tests, and it also shows how prevalent they were during the early 1980s, springing up throughout the United States. Hinting at the ubiquity of such facilities, one ad from a laboratory with branches in a number of southwestern locations contended that "All Cytotoxic Labs Are Not Created Equal!" National Allergy Clinics, an organization based in Beverly Hills, even promised to help would-be laboratories get established:

> GET RICH! BE FIRST in your area to open a very lucrative allergy testing center—an ALL-CASH-UP-FRONT money-maker which uses a scientific breakthrough—a blood test that charts 245 food allergies simply and efficiently. Not a franchise, but we train, support, and assist you. $30,000 capital outlay.* ABSOLUTE PROOF of marvelous earnings by visiting our successful operation at our corporate headquarters.
>
> * Plus some additional start-up costs.[112]

Although this ad, published in the *Wall Street Journal*, was the most blatant attempt to capitalize on the testing craze, other advertisements for such testing similarly appear to have been thinly disguised attempts to part desperate, gullible patients, and possibly some physicians, from their money.[113] Such was a far cry from the earnest appeals made by the likes of Theron Randolph and Ben Feingold about the hazards posed by industrial and food chemicals. Nevertheless, orthodox allergists typically lumped clinical ecology together with the purveyors of cytotoxic tests and other questionable products in their efforts to protect the legitimacy of allergy.

The AAA's reaction to clinical ecology, which included such dubious laboratories, was varied and robust, ranging from responding to media stories to targeting individual practitioners. While its executive director, Donald McNeil, investigated the possibility of republishing an article in *Women's Wear Daily* that presented a succinct and sympathetic version of its position on many issues, the AAA's president, Raymond Slavin, wrote the senior producer of *CBS Morning News*, complaining that the program had described environmental illness as "an exciting new concept."[114] Other actions included lobbying the AMA to prevent physicians from earning continuing education credit for taking courses in clinical ecology.[115] Most such activities fell under the auspices of the AAA's Committee on Abusive Practices, which was informed about the claims in advertisements by allergists throughout the country. When a suspicious practitioner was identified, the committee responded vigorously through a range of channels, including the media, regulatory agencies (such as state medical boards), and governmental bodies (such as the FDA).

An example of such retaliation can be found in the case of Yehuda Barsel, a New Jersey–based physician who had written a short article for the *Jewish Times* on July 19, 1984, about the hidden allergies affecting 100 million Americans. He contended that most pediatricians were not willing to diagnose allergies in young children, leaving them with "annoying, painful, and even debilitating allergy symptoms."[116] Barsel had also advertised his "dramatic breakthrough" in the *Daily Register* of Shrewsbury, New Jersey, in July 1982, claiming that it helped "90% of the people 90% of the time" and could identify the hidden causes of hyperactivity, rashes, migraine, asthma, and assorted aches and pains. His "method" apparently combined RAST, cytotoxic testing, and the use of elimination and rotary diets.[117] After the publication of the *Jewish Times* article, Charles G. Blumstein wrote to Leon Brown, the editor of the newspaper and one of his patients, arguing that the paper should not have published the opinions of a physician who had a "poor" reputation and practiced techniques not recognized by "scientific authorities."

Blumstein also sent a copy of his letter to the AAA, which had already been investigating Barsel and his status with the New Jersey State Medical Board, the New Jersey Medical Society, and the Middlesex County Medical Society. Although the president of the board, Frederic Schulaner, admitted that Barsel "had not broken any laws," the board "would be glad to work with the AAA in any way possible to deter Dr. Barsel's efforts." Interestingly, in this case, Schulaner suspected that individual New Jersey allergists' attempts to counter Barsel in the media had backfired, merely generating more publicity for him. When the New Jersey State Board of Medical Examiners began an independent review into Barsel's activities in 1982, the AAA provided it with a selection of articles in the *Journal of Allergy and Clinical Immunology* (*JACI*) that undermined Barsel's claims, enclosed details about the AMA's policy on ethical standards, and offered to provide an out-of-state medical expert witness to speak against him. Although Barsel's article suggests that such efforts went unrewarded, other practitioners were successfully reprimanded in other states for "repeated negligent acts in the diagnosis and treatment of allergic conditions."[118]

In addition to taking action against individuals or specific articles that went against its conceptualization of allergy, the AAA employed broader measures to state its concerns. When the FDA and the Health Care Financing Administration (HCFA) announced that they would investigate cytotoxic testing, the AAA designed a letter that parents of children with food allergies could mail to their senators (or use in a phone call) to encourage them to support the initiative. In the bottom-right-hand corner of the letter was a copy of the "GET RICH!" advertisement from the *Wall Street Journal*. Citing the precarious position of the Medicare program, the letter declared that it was "wrong to weaken Medicare . . . by paying for unproven or unscientific procedures."[119] In 1985, when the FDA and HCFA announced that such tests were a "unproven diagnostic procedure," the AAAI sent a news release to every newspaper in the country summarizing the decision and declaring its support.

At roughly the same time, Raymond Slavin, the AAAI's president, also contributed to an article in *Town and Country* that, in addition to highlighting new drugs that could fight allergy, downplayed the significance of food allergies. Slavin advised readers how to "steer clear of quacks," meaning anyone who practiced allergy who was not a board-certified allergist, and "useless tests," such as cytotoxic testing, sublingual testing, and skin titration.[120] In response to the article, Helen Krause and Jerome G. Goldstein, members of the American Academy of Otolaryngology (AAO), wrote to Slavin, complaining about the article's tone and what it implied about their discipline, since they fit into the category of physicians who practiced allergy but were not allergists, and since they often used the tests that Slavin rubbished. The otolaryngologists were particularly annoyed that Slavin's comments went against a joint statement that the two societies had recently drawn up in an attempt to resolve their differences. Describing Slavin's implication that otolaryngologists were quacks as "undignified," "unprofessional," and "dishonest," Goldstein added that his "condemnation" of such tests was "downright inflammatory as well as inaccurate." Slavin replied angrily, retorting that "if your society took offense at such statements they would be in for many disappointments in the future."[121]

The correspondence between Slavin and the two otolaryngologists highlights how personal the debates surrounding food allergy, clinical ecology, and testing could be. On the one hand, such hostile reactions were under-standable. Many allergy-testing laboratories and physicians promising cure-alls were essentially snake-oil salesmen. The AAAI was also bombarded with venomous letters from patients and practitioners who opposed its views of clinical ecology, as well as flooded the society with numerous requests for more information about food allergies and MCS.[122] Similarly, the legal representatives of some clinical ecologists could be overbearing, leading Donald McNeil, an AAAI executive, to ask the SCE's attorney if it would be possible to impose an injunction banning such lawyers from sending the AAAI endless missives.[123] Other advocates of clinical ecology on whom the AAAI kept tabs appear simply to have been unbalanced. For instance, the Hawaii-based artist and writer Carol Barr, author of the *International Allergy Workbook* ("Dedicated to the memory of the young Tsarevitch Alexis of Russia, 1903–1913, written in the belief that hemophilia was and still is an allergic reaction"), believed that the consumption of berries early in life was a prominent factor in the height of individuals.[124] She also advised the AAAI in correspondence that "if any of you people wish to speak to me; make an appointment in writing so there will be no misunderstanding. Do not walk up to me in the street asking all sorts of questions without identifying your-selves. MAKE AN APPOINTMENT IN WRITING," which was quite an odd re-quest for someone living in Captain Cook, Hawaii.[125]

But on the other hand, the AAAI's proclivity to cite established clinicians, such as Randolph and Feingold, together with cranks and quacks was un-fair and misleading. The biases in this respect reflected not only its concern about allergy's status but also its ties to food, pharmaceutical, and chemical corporations, with which the AAAI was allied in the fight against clinical ecology. Companies representing these industries funded AAAI conferences, publications, and training, working with the association to convince the public that its restricted definition of food allergy was indeed correct. One letter to the AAAI from the food industry lobby group, the International Food Information Council (IFIC), discussed their "mutual efforts to com-municate with the public in the area of food allergy," correcting "frustrat-ing" and "outlandish claims" put forth in the media. Then in 1988, Merrell Dow Pharmaceuticals sponsored an advertising supplement for the AAAI in *Time*, which among other things made clear its views on food allergy.[126] The AAAI's attitude toward clinical ecology and food allergy, therefore, was not purely ideological; it was also connected to the economics of allergy.

The antagonism between orthodox allergists and clinical ecology finally came to a head in 1984, when the Texas clinical ecologist William Rea (b. 1935) launched an antitrust suit against the AAAI, the ACA, and the Joint Council of Allergy and Immunology (JCAI), in addition to the Prudential and Aetna insurance companies. Rea, a thoracic and cardiovascular surgeon, had established his Dallas-based Environmental Health Center in 1974 as an outpatient facility specializing in MCS diagnosis and treatment. Representing the interests of both clinical ecologists and their patients, Rea's class-action lawsuit contested that the parties named had systematically excluded clinical ecologists from fair compensation by colluding to make sure that their services were not covered under health insurance. The AAAI, in particular, had "attempted to improve its market position through means other than lawful competition."[127] For his part, Rea claimed damages in excess of $1 million in lost payments and business; the claims made by patients ranged from just over $1,000 to more than $62,000.

It did not take long for the case against the AAAI, the ACA, and the JCAI to be dismissed on jurisdictional technicalities. The remaining defendants, Prudential and Aetna, based their defense on the argument that clinical ecology did "not have a commonly understood meaning the medical community," a claim that the companies backed up with affidavits from allergists and immunologists. Since there was no board-certified training for clinical ecology, there was no such thing as a clinical ecologist and, therefore, the plaintiffs did not meet "the threshold requirements of showing the existence of a recognizable and identifiable class."[128] Paradoxically, Rea helped establish this claim himself by describing clinical ecology in an earlier court case as a "point of view" rather than a medical specialty.[129] In February 1985, the case was dismissed on these grounds, much to the relief of the defendants, and effectively determining that under law there was no such thing as clinical ecology.

• • •

ALTHOUGH THE COURT RULED IN FAVOR of the AAAI and the other defendants, the decision ultimately rested on a technicality—that is, whether clinical ecology was indeed "recognizable and identifiable" as an entity that could launch a class-action suit. Deeming that it was not, the court was never in the position to judge whether the defendants had conspired against William Rea and other clinical ecologists and their patients. John E. Salvaggio, president of the AAAI, may have described the result as "the best news I've heard all year concerning our field," but the case ultimately failed to deter patients from turning to environmental medicine and from Rea.[130] While Theron Randolph effectively retired from practice in 1986 at the age of eighty, he remained adamant that his approach to food allergies and other environmental illness was valid. As for allergists who insisted on the "immunologically restricted interpretation of allergy," they were "stuck in a trap of their own making. There are numerous mechanisms in allergy. It's ridiculous to limit the concept of hypersensitivity to the one mechanism of IgE. They're trying to make it an exclusive practice. They won't give up. Why? Because they are blockheads."[131] Other clinical ecologists and food allergists, such as Rea, William Crook, and Doris Rapp, continued to practice on the fringes of medicine; Rea was charged by the Texas Medical Board in 2007 for a range of malpractices.

In turn, the AAAI continued to monitor the claims and practices of clinical ecologists, making its opinions clear in position statements and in the media, and taking more aggressive action when it deemed appropriate. Despite fending off clinical ecology in the courts and despite the apparent immunological revolution ushered in by the discovery of IgE, clinical allergy remained somewhat static. According to Anthony S. Fauci (b. 1940), director of the National Institute of Allergy and Infectious Diseases (NIAID), writing in *Annals of Allergy* shortly after the Rea verdict, one of the questions that allergists had to ask themselves was "whether the rapidly evolving technology and fundamental breakthroughs in knowledge are being creatively and effectively translated into clinical applications." Hinting that they had not yet done so, Fauci suggested that the discipline of allergy needed to "take stock" in order to "wisely avail ourselves of the extraordinary opportunities before us" and "improve therapies which will bring greater benefit to patients."[132] The continued demand for alternative, unorthodox, and even sham remedies offered by the wide range of practitioners cast under the banner of clinical ecology suggested that many patients continued to miss out on such benefits. That many such tests had been inspired by the discovery of IgE and the development of RAST, both underlying the idea that testing for allergy could be a simple, in vitro, mail-order procedure, also dimmed the glow of the immunological revolution depicted by Fauci.

Although the deeper significance of IgE was overlooked by allergists and caused clinicians as many problems as it solved, IgE's ideological importance for orthodox allergists cannot be overstated. From 1966 on, it served as a standard, an emblem signifying all that was scientific and respectable about allergy, providing irrefutable proof of allergy's immunological nature. And, more so than any other allergic phenomenon, it was food allergy that was subject to the IgE crucible, distinguishing true allergy from mere intolerance, bona fide allergist from charlatan, and legitimate allergy sufferer from hypochondriac. Practically, the impact of IgE was limited; theoretically, its effect was enormous.

Since IgE was associated only with the reactions caused by a small number of foods, it effectively pushed food allergies to the sidelines, at least for orthodox allergists. But this soon changed in the 1990s, with the sudden emergence of an apparently new phenomenon in allergy: anaphylactic peanut allergy. Peanut allergy—a classic, potentially deadly, Type 1, IgE-mediated allergy—allowed orthodox allergists to take one step farther in the endless debates about food allergy, for it permitted them to reclaim food allergy for themselves. Even more so than promoting IgE as the litmus paper of allergy and fighting off the presumed threats of food allergists and clinical ecologists, it was peanut allergy—a true immunological explosion—that finally gave allergists the scientific legitimacy, public profile, and medical status that they had always desired.

SIX

The Problem
with Peanuts

IN HIS SYNDICATED COLUMN published on June 5, 1972, the Franco-American nutritionist Jean Mayer (1920–1993) reprinted a letter he had received from Chester Gryzbinski of Dedham, Massachusetts. Gryzbinski described how his ten-year-old son, Michael, had been invited by a friend to go to his house and eat some Butterfinger ice cream. Michael, who was allergic to peanuts, was accustomed to checking labels, and he examined the tub carefully. There were no ingredients identified, simply a picture of a Butterfinger chocolate bar, so Michael assumed that the ice cream was safe. Tragically, the manufacturers had whipped peanut butter into the ice cream. Feeling unwell, Michael soon returned home, where he quickly went into anaphylactic shock. He was dead within minutes.[1]

As Gryzbinski explained to Mayer:

> The reason I am writing this letter to your office . . . is my wife's and my hope that this tragedy does not happen again to other people who have this allergy, and that the container would be marked with the contents spelled out instead of only the picture of a candy bar. We intend NO legal action against this ice cream company, but only wish that they can see their way clear to change the container cover and identify the contents.[2]

For his part, Mayer wondered about what American authorities were doing to prevent such tragedies. While some "industries oppose labeling vigorously—ostensibly because the public would 'be confused,'" government agencies, such as the FDA, were "curiously unwilling to enter the arena."[3] As Mayer, who had worked with the Harvard nutritionist Frederick Stare (co-author of *Panic in the Pantry*), was well aware, this was partly due to the fact that much of the pressure for food ingredient labeling had not come from the parents of allergic children but from consumer advocates, such as Ralph Nader (b. 1934) and Beatrice Trum Hunter, who were more concerned about potentially harmful food chemicals.[4] The Gryzbinski case was different. It did not involve "the full chemical names of certain ingredients," but "natural contents" that might nevertheless go unnoticed when children were left to their own devices. Although the FDA had tabled a bill targeting the issue, Mayer dismissed it as "weak," and a number of concerned congressmen, led by Representative Benjamin S. Rosenthal (D-N.Y.), introduced tougher bills into the House and Senate. Mayer urged "aroused citizens" to exert "vigorous pressure" on their representatives in order to make sure that the bills would be passed into law.[5] Unfortunately for its proponents, nothing came of it.[6]

And nothing much was made of peanut allergy at the time, either. The odd case, such as the one reported by Mayer, may have made a headline or two, but for the most part, peanut allergy simply did not register in the mainstream media. Similarly, instances of fatal or near-fatal peanut allergies were rarely mentioned in medical literature.[7] Although Michael Gryzbinski's death demonstrates that this was not quite the case, the column correctly inferred that life-threatening peanut allergies were breathtakingly rare. Similarly, peanut allergy rarely featured in the activities or communications of both the AAAI and the ACA prior to the 1990s, though the exceptions do provide some insights. One letter to the AAAI from a Maine internist, written in 1978, requested more information about such allergies:

> I have recently had a patient who is quite sensitive to peanuts and who had such a severe anaphylactic reaction to hors d'oeuvres cooked in peanut butter oil that he nearly died. He has stated to me that many packages of do-nuts state that they have been cooked in peanut butter oil. I have given him a Hollister-Stier Anakit [epinephrine syringe] and of course instructions to stay away from all food fried in oil. I would like more help and advice regarding this situation.[8]

This letter is interesting, partly because of a minor debate that would emerge about the allergenicity of peanut oil, but more significantly because it hints at the ubiquity of peanuts and peanut products in the food supply.[9] In general, though, such cases were rare and did not, in fact, generate much attention. The AAAAI's apparent lack of interest in peanut allergy is also highlighted by its unwillingness to respond to a letter from a USDA food scientist about the unlabeled use of peanut meal in hamburgers and other foods. The scientist, who was allergic to peanuts himself, wrote back complaining that he had been ignored, but no subsequent response was recorded, as usually was the case with AAAAI correspondences.[10]

Peanuts, it seems, were perceived much the same as other food allergens, substances to which orthodox allergists were unwilling to draw attention. A pair of letters written by Charles D. May, chairman of AAA's Food Allergy Committee, during the late 1970s, for instance, imply that ignoring the issue altogether was the preferred approach.[11] In the first letter, May described being at a loss to find any worthwhile activity that his committee might undertake; the second letter, to Roberta Buckley, the AAA president at the time, urged that it be discontinued. While the "heterogeneous" composition of the committee, including both food allergists and orthodox allergists, was partly behind May's suggestion, his letters indicate the widespread belief that the less attention afforded to the subject, the better.[12]

By the 1990s, however, the AAAAI's attitude toward food allergy could not have been more different. Far from being a topic to be snubbed, food allergy was a major public-health issue, with the association taking a major role in raising awareness of and taking action about it. Of course, it was not just any food allergy the AAAAI had in mind; it was IgE-mediated, anaphylactic reactions to peanuts and a small number of other foods.[13] More than any other food allergen, peanuts became synonymous with food allergy and the subject of grassroots activism, voluntary industry action, legislation, and extensive media coverage. Much as orthodox allergists had heralded the emergence of IgE for giving allergy scientific legitimacy, peanuts made food allergy respectable, thrusting it into the spotlight like never before. Peanut allergy made allergy matter.

This chapter explores the process by which this remarkable transformation took place. Unlike other developments in the history of food allergy—which were dominated by ideological debates among physicians, the

clinical challenges of diagnosis and treatment, and the politics and economics of allergy—patients and parents were instrumental in putting the spotlight on peanut allergy by raising awareness, monitoring for peanut contamination, lobbying for better labels, and raising funds for research. Concurrently, allergy associations and the food industry were also able to harness
public concern about and interest in peanut allergy in order to shape understandings of food allergy in ways that were in their own interests. While
some of the proactive measures taken by the food industry were designed
to limit its liability in the case of accidental exposure, peanut allergy also
helped to distract from potentially bigger issues, including the amount of
food additives, sugar, salt, and saturated fat in packaged food. Similarly, orthodox allergists, represented by the AAAAI, worked with the food industry to reinforce their narrow definition of food allergy, a definition that was
epitomized by peanut allergy. Forgotten in the focus on the acute, anaphylactic reactions were the chronic, delayed, lingering, and much more mysterious reactions to foods that food allergists had long argued were more common and problematic. Although some of these patients' problems came to
be understood in terms of intolerances to lactose or gluten, symptoms connected to food additives or refined foods continued to be viewed with sus-
picion in the face of mounting evidence that they could be harmful. Despite
making food allergy a legitimate health concern, the rise of peanut allergy
also helped to transform food allergy into a very specific, attenuated, and
limited phenomenon, adhering to the way orthodox allergists had defined
it all along.

ENTER THE PEANUT

Unlike peanut allergy, peanuts are nothing new. Archaeological evidence
suggests that peanuts, which are legumes, not nuts, were grown in South
America as early as 3000 B.C.E. and possibly earlier, which makes them
one of the first cultivated plants. According to the food historian Andrew F.
Smith, peanuts were so common in what is now coastal Peru from around
500 B.C.E. to 100 C.E. that "archaeologists have exclaimed that some sites . . .
looked like poorly swept baseball stadiums with peanut shells scattered
about."[14] Brought to Africa by Europeans during the early sixteenth century,
peanuts largely replaced the Bambara groundnut, which had been cultivated in West Africa for thousands of years.[15] Later in the century, they were

brought to Asia; China, now the world's largest producer of peanuts, was introduced to the legume in the early seventeenth century. Rather than coming to North America from South America, peanuts first came to the American South in the eighteenth century from Africa, as a by-product of the slave trade.[16] The sandy soil of the southeastern United States would prove ideal for their cultivation.

By the late nineteenth century, peanuts (otherwise known as groundnuts, monkey nuts, or goobers) began to take on economic, social, cultural, and even political significance in the American South. As Smith describes, the Civil War enhanced the importance of peanuts for a number of reasons. The blockade of whale oil meant that peanut oil was turned to as a lubricant for machines. Peanut oil was also burned in lamps, utilized in medications, and used extensively in cooking, becoming a staple food for soldiers. As stanzas from the Civil War–era song "Eating Goober Peas" suggests, peanuts had become a staple associated with the South and also a snack that accompanied leisurely pursuits and good company:

Sitting by the roadside on a summer day
Chatting with my messmates, passing time away,
Lying in the shadow underneath trees
Goodness how delicious, eating goober peas! . . .
I wish this war was over, when free from rags and fleas
We'd kiss our wives and sweethearts and gobble goober peas![17]

Peanuts also became associated with other aspects of American culture. They were hawked by Italian street vendors in New York City, and munched at circuses, fair grounds, and baseball games. Economically, they served as an agricultural alternative to cotton in the South, particularly after the calamitous boll weevil infestations of the early twentieth century.[18] When improved agricultural technologies, which allowed peanuts to be planted and harvested mechanically, were developed around 1900, it became possible for the legume to become an important and profitable crop, one that attracted both farmers and the food industry.[19]

With the invention of peanut butter in the mid-1890s (either by the Michigan health-food pioneer John Harvey Kellogg, who saw it as a health food, or by George A. Bayle, a St. Louis food manufacturer who established it as a snack food), the prominence of the peanut grew even more.[20] As soon as peanuts were being ground into butter, people were spreading it on bread and the childhood essential, the peanut-butter-and-jelly sandwich, made its first appearance in 1901.[21] Consumer demand for the sticky stuff escalated rapidly in the first two decades of the twentieth century. While 2 million pounds of peanut butter were produced in 1899, by the end of the First World War the total was 158 million pounds, partly because the U.S. government had encouraged people to eat more peanuts and less wheat so that the latter could be sent to the European allies as part of the war effort.[22] Given the high nutritional value of peanuts, it is perhaps unfortunate that the government did not send them instead. Following the war, peanut butter was hydrogenated in order to make it smoother, more spreadable, and less perishable. As author Jon Krampner describes, what had been a regionally produced food now could be manufactured nationally and distributed throughout North America by major food companies. By the Second World War, peanut butter was widely marketed as an efficient and nutritious component of a good lunch, especially for children.[23] As one advertisement declared: "Hey, Mrs. America! Peter Pan peanut butter makes the eating-est lunch boxes!" Assuring mothers that the proteins found in its product would "help children build husky bodies," the ad suggested a number of novel peanut butter pairings, including chopped dates, raisins, bacon, celery, and olives.[24] Peanut butter had become part of the culinary landscape, primarily in the United States but also in a number of other countries, including Canada and the Netherlands, where the per capita rates of consumption were even higher.[25]

Peanuts have also packed a political punch, perhaps best exemplified by the electoral vicissitudes of President Jimmy Carter (b. 1924), a Georgia peanut farmer. Although Carter "adroitly used his connection to America's beloved food to bolster his public image" during the 1976 election campaign—and boosting the profile of the peanut industry in the process—the effects of a slumping economy plus a severe drought on the 1980 peanut crop contributed to his undoing.[26] When the drought's catastrophic effect on peanut yields became apparent, peanut butter producers sensibly went to the president for support, hoping that the administration would lift restrictive peanut import quotas in order to provide more peanuts for peanut butter production. In the midst of his campaign against Ronald Reagan (1911–2004), the former peanut farmer refused, not wanting to appear as if he were buying support. The election was lost, the price of peanuts skyrocketed, and consumers struggled to find enough peanut butter to satisfy their cravings. Even the USDA had to switch from peanut butter to cheese sandwiches in its school-lunch programs.[27]

Although crops recovered the following year, the 1980 peanut crisis foreshadowed other troubles for the peanut industry, related in part to changing ideas about whether peanuts were actually healthy. In health terms, peanuts are somewhat paradoxical. On the one hand, and as the National Peanut Council of America (NPCA) often stresses, peanuts are crammed full of nutrients, including protein, fiber, phosphorus, sodium, potassium, magnesium, thiamine, niacin, folic acid, vitamin E, polyphenols, antioxidants, and fats (more of the "good" variety than the "bad").[28] Peanuts have also been among the world's most versatile foodstuffs. While peanut oil, given its high smoke point, resistance to rancidity, and low levels of saturated fat, is found in kitchens across the globe, peanuts, peanut butter, and peanut flour have also been used into numerous processed foods, including candies, cakes, cookies, sauces, and ice cream.[29] When these beneficial properties are considered, it is no surprise that peanuts continue to be a major global food crop, especially in the developing world, where they are seen as a key weapon in fighting malnutrition.[30]

On the other hand, peanuts also have negative health connotations. Putting allergy to one side, people can have too much of a good thing when it comes to peanuts, particularly in North America. Epitomized by Elvis Presley's fried peanut-butter-and-banana sandwich (which often included slices of bacon), peanut butter has been associated with binge eating and excess, the favorite sandwich spread for the gluttonous midnight snacker. And not all peanut butters are created equal. While some consist only of peanuts, others contain additional sugar and oils, adding to their caloric content. During the 1950s, debates about how much of these supplementary products could be included in peanut butter led to the FDA's so-called Peanut Butter Hearings, which affirmed that the product had to contain at least 90 percent peanuts and no more than 55 percent fat.[31] Other health concerns connected to peanuts have been related to possible contaminants, including alfatoxin, produced by a mold that grows on peanut shells, and salmonella, both of which have resulted in major food recalls.[32] By the early 1990s, as the specter of peanut allergy was looming, health concerns about peanut butter, particularly its fat content, contributed to plummeting sales. In response, the American Peanut Shellers Association founded the Peanut Institute to promote peanut-friendly nutrition research and, despite the emergence of peanut allergy, sales of peanut butter rebounded, with 1.2 billion pounds of it consumed in 2010 and 2011.

Ironically, it has been one of the peanut's most beneficial qualities, along with its ubiquity, that has made it such a potent allergen, and one difficult to avoid. The proteins in peanuts that make them so nutritious are also highly allergenic, meaning that highly sensitive people can react to exceedingly small amounts of peanut.[33] Such potency, combined with the widespread use of peanuts in processed foods, has resulted in the danger of "peanut contamination," a problem for both allergy sufferers and the food industry. In other words, certain foods might not contain peanuts, but if they are produced in a facility in which peanuts are used, such products run the risk of being contaminated by infinitesimal peanut particles.[34] As early as 1990, researchers were designing tests to quantify the trace amounts of peanut allergens in such manufacturing plants, hoping to avoid accidental exposures.[35] Even airborne peanut dust was believed by many to elicit anaphylaxis in highly sensitive individuals. According to two British allergists, A. W. Frankland and R. S. H. Pumphrey, reactions could be triggered by the most innocent of exposures: "A few million molecules of peanut butter which becomes airborne when a parent eats it may be enough to sensitize a young child to the food, so that the first time it eats peanut (ground-nut), it will experience an allergic reaction."[36] The fear of such a reaction, moreover, could psychosomatically transform a mild reaction into full-blown anaphylaxis.[37]

A robust allergen that causes unquestionable and deadly symptoms, a cultural and political symbol, a historical driver of the southern economy, a staple food consumed in abundance by both children and adults in a wide range of settings (breakfast, lunch, and dinner included), and a hidden ingredient in many other foods, the peanut has all the attributes to become an extraordinary allergen, one that has baffled physicians, frightened parents, and divided opinion for many years. But, despite all this, peanuts were not a problem for allergists for most of the twentieth century. How did they become so? Just as the societal impact of the peanut was multifarious and far-reaching, the issues of how and why it became a notorious allergen would be one that involved the interests of many parties connected to the experience and practice of allergy.

POTENT PEANUTS

In 1982, just as American peanut crop was recovering, an article appeared in *Annals of Allergy* that threatened to cast another shadow over the troubled peanut industry. In one of the last articles written by the New York allergist Joseph Fries (1902–1982), peanut allergy was portrayed, in allergy terms, as a veritable sleeping giant. Fries, who had been an associate editor of *Annals of Allergy* and the *Journal of Dermatology*, had written widely since the 1950s on many allergy topics, often downplaying the significance of food allergies and the effectiveness of elimination diets. Recently, he had weighed in on the issue of chocolate allergy, claiming that "pervasive mistrust" of chocolate was misplaced, and the Feingold diet, which he insinuated was typical of the sort of "food faddism" that abounded in contemporary society.[38] One exception to this faddism, according to Fries, however, was the soy bean, the use of which had become widespread in processed and vegetarian foods. As early as 1971, Fries had warned that allergies to soy were bound to increase due to its ubiquity, and, ten years later, his prediction appeared to be correct.[39] Eleven years later, in 1982, Fries made a similarly prescient divination about peanuts. Peanuts were "potent antigens," but "just how potent has never been fully explored."[40] Strangely, there had been "no documentation of fatal or near-fatal anaphylaxis reactions in the medical literature, although explosive allergic reactions to the ingestion of botanically related chickpea (garbanzo bean) and pinto bean have been described."[41] This was despite the fact that peanuts were often—though not always—mentioned as a common allergen by orthodox allergists. Although Jean Mayer's column about Michael Gryzbinski indicated that fatal peanut anaphylaxis was not completely unknown, allergists were more likely to be concerned about the severity of seafood, milk, or egg allergies. This state of affairs, Fries prognosticated, was likely to change, given the increased use of peanuts in food production, made possible by advancements in food-processing technology. Having said this, however, Fries also hinted that severe anaphylactic reactions to peanuts had also been underreported, partly because of "a natural disinclination to report an unfortunate experience."[42]

While Fries's predictions about the mushrooming prevalence of peanut allergy were correct—indeed, more correct that he would have imagined—his suggestions about the reasons for such increases were not as well founded. Peanuts were increasingly used in food production, but, as Andrew Smith and Jon Krampner indicate, this had been a trend dating back to the turn of the century, with the hydrogenation of peanut butter in the 1920s proving to be the most important development in the process. If anything, given the peanut crop failure of 1980, the escalating cost of suitable land and associated economic pressures in agriculture, and the concerns about the fat content in peanut butter that would follow, the prominence of peanuts in food production, particularly in the United States, was more likely to plateau rather than escalate, even without the advent of peanut allergy and the complications posed by cross-contamination.[43]

Fries's point about physicians not wanting to report an "unfortunate experience" was similarly questionable. Both orthodox allergists and food allergists had long been willing to describe strange and severe reactions to food, with the former being particularly eager to discuss cases of anaphylaxis, or "true" food allergy. Such was the case even when it was allergists' own misguided attempts to test for or desensitize food allergies that caused such reactions. While foods, insect stings, and foreign sera were among the long-standing offenders, the widespread use of penicillin in the postwar years presented another type of potentially fatal anaphylactic reaction.[44] In some ways, the stranger the reaction was, the more likely it was to attract attention, as a *New York Times* article suggests:

It was a little thing, presumably harmless; a few drops of red pigment from guinea pig blood injected into the skin. Yet, in just 16 minutes, the healthy young woman who received it was dead. She was a volunteer in a medical experiment thought to be entirely safe, but her body reacted violently. Within minutes she complained of headache and began to wheeze. Her skin turned blue. Despite everything doctors could do for her in those remaining few minutes, she died.

The cause was an immunologic reaction gone wild. Her body's internal defense system had reacted too powerfully . . . to an intrusion of something foreign. That reaction described as anaphylactic shock kills an estimated 30 persons a year from such trivial causes as bee stings; and kills a substantially larger number who react violently to antibiotics such as penicillin.[45]

Although it is notable that the journalist who reported this story did not list foods as particularly anaphylactic, allergists certainly did, often highlighting the dangers of skin testing with certain food allergens. Some allergists, such as Ben Feingold, mentioned nuts (not peanuts) as potentially dangerous, but instances of fatal reactions to peanuts were remarkably scarce.[46]

Quibbles about Fries's analysis notwithstanding, by the late 1980s his general prediction about mounting cases of peanut allergy was beginning to be proved correct. Shortly after the publication of his article, more studies emerged that analyzed various aspects of peanut allergens, including the proteins found in peanuts; the tests that were best for diagnosis; and the effect of breast-feeding on infants becoming allergic to peanuts and other IgE-mediated food allergens.[47] None of these discussed fatalities, however. Then, in 1988, an article appeared in the *CMAJ* that not only provided an early example of a peanut allergy death but also highlighted how careful allergy sufferers had to be in order to avoid accidental exposure.[48] The victim was a twenty-four-year-old Ontario woman who was well aware of the severity of her peanut allergy; having once been admitted to a hospital following an anaphylactic reaction, she routinely carried an epinephrine syringe with her. On this occasion, a catered reception, she had eaten a bakery-produced cake topped with hazelnuts and almond icing (marzipan), neither to which she was allergic. Within minutes, she began to have breathing troubles, vomited, and died, without having the chance to use her epinephrine. Upon investigation, it was determined that peanut oil had been used in the preparation of both the cake and the icing; the tiny amount of peanut proteins found in the latter was eventually blamed for the death. As the coroner eventually discovered, almond icing was often made by mixing almond paste with peanuts, labeled in this instance as "groundnuts." Staff at the bakery had not been aware that "groundnuts" were synonymous with "peanuts," and, as a result, the catering staff had not been informed that the cake would be dangerous to those with peanut allergy. In concluding their article, the authors advised that restaurants and caterers should provide more comprehensive labels.

As Edmonton's AC/DC concert furor and other Canadian developments suggest, it was somewhat fitting that one of the first instances of a fatal peanut allergy reaction was reported in Canada, where high rates of anaphylactic allergies, sensational media stories, and grassroots activism have prompted some of the world's most proactive responses. A letter to the editor of the *CMAJ* that same year also described the death of a teenager who succumbed to anaphylaxis after eating an apple turnover that contained

ground hazelnuts, to which she was allergic. Foreshadowing Canadian legislative action against accidental anaphylaxis, the writer added that he and
others had successfully encouraged a parliamentarian, Sheila Copps (b.
1952), to table a private member's bill aimed at improving the labeling of
such products.[49]

It did not take long for American fatalities to be reported as well. A month
after the Canadian story, a review appeared in *JAMA* that documented seven
deaths due to food anaphylaxis. Noting that there was "virtually no data on
the incidence" of such fatal reactions, the authors proceeded to document
their cases.[50] Of the seven cases, four were blamed on peanuts, with pecans,
crab, and fish being the other culprits. Although five of the seven were children or teenagers, the deaths of two adults highlighted for the authors that
individuals did not always grow out of such allergies, as they might for others, a characteristic of peanut allergy still remarked on today. Also notable
was the fact that six of the seven deaths occurred away from home where
sufferers had less control over what they ate. The source of the allergen in
the case of an eighteen-year-old college student, for instance, was peanut
butter that was used to thicken chili, a dish not normally expected to contain peanuts.[51]

Similar studies followed swiftly. A review conducted by a Rhode Island
allergist, Guy Settipane (1930–2004), described the deaths of seven asthmatics who were also allergic to peanuts; another article reported six fatalities
(three to peanuts, two to other nuts, and one to eggs) and seven near-fatal
reactions in children and adolescents.[52] As the authors of the latter study
indicated, such cases were exceptionally rare, so much so that there was no
code for them in the *International Classification of Diseases*. Moreover, in
the six fatalities, none of the patients, or their parents, had been aware of
the deadly allergen in the food they had eaten, and even though all of them
were asthmatic, not one had experienced a near-fatal reaction before. Many
of the parents, according to the authors, "did not appreciate the potential
severity of allergic reactions."[53] Four of the six fatal reactions had occurred
in schools, foreshadowing a site where action against anaphylactic allergies
would soon be taken, and many of those who had survived had used epinephrine. In conclusion, the authors asserted that anaphylactic food allergy
had escalated in recent years and urged that parents, schools, and other institutions become better educated about it.[54]

By the early 1990s, allergy associations, such as the AAAI, also began to take notice of food anaphylaxis. Unlike chronic food allergies, the AAAI found it impossible to ignore these reactions. A letter from Timothy J. Sullivan, the incoming chairman of its Food and Drug Interest Section, to the AAAI president, William A. Pierson (1934–2011), described how the section's 1990 and 1991 meetings had featured lively discussions about anaphylaxis and its looming significance for allergists. In addition to changing the name of the group to the Food and Drug Reactions and Anaphylaxis Interest Section, Sullivan recommended that the AAAI begin "to monitor fatal and near fatal anaphylaxis, and to emphasize the importance of this lethal allergic disease to physicians and the public."[55] Anaphylaxis, concluded Sullivan, was "a disease that should be a prominent focus of the Academy [AAAI]."[56] Soon it and other allergy associations began to take anaphylaxis much more seriously, making the condition central to their efforts. What really spurred allergists into action was the pressure of another group affected much more intimately by anaphylactic food allergies: parents.[57]

POTENT PARENTS

The role of parents in raising awareness about food anaphylaxis and, consequently, transforming it from a clinical curiosity to a public-health phenomenon is subtly illustrated in the story of Kate Brodsky. Kate was the eighteen-year-old anonymously depicted in the *JAMA* article about the college student who had eaten peanut butter hidden in chili. When she died on February 18, 1986, it was not *JAMA* or an allergy journal that initially reported her story but, as with the tragic death of Michael Gryzbinski, a newspaper: the *New York Times*. Kate was not merely a statistic in a medical journal but a nationally ranked squash player and freshman at Brown University, who had eaten only a few spoonfuls of chili when her fatal reaction began. According to her mother, Barbara, "She had known she was allergic to nuts since she was 2 or 3. . . . She couldn't stand the smell of peanuts and she consciously avoided any food that had nuts in it. Who would expect peanut butter in chili?"[58] When compared with the relatively laconic medical article, which actually apportioned some blame to the student (believing her reaction to be mild, she had initially refused to be admitted to hospital), the newspaper's vivid, sympathetic depiction of Kate Brodsky's tragic death, particularly her mother's poignant bafflement, provides an indication of how parents' accounts could be influential.[59] Parents' anaphylaxis anecdotes made for good media stories, and they also influenced allergists, school boards, governments, and the food industry to take the issue seriously, in a way as yet unprecedented in the history of food allergy.

The effectiveness of parents in making an impact on these often self-interested and recalcitrant groups was due in part to their ability to organize. Today there are dozens of associations and networks around the world run by food allergy sufferers and parents, but two early initiatives, which continue to influence understandings of and action against anaphylaxis, stand out. They are the Virginia-based Food Allergy Network (FAN), later known as the Food Allergy and Anaphylaxis Network (FAAN), which recently merged with the Food Allergy Initiative (FAI) to become Food Allergy Research and Education (FARE), and the Anaphylaxis Campaign (AC), founded in the United Kingdom in 1994.[60] Although both of these organizations began largely on the initiative of individual parents (Anne Muñoz-Furlong, in the case of FAN, and David Reading, with respect to AC), they quickly made inroads into both organized allergy and the food industry. On the surface, both Muñoz-Furlong and Reading became interested in allergy activism because they were parents of children with food allergies, but the specifics of their experiences were very different. Although Reading's teenage daughter died from peanut allergy–induced anaphylaxis in October 1993, Muñoz-Furlong was the parent of a daughter whose milk and egg allergies caused chronic health problems rather than anaphylactic symptoms.[61] Nevertheless, what Reading and Muñoz-Furlong did have in common was considerable media experience; Muñoz-Furlong wrote for *Time*, and Reading had worked as a writer and editor for thirty-four years, including for a prominent food and drink journal.[62] Moreover, both worked effectively with the media, organized allergy, and the food industry to increase awareness, raise funding for research, and protect those susceptible to anaphylactic allergies.

For Muñoz-Furlong, it was the desire to reach out to and inform other parents struggling with food allergies that spurred her to create FAN. Almost as soon as her youngest daughter, Mariel, was born, she began to present "classic food allergy symptoms," including hives, projectile vomiting, cramping, and rhinitis, though Muñoz-Furlong did not recognize such indications as allergic at the time.[63] Concerned that Mariel was not getting enough to eat, Muñoz-Furlong would feed her more, merely exacerbating the symptoms. Struggling and concerned, she took her daughter from one physician to another, without much success, before arriving at the Children's Hospital in Washington, D.C., where Mariel was diagnosed with milk and egg allergies. Advised simply to avoid these foods, Muñoz-Furlong went home relieved but also bemused about how to feed her daughter in the future.[64]

As with many parents dealing with food sensitivities, Muñoz-Furlong did not receive a great deal of support initially from family and friends.[65] While some, like her, were unfamiliar with such conditions, others flatly disbelieved that an egg or some milk could cause such problems. When Mariel was ready for preschool, Muñoz-Furlong struggled to find her a place because many facilities were unwilling to take allergic children. Even when she did find a suitable preschool, some parents were unsympathetic. On one occasion, a mother, who knew of Mariel's allergies, brought in cupcakes and ice cream for all the children. Mariel was left with crackers and water. In the midst of such skepticism and apathy, Muñoz-Furlong was forced to go against her predilection to avoid conflict and became assertive, taking full control of her daughter's diet. Relying on her journalism background, she began researching food allergies and immunology as well as the byzantine world of food labels and ingredients. She figured out how to make cupcakes without eggs or milk; learned that certain chemicals, such as ammonium caseinate, were effectively synonymous with milk; and, once her family life had stabilized somewhat, began to write articles on food allergy for parenting magazines.[66]

When Muñoz-Furlong's articles began to appear in print, she started to receive letters from parents who also were coping with allergic children. Encouraged that her efforts were being appreciated, Muñoz-Furlong came up with other ways in which to reach out to parents, including a newsletter, *Food Allergy News*, in which both scientific and practical information about food allergies was presented, and creating wallet-size laminated cards with instructions on how to interpret food labels.[67] After the first edition of *Food Allergy News* was published in 1990, Muñoz-Furlong decided to attend the ACA conference, leaving some of the newsletters in the exhibition hall. Before long, she had people asking her about becoming members and, in 1991, FAN was born.

FAN, ALLERGISTS, AND INDUSTRY

From the outset, Muñoz-Furlong received tremendous support from the allergy community, starting with Hugh Sampson, who soon became the director of FAN's medical advisory board. Sampson checked over Muñoz-Furlong's articles to be sure that they were scientifically accurate, a function the advisory board also took on. Of course, not everyone agreed about what counted as legitimate allergy knowledge. Instead of delving into such thorny issues, Muñoz-Furlong decided early on to focus solely on the top eight food allergens (milk, egg, peanut, soy, fish, shellfish, wheat, and tree nut) and avoid discussion of food chemicals and other controversial allergens altogether.[68] On the one hand, this pragmatic choice simultaneously gave FAN a more precise focus and made it easier for orthodox allergists and the food and restaurant industries to support its efforts. Severe food allergy sufferers, parents, allergists, and industry all had to cooperate in order to combat the threat posed to them by anaphylactic food allergies, as the title of Muñoz-Furlong's regular editorial in *Food Allergy News*—"We're All in This Together!"—suggested. But on the other hand, the decision to downplay the role of chronic food allergies caused by less common and more controversial ingredients (such as food additives) meant that many others were excluded. Chronic sufferers, clinical ecologists, and many traditional food allergists were not, in fact, all in it together with FAN. While FAN's emphasis on severe allergies helped it achieve its own laudable objectives, it also effectively helped marginalize those who espoused more liberal definitions of allergy.

Due in part to FAN's approach to food allergy, which was sympathetic to its own, the AAAI quickly became a key ally. Before long, it, along with other interested organizations, was funding many of FAN's projects, including providing $23,600 in 1992 to produce a "patient education" video on anaphylaxis called *It Only Takes One Bite: Food Allergy and Anaphylaxis*, and $21,800 in 1996 for the School Food Allergy Program, an awareness initiative for schools.[69] In addition to writing columns for *Food Allergy News*, which typically accorded with orthodox definitions of allergy, the allergists and allergy associations worked with FAN to produce reports on specific aspects of food allergy, usually co-authored by Muñoz-Furlong and a leading allergist. Covering topics ranging from *Food Allergy and Atopic Dermatitis* (eczema) to *Off to School with Food Allergies*, such reports were aimed at parents and offered information, advice, and the contact details of support groups, medical associations, and companies selling hypoallergenic products.[70]

Food Allergy and Atopic Dermatitis (1992), in particular, also provides an indication of the way FAN liaised with the food industry, in that it was funded by the International Life Sciences Institute (ILSI), essentially a lobby group for the food, drug, and chemical industries. ILSI was founded in 1978 as a branch of the Nutrition Foundation, which had been involved in discrediting both *Silent Spring* and the Feingold diet, among other initiatives, and which it nominally replaced during the mid-1980s.[71] From FAN's perspective, especially given that it was in its infancy, funding from ILSI might not have seemed to be particularly problematic. FAN was not interested in highlighting the food chemicals that ILSI traditionally defended, and Muñoz-Furlong was convinced that her blossoming organization would have to cooperate with the food industry if food production and labeling were to become more allergy-friendly. Although *Food Allergy and Atopic Dermatitis* recommended a number of allergy drugs and hypoallergenic products, the overall tone of the booklet was not particularly biased toward industry interests. The only hint of ILSI's hostility to clinical ecology and liberal approaches to food allergy was found in a statement at the end, where it was suggested that parents often overestimated the number of foods to which their children were allergic.

Perceived in another way, however, FAN's flirtation with food industry interests, whatever the rationale, did indicate its stance on the food allergy debates that had raged for most of the twentieth century. Although it was a grassroots, parent-based organization in one sense, in other ways its approach was top–down, relaying a version of food allergy that was acceptable to orthodox allergists, conservative medical associations, and the food, chemical, and drug industries. As discussed earlier, the AAAI had regularly courted the affections of such interests, as demonstrated by the activities of its Related Industries Committee.[72] The pharmaceutical industry was a primary target. One 1990 letter from Jordan N. Fink, a past president, to then-president John A. Anderson encouraged him to promote more regional allergy conferences paid for by "our Pharmaceutical friends." Having recently attended such a meeting in Wisconsin, fully funded by "local pharmaceutical reps," Fink believed that more such occasions would benefit all parties involved.[73]

Not everyone, however, viewed such partnerships so positively. A story published in *Time* less than a month before had warned that pharmaceutical companies were exerting undue pressures on physicians to use their products. Seldane, an allergy medication manufactured by the generous AAAI donor Marion Merell Dow, was one of the products highlighted.[74] Two years later, the *New England Journal of Medicine* (*NEJM*) also criticized the publication of the proceedings of industry-sponsored symposia, stating that journals tended to abandon any notion of peer review in such articles, rendering them into de facto promotional materials.[75] Despite such concerns, by 1991, the AAAI had succeeded in achieving its goal of $1 million in sponsorship from the pharmaceutical industry; by 1995, on the back of aggressive fund-raising by the Related Industries Committee, this amount had tripled. While this may not have been an usual amount of support for a medical organization, it is indicative of the symbiotic relationship between the two parties and the AAAI's active pursuit of stronger links.[76]

The pharmaceutical industry's support of organized allergy also entrenched the expectation that allergies, including anaphylactic food allergies, were conditions not just to be prevented through education, awareness, and improved labeling but also to be treated with pharmaceutical products, such as steroids and epinephrine/adrenaline injectors. There was money to be made from the increasing prevalence of allergy. This "global economy of allergy" was nothing new, but with fears of food anaphylaxis escalating during the early 1990s, it took on an added intensity, which has not abated since.[77] When an unprecedented number of adrenaline pens (250,000) in the United Kingdom were set to expire in late 2009, for example, it made headline news, with AC and Allergy UK warning that thousands of allergy sufferers were at risk.[78] Even more recently, President Obama signed the School Access to Epinephrine Act, which will provide financial incentives for schools that keep stockpiles of epinephrine.[79] Although such legislation is undoubtedly in the interest of young allergy sufferers and their parents— it was inspired, in fact, by the deaths of two girls as a result of food allergies and spearheaded by FARE—it will also be a boon to the pharmaceutical industry.

In addition to working with pharmaceutical companies, the AAAI consolidated its connections with the food industry during the early 1990s, as FAN and peanut allergy began to emerge. In 1992, for example, it decided to work with IFIC to produce a pamphlet designed to educate the general public about food allergy. As were many such organizations, IFIC, which was founded in 1985 and published the *Food Insight* newsletter, was not officially a lobby group, and ostensibly existed only to provide science-based information about food safety and nutrition. A quick look at its funders (including Coca-Cola, Monsanto, and DuPont), activities, and general message suggested otherwise. With regard to the pamphlet, a letter outlining the agreement between the AAAI and IFIC describes how the booklet would "be written and edited by members of both organizations and will not be published unless both organization approve the final product."[80] Although the perspectives of the AAAI and IFIC with respect to food allergy were not particularly different, the former's willingness to go along with such an agreement, in addition to its ties with pharmaceutical companies, raises questions about the influence that various industries had on AAAI policies and position statements with respect to food allergy. When juxtaposed against the outright hostility that characterized its dealings with clinical ecologists by the 1980s, the AAAI's relationship with industry was very warm indeed.

Subsequent pamphlets were produced, which were also endorsed by FAN, indicating that it, too, had to empathize with the food industry if it was to convince the industry to change its practices in ways that would protect food allergy sufferers.[81] Despite Muñoz-Furlong's willingness to cooperate, the food industry was initially suspicious of her overtures, fearing that she would ultimately take "them to task," as had so many other consumer groups.[82] Eventually, however, they realized that Muñoz-Furlong was genuinely interested in forging a partnership that would be mutually beneficial. While parents would feel that their children were better protected by clearer labels and less allergen contamination, the food industry would have less to fear from potential litigation. FAN was also quick to praise food producers in *Food Allergy News* when they voluntarily removed a product contaminated with an unlabeled allergen. Although Muñoz-Furlong was frustrated by how slowly practices changed, eventually she and FAN convinced the food industry to join forces with them. Among FAN's first industry allies were General Mills and Disney, two corporations that depended enormously on appearing to be child-friendly. While General Mills quickly changed its labeling practices and, along with Hershey, created an in-house video to educate employees about food allergies, Disney created posters for display in hospital cafeterias and other public eating spaces that warned about food allergies.

Less supportive initially was the restaurant industry, partly because it was difficult to train staff sufficiently in such a high turnover industry and also because restaurants also felt pressured by other health campaigns, such as those targeting heart disease. In 1986, for example, Senator John Chafee (R-R.I., 1922–1999) convinced fast-food restaurants to list the nutritional components of the foods they served in an attempt to promote cardiovascular health. Following Kate Brodsky's fatal anaphylaxis the same year, the AAAI wrote to Chafee urging him to consider including common allergens as well.[83] At that time, nothing materialized, but six years later, with awareness of peanut anaphylaxis rising, the AAAI and FAN again targeted the restaurant industry, specifically the National Restaurant Association (NRA). This time, they received a more favorable response. The NRA agreed to work with FAN to launch the Restaurant Food Allergy Awareness Program, which involved sending a pamphlet titled *What You Need to Know About Food Allergies* to eighteen thousand restaurants across the United States.[84] Although producing more informative menus was not necessarily one of the recommendations, the pamphlet did provide advice about foods that often contained hidden food allergens, how to deal with allergic customers, and what to do in the case of an anaphylactic reaction.[85] For its part, FAN instructed its members via *Food Allergy News* how to request allergen-free foods and which menu options were likely to be safe. Those with severe food allergies also had a role to play in educating restaurants about how to protect themselves and other allergy sufferers.

TAKING ON PEANUTS

As with FAN's overall objectives and the AAAAI's approach to food allergies, anaphylaxis-inducing allergies were privileged in such cooperative ventures. FAN's limited mandate, which concentrated solely on IgE-mediated allergies, made it much easier for it to convince the food industry to change. Not only did this focus restrict discussion to the eight top food allergens, but the severe, immediate nature of such reactions also clarified matters for restaurants and food producers. Unlike a delayed reaction to a controversial food additive, such as monosodium glutamate (MSG), which could manifest itself in a chronic symptom such as headache and was associated with innumerable causes, anaphylaxis was a discrete, acute, and frightening response, the causes for which were easy to identify.[86] And among the eight food allergens, peanuts were singled out as the most severe and targeted for prophylactic action.

There are a number of reasons for why this was the case. Compared with those of most other allergens, the symptoms that peanuts induced were exceptionally severe and could be triggered by minute quantities of peanut protein. More to the point, they were disproportionately fatal, when compared with other anaphylactic allergies. Whether it was reported in *Food Allergy News*, in the mainstream media, or by word of mouth, the speed, ferocity, and lethality of peanut allergy presented a compelling case for action. The stories parents described of such fatalities were similarly difficult to ignore, as the case of twenty-one-year-old Sarah Weaver exemplifies. In the summer of 1996, Sarah and her family had been at a wedding in New York City that culminated in a buffet dinner. Not finding the buffet particularly appetizing, Sarah decided to pick up something on their way back home. Just before she left, however, one of the caterers came out with a tray of cookies. Sarah asked if they contained peanuts and, being assured that they did not, ate one. Minutes later, her stomach began to feel upset, and by the time she and her family got outside she had become asthmatic, with the signs of cyanosis appearing on her ears. Without epinephrine to hand, they waited for an ambulance, the first of which did not have any epinephrine available. Sarah soon lost consciousness, suffered cardiac arrest, and died the following day. The chance nature of Sarah's accidental reaction, juxtaposed against what was supposed to be a joyous wedding, made her death, as with so many similar fatalities, even more difficult for other parents, allergists, politicians, and the food industry to downplay, let alone ignore.[87]

According to Muñoz-Furlong, fear of such reactions made the parents of children with peanut allergy especially vociferous with respect to protecting their children, even if it meant banning peanuts from public places.[88] In order to get a better sense of peanut allergy mortality and morbidity, FAN, along with its medical board, began tabulating a voluntary nut registry, which kept track of the experiences of peanut- and nut allergy sufferers and the circumstances surrounding fatalities, such as age, gender, when and where nuts were consumed, and if epinephrine had been administered.[89] Among the findings presented in one of the first reports on fatalities was that peanut and nut allergies accounted for 94 percent of fatalities (and peanuts 62 percent of that) in a sample of thirty-two cases, but that children, adolescents, and young adults, like Sarah Weaver, were most likely to succumb to fatal nut anaphylaxis, making the cases all the more tragic. Fatalities were also most likely (85 percent) to occur away from home—at school, in restaurants, or at other people's homes—making education, better labeling of all foods, and possibly banning peanuts from certain places even more appropriate.[90]

If peanut anaphylaxis was not senseless and captivating enough in itself, a series of strange cases soon emerged that made it appear even more bizarre. A Quebec teenager died after kissing her boyfriend, who had recently eaten a peanut butter sandwich. Although the coroner was unable to confirm that the sandwich had definitively been responsible, the notion of a deadly, anaphylactic kiss proved irresistible to the international media.[91] Another Quebec case involved an eighty-year-old woman who became allergic to peanuts after receiving a blood transfusion from someone who was allergic; this then raised questions about whether blood donors should be screened for such allergies.[92] Such strange and salacious means of transmitting peanut allergens and peanut allergy made the condition irresistible to the media and further expanded the scope of the risk posed by peanuts, thus justifying assertive responses. Peanut allergy, unlike other severe food allergies, was also a new phenomenon. As such, research on the prevalence and severity of peanut allergy was limited, adding to speculation in the media, the Internet, and elsewhere.

Finally, and partly due to anthropomorphic characters like Planter's Mr. Peanut, peanuts are readily recognizable and fairly easy to demonize, as graphic depictions of peanut allergy often illustrate. Peanuts are not as ubiquitous as milk, eggs, or wheat but not quite as avoidable as fish. Peanuts are also, especially in the form of peanut butter, kid food, "an American icon" associated with children, who are especially vulnerable to accidental exposures.[93] Peanut butter sandwiches are stuffed into millions of school lunchboxes, and peanuts are found in numerous other foods aimed specifically at children.

All these factors make it possible for peanuts to be regarded as a serious enough risk to public health to legitimize banning them from public places where accidental exposures are most likely, much like smoking bans in restaurants, on airplanes, and in other public spaces. Schools, child-care facilities, airplanes, and sports venues are the spaces most commonly targeted, but many other measures have also been taken to deal with the problem.[94] While some responses, such as creating T-shirts for allergic children to wear that highlight what not to feed them, are relatively simple and un-obtrusive (although they might be embarrassing for the wearer), others are more elaborate. In one case, a nut-sniffing dog is used by parents to protect their seven-year-old girl from accidental exposure.[95]

The threat posed to peanut allergy sufferers from bullies who might use peanuts to intimidate their victims is also being treated seriously. According to a 2013 survey of 251 food allergy sufferers in *Pediatrics*, one-third of children reported being bullied for their allergies, with only half of the parents being aware of what was going on.[96] One Australian example involved Daniel Browne, a thirteen-year-old peanut allergy sufferer, whose assailant began his assault by throwing a peanut butter sandwich at his face. Following this, the bully waved another sandwich under his victim's nose, and shortly thereafter Daniel went into anaphylaxis. Although the reaction was severe, the quick arrival of an ambulance, copious amounts of adrenaline, and hours of intensive care helped the teenager to pull through.[97] In the United Kingdom, Paul Bentley, a former employee of Kinnerton Confectionary, was charged with scattering peanuts throughout the "nut-free" section of the company's production line after a dispute. Bentley was acquitted, but the factory still had to be decontaminated at the cost of £1.2 million (more than $2 million).[98]

According to Clive Beecham, Kinnerton's managing director, the company decided to segregate a nut-free section after being "harangued by a child's mother about a Teletubbies chocolate bar they produced which carried a 'may contain traces of nuts' warning on the wrapper." Such labels, designed to assuage producers' fears about litigation, were not of much help to parents, particularly when they appeared almost automatically on packaged foods. Agreeing with her that they could not justify making products aimed at children in a "potentially lethal environment," the company decided to separate the plant into two sections, at the cost of over £1 million ($1.7 million). Everything, including tools, clothing, kitchens, changing areas, and first aid rooms, was duplicated and color-coded to prevent contamination, and a testing regimen was put in place to ensure that no traces of peanut, almond, or hazelnut came into or out of the nut-free zone.[99]

Such measures have been replicated in other facilities in the United Kingdom, Canada, and the United States, with the "nut-free" label being seen by many companies, including Mars Canada, as a marketing tool. In 2006, Mars Canada began a major advertising campaign stating that its chocolate bars were produced in a completely nut-free environment. To parents desperate for a "safe" candy bar in the midst of peanut-packed Snickers, Reese's Pieces, and Peanut M&M's, such a campaign was a blessing. To marketing experts, the move was probably interpreted variously as clever or cynical. But to a growing number of critics—and particularly in the context of peanut bans in schools, on airplanes, and at AC/DC concerts—such strategies are seen as excessive at best and, at worst, a worrying sign of either misplaced priorities or the panic-induced restriction of civil liberties. According to a Harvard medical sociologist and attending physician, Nicholas A. Christakis, in a widely publicized *British Medical Journal* (*BMJ*) editorial "This Allergies Hysteria Is Just Nuts," peanut bans are "an overabundance of caution . . . a gross overreaction to the magnitude of the threat" and a "charade . . . making things worse."[100] Attempting to demonstrate the degree of this "epidemic hysteria," Christakis has relied on some familiar chestnuts, comparing the 150 annual deaths in the United States from food anaphylaxis with the 100 deaths annually from lightning strikes and, bizarrely, the 50 deaths a year from bee stings (one would have thought he would have steered away from other anaphylactic fatalities). He also highlights in comparison the 45,000 deaths due to motor vehicle collisions, 1,300 deaths from gunshot wounds, 2,000 deaths by drowning, and the fact that thousands of children are admitted to hospital for head injuries incurred during sports activities. He does not deny the existence of peanut allergy, or the fact that thousands of people have found themselves in the hospital because of it, but he also argues that the wholesale avoidance of peanuts actually would result in *more* peanut allergy because large numbers of children would never be exposed to them. Hysterical fear of peanuts compounds the problem by encouraging parents to have their children tested, with the result that they would be diagnosed with "mild and meaningless 'allergies' to nuts." Ultimately, a vicious cycle of "anxiety, draconian measures, and increasing prevalence to nut allergies" has been created. The technical term for this phenomenon is "mass psychogenic illness," and, according to Christakis, that in itself has to be cured.[101]

Although the polemical tone of Christakis's article, perhaps more suited to AC/DC fans, suggests that he was being deliberately provocative, his arguments contain many inconsistencies. For a start, Christakis's focus on peanut bans overlooks the fact that education, awareness, and developing action plans for anaphylaxis are also key, less restrictive aspects of tackling the threat posed by peanut allergy. Parents even enroll their children in relatively risky desensitization trials in order to lower their sensitization to peanuts, demonstrating their willingness to take ownership over the condition. Moreover, as Muñoz-Furlong claims, not all parents of children with peanut allergy desire peanut bans, believing that educating their children and others to be vigilant—and to always carry an epinephrine injector—is a better approach.[102] Christakis's suggestion that peanut bans make the general childhood population more sensitive to peanuts also glosses over the fact that nonallergic children can eat whatever they want at home and in most public places, but that overall consumption of peanut products has increased in the United States and globally.[103] Although fear of peanut allergy might compel more parents to have their children tested, the potency of peanut allergy—plus the fact that a history of mild reactions does not preclude the possibility of a severe response—suggests that there is no such thing as a "mild and meaningless" peanut allergy, particularly if it is diagnosed in a person with asthma.[104] Moreover, since the scientific evidence about what triggers the rise in peanut allergies is limited, any such epidemiologic assumptions are imprudent at best.

Finally, Christakis's rather blunt comparison of deaths from peanut allergy with those from other causes smacks of illogic and insensitivity. Unlike the risks posed by lightning, gunshots, and motor vehicles, deaths from peanut anaphylaxis endanger only the allergic. As such, Christakis's epidemiological statistics do not compare like with like; the risk of mortality from lightning for the general population, for instance, is far less than the risk posed to the peanut allergy sufferer by fatal anaphylaxis. His argument about gunshots, even in the gun-happy United States, similarly fails to hold up under scrutiny, since the risk of being killed by a bullet disproportionately affects only certain populations within American society, particularly those who insist on keeping guns in their homes. Christakis might well have countered that a peanut allergy sufferer is still more likely to be killed in a car crash than by a peanut, but then this says more about what little society does to prevent road deaths than what it should do about peanut allergy. Furthermore, Christakis's conflation of the general population with peanut allergy sufferers in relaying such statistics also overlooks the simple fact that the two groups are speciously different and that, as a vulnerable population, it is invariably humane to take certain measures to protect them. Western societies have taken considerable steps since the 1980s to make life easier for those confined to wheelchairs, to give but one example. Why should they not attempt to do the same to prevent accidental exposure to peanuts?

All of this is not to say that the responses to peanut allergy are excessive, at least when compared with other threats to public health, particularly those affecting a greater percentage of the population. Asthma is an allergic disease that results in far more mortality and morbidity than peanut allergies, with more than 3,400 deaths and nearly 500,000 hospitalizations annually in the United States.[105] Unlike peanut allergy, which essentially involves avoiding peanuts, asthma is a truly chronic condition with which sufferers must cope on a daily basis. Although pollution from various sources and poor housing have long been acknowledged as a contributing factor in these statistics, steps to reduce exposure to pollutants and improve housing have been less aggressive and less voluntary than those taken to combat accidental exposure to peanuts, especially when the relative scope of the problem is taken into consideration. Why has this been the case? Gregg Mitman argues that the reasons involve the reluctance of organized medicine and the pharmaceutical industry to turn their focus away from producing profitable drugs and inhalers, as well as the difficulty in convincing industrial polluters, consumers, and government that there is indeed a link between pollution, poor housing, and asthma, and that it is incumbent on society to take action.[106] Unlike peanut allergy, around which the interests of patients, parents, orthodox allergy, and the food industry have coalesced, asthma divides the opinions of those who experience it, treat it, provide drugs for it, and exacerbate it, even though more aggressive prophylactic responses would have a far greater positive impact in public-health terms. But as the longer history of food allergy suggests, this does not have to be the case. Other divisive allergy theories, such as the link between food additives and behavioral problems, were lampooned extensively during the 1970s and 1980s, only to be reassessed more positively in certain contexts in the years that followed. Both the food-additive and peanut allergy examples suggest that it has been a combination of lobbying from patient groups combined with gradual or immediate acknowledgment by organized medicine, the food industry, and other interested parties that have resulted in change.[107] Instead of criticizing or ridiculing the muscular measures employed to prevent accidental peanut anaphylaxis, perhaps those interested in public health more broadly should take lessons from it.

WHY PEANUTS?

Despite all the success food allergy support groups, organized allergy, and the food industry have had in raising awareness about peanut allergy and instituting steps to prevent accidental deaths during the past quarter century, the number of fatalities continues to increase.[108] The uncomfortable reason is that more people are becoming allergic to peanuts, and severely so. Why is this the case? Although theories abound, there is little consensus and, even more worrying, not a great deal of interest in pursuing the matter, at least when compared with the energy expended by allergists in raising awareness about anaphylaxis, promoting the availability of epinephrine injectors, and lobbying the food industry. This has occurred despite the efforts of FAN, later FAAN, and now FARE in making a cure for food allergy a key priority. By the mid-1990s, FAN and other food allergy groups began offering grants to researchers in the hope of determining what specifically caused the epidemic. One fund-raising initiative started in the first decade of the twenty-first century was an annual walk, similar to those organized by other health campaigns. Supporters were asked to "Walk for Food Allergy: Moving Toward a Cure." While some of this research was dedicated toward therapies and treatments, determining what was causing the increase in such allergies has also been a central question. But although the question has been around, waiting for an answer, for twenty-five years, by November 2013 when FARE released *A Vision and Plan for Food Allergy Research*, the association had to admit: "Relatively little is understood today about the underlying causes, mechanisms, and natural history of food allergy."[109]

When many of the hypotheses are put forward for the increase in food allergies and examined (especially in the case of peanut allergy), the reasons for this apparent lack of understanding becomes clear. While a small number of theories, such as the suggestion that the roasting of peanuts makes them more allergenic (peanuts are typically roasted in Western countries where peanut allergy is rife, rather than boiled, which is the practice in Asia and Africa where it is uncommon), have not been particularly contentious, most other theories have divided opinion or have been stubbornly resistant to verification.[110] Among the most long-standing speculations, dating back at least to the 1920s, has revolved around whether foods consumed by pregnant or breast-feeding women could induce food allergies in their children.[111]

Although the advice for many years to British women, for instance, was to avoid peanuts, the Food Standards Agency (FSA) reversed its policy in 2009.[112] A Canadian study the following year, however, provided contrary evidence, suggesting, yet again, that consuming peanuts during pregnancy and breast-feeding did constitute a risk factor.[113] Two years later, a Danish team reported conversely that consuming peanuts and other nuts during pregnancy could actually prevent allergies, muddying the debate even more.[114]

Breast-feeding, a loaded topic by itself, connected to peanut allergy in other ways. One of the reasons put forth by organizations ranging from La Leche League to UNICEF for encouraging mothers to nurse their babies is that breast-feeding is good for infant immunological health. Adding to this claim is the assertion that the soy used in artificial formulas could also trigger peanut allergy, because the soybean is a relative of the peanut.[115] Flying in the face of this advice, however, is other evidence that breast-feeding may in fact contribute to allergic disease in infants. Two Canadian researchers, Joanne Duncan and Malcolm Sears, questioned in their provocatively titled article "Breastfeeding and Allergies: Time for a Change in Paradigm?" whether breast-feeding does indeed result in a reduction of allergic disease in the long term.[116] Although they do not discourage breast-feeding, the researchers warn that advocating its immunological benefits might be misleading. Making matters more confusing is that the debate has been regularly reported in the media, leaving mothers in a quandary over whether to consume what is a highly nutritious food during a critical period in their baby's development.

The equally contentious "hygiene hypothesis" has more to do with the environment in which children grow up. There has long been an undercurrent of allergy research connecting helminthic infections to the emergence of allergy as a disease of Western civilization. In 1989, this idea was expanded to encompass other infections, suggesting that since children live in pristine, antiseptic environments and thus are not exposed to many pathogens, their immune systems are ill prepared to determine harmful proteins from harmful or nutritious ones.[117] Or, to use the formulation of Frank Macfarlane Burnet, their systems are unable to determine self from non-self. Some go even further, arguing that the very chemicals used to disinfect households also adversely affect children's immune systems. Perceived in this way, allergy is even deeper entrenched as a disease of civilization.[118] Given the way the hygiene hypothesis mirrors similar clinical ecology theories about the link between the environment and the emergence of allergic disease, it is not surprising that many orthodox allergists are loath to put it to the test.

But if anything has the potential to top the hygiene hypothesis and breast-feeding for controversy, it is the theory linking peanut allergy with vaccination. Heather Fraser, a Canadian historian, author, and mother of a child with peanut allergy, explores this theory, carefully tracing the emergence of peanut allergy and assessing the various explanations for its recent proliferation.[119] Fraser argues that most hypotheses, ranging from hygiene to helminths, do not adequately explain the sudden rise in peanut allergy during the 1990s. The timing simply does not fit. What does coincide closer with the emergence of the peanut allergy epidemic, according to Fraser, is the rapid uptake of certain vaccines that use peanut oil as an adjuvant to prolong its effectiveness.

Fraser explains that after the Second World War, peanut oil replaced cottonseed oil (another potent allergen) as an adjuvant in penicillin. The peanut oil coated the penicillin, which was already combined with beeswax, allowing it to be released more slowly into the bloodstream.[120] Although Fraser speculates that some people acquired peanut allergy after being prescribed penicillin, the condition remained rare. A further development occurred in 1964, when the pharmaceutical giant Merck announced in the *New York Times* that it would begin using a new peanut oil adjuvant (Adjuvant 65) in a series of vaccines it was producing. Adjuvant 65 would not only produce the same gradual release as in penicillin but also stimulate the production of antibodies.[121] Again, an epidemic of peanut allergy did not occur, although Fraser claims that doctors did notice more children with peanut allergies.[122] There was concern then about the safety of such adjuvants and their propensity to induce hypersensitivity and other conditions in patients, resulting in a number of lawsuits. Although Adjuvant 65 was approved for use in the United Kingdom, it failed to get approval in the United States and was not used during the late 1970s or the 1980s. With more lawsuits being launched during the 1980s and many pharmaceutical companies abandoning the production of vaccines altogether, President Reagan signed the National Childhood Vaccine Injury Act in 1986, which made vaccination litigation more difficult. With the act in place, pharmaceutical companies could revisit the idea of making vaccines, but they did so more secretively, not heralding grand announcements in the *New York Times* about the ingredients found in their products. Parents and patients were left in the dark.

Then, during the early 1990s, alongside the proliferation of peanut allergy, a number of developments occurred that spurred vaccine production. In an attempt to boost the take-up of vaccines in preschool-aged children, which had fallen to approximately 60 percent, the first Bush administration announced its goal of raising national vaccination levels in preschoolers to 90 percent by 2000.[123] Among the new vaccines developed to achieve this aim were ones for *Haemoiphilus influenzae* type b (Hib). The Hib vaccine was combined with others to provide a conjugate vaccine covering a number of other infections in order to make vaccination more efficient. The new vaccines proved to be popular not only in the United States but also Canada, Great Britain, and other Western countries. But did they contain peanut oil? By law concerning trade secrets, American, Canadian, and British manufacturers do not have to disclose such information. Moreover, there is also the possibility that Hib proteins, combined with those found in other vaccines, could trigger sensitivity to Hib. Since Hib and peanut protein molecules are roughly the same size, there is a potential for cross-reactivity: in other words, antibodies reacting to Hib might also respond to peanut. Other peanut allergy–inducing examples of cross-reactivity are possible as well. Although many questions remain unanswered, the bottom line for Fraser is that there is a connection between vaccine use and the rise of peanut allergy, one that requires much more investigation.[124]

Fraser's thoughtful, meticulous study, unlike many polemical, paranoid anti-vaccination manifestos, is provocative and compelling. By implicating vaccines, it brings allergy full circle, back to Clemens von Pirquet's initial investigations of serum sickness. But it also pokes a hypodermic needle into venerable debates about vaccination, which have recently escalated due to Andrew Wakefield's hypothesis about the link between mumps, measles, and rubella (MMR) vaccination and autism. Fearing that MMR could cause autism, thousands of parents shy away from the vaccine, resulting in measles outbreaks in places such as South Wales in 2013 and Ohio in 2014. Although many in the medical profession reject Wakefield's theory, a quick stroll through the Internet indicates that such anti-vaccination theories remain popular on the fringes of medicine. Moreover, there is some speculation about the relationship between autism and gastrointestinal problems, including allergy.[125] But instead of taking on Fraser headfirst, allergists have chosen to ignore her, possibly because she is not a physician and certainly because it involves vaccination, a topic so toxic that no sensible researcher dares tackle it.[126] When asked a question about whether peanut antigen could be found in vaccines, a spokesperson for the AAAAI (which at least published an answer on its Web site) merely stated:

> The issue of peanut antigen in vaccines, at least according to my assessment of the reading material available, is similar to the issue of adverse effects of mercury in vaccines. It seems to be fueled by consumer message boards and consumer-oriented websites. These websites and consumer message boards, as best I can tell, claim that small amounts of peanut allergen contaminate vaccines and are not listed as an ingredient in the package insert. I personally have not been able to find any confirmation in the medical literature of contamination of vaccines by peanut antigen.[127]

What this statement suggests is that there is probably nothing to it . . . the people discussing it are cranks . . . and if no serious scientist is researching it, it is likely nothing to worry about. For an organization that has dedicated so much time, money, and effort to raising awareness about peanut allergy, one would think the AAAAI might be slightly more curious.

●●●

APPROXIMATELY ONE HUNDRED YEARS after the London physician Alfred T. Schofield described using pills containing small amounts of egg to desensitize his patients to egg allergy in 1908, trials began in Cambridge to attempt to desensitize children with severe peanut allergy. For most of the century between Schofield's reported successes and the Cambridge experiments, food allergists shied away from desensitization, partly because it did not appear to be particularly effective but also because it was dangerous. By employing twenty-first-century technology and by using antihistamines and adrenaline in order to suppress the children's immune systems, the Cambridge researchers could desensitize their subjects using oral immunotherapy (OIT), beginning with infinitesimally small amounts of peanut protein (5 mg). By the end of the trial, three out of the four patients could consume up to twelve peanuts without a reaction. They were then instructed to keep up a desensitization regimen at home in order to maintain their resistance.[128] Peanut butter sandwiches might not suddenly show up on the menu, but, if one of these children accidentally ingests a peanut, she would be less likely to go into severe anaphylaxis. Similar trials have been launched elsewhere to test OIT, as well as sublingual desensitization, in which a liquid peanut extract is placed under the tongue but not ingested. Although arguments are already beginning about which of these approaches is preferable, and although some caution that the research is in its early stages, it appears that hope is in sight for peanut allergy sufferers and their families.[129]

It is somewhat fitting that allergy researchers had to go back one hundred years in order to seek out a solution for peanut allergy. Considered to be "witchcraft, fad, or a racket" by most orthodox allergists, peanut allergy has pushed anaphylactic food allergy into the spotlight like never before. Frightening, bizarre, controversial, confounding, and ubiquitous: allergy to the humble peanut forces physicians, parents, educators, politicians, and the food industry to reassess how far society should go to protect those vulnerable to rare, but very real, anaphylactic emergencies. Whether it be banning peanuts from places like Commonwealth Stadium, changing food production practices, or enrolling children in potentially fatal peanut desensitization trials, peanut allergy is deadly serious and should be treated as such. Fomenting both bottom–up and top–down pressure for increased awareness and prophylactic action, peanut allergy is a remarkable example of how societies have adapted rapidly and significantly to address the threats to health faced by a small, but vulnerable, group of people. Although such responses might correctly be described as excessive as an anaphylactic reaction itself, they provide hope to others striving to instill preventive measures in the interest of health. The willingness to ban peanuts from a huge, open-air stadium might be somewhat over the top, but it is also a humane, empathetic response to a potential threat.

All this attention, profile, and action, however, comes at a cost. For those suffering from chronic allergies, peanut allergy does little more than to reinforce the notion that their non-anaphylactic symptoms are illegitimate, mere intolerance at best, and psychosomatic at worst. Terms such as "lactose intolerance" and "gluten intolerant" may provide some patients with more authoritative terminology to describe their ailments, and one can now find gluten-free breads, cookies, cereals, and cakes at many food stores and bakeries. Nonetheless, such sufferers continue to be perceived somewhat suspiciously, as if their symptoms are somehow, indeed, all in their minds. It is much easier to dismiss the gastrointestinal complaints of a middle-aged woman than it is to question a child with a severe anaphylactic allergy to peanuts or one of the seven other recognized major food allergens. With peanut allergy, the long-stated desire of orthodox allergists to restrict the definition of food allergy has finally become a reality.

Conclusion

IN A PROVOCATIVE 1997 ARTICLE, the biophysicist Richard Cone and the anthropologist Emily Martin described how human bodies were increasingly in disharmony with the environment, resulting in epidemic levels of autoimmune disease, including not only allergy and asthma but also multiple sclerosis, arthritis, lupus erythematosus, and diabetes.[1] One of the reasons for this upsurge in immune pathology, according to the authors, had to do with diet. Unlike in the past, when most people were more likely to consume seasonal and local fruits and vegetables as well as a wider range of animal tissues, the modern diet, and especially that of the urban poor, consisted increasingly of a limited range of fats, sugars, and starches, often found in the form of processed foods produced in faraway places. One consequence of this change in diet was that people were less likely to come in contact with proteins that matched those found in the body and were essential for health. By not eating chicken stock prepared by boiling the entire chicken, including bones, tendons, and other tissues, for example, an individual's immune system would be less likely to recognize its own connective tissue and usher an immune response against it, otherwise known as arthritis. By not eating local honey, a person would have less exposure to harmless airborne proteins found in the local atmosphere, including pollens, dust, and molds, meaning that her immune system might react to such inhalants in the form of asthma or hay fever. Pesticides and preservatives exacerbated the problem by acting as adjuvants, tricking the immune system into thinking that a harmless food protein, such as lactose, was actually toxic and required an immune response.

In the two decades since Cone and Martin's article was published, it has been regularly cited and reproduced in science studies literature but has been completely ignored by medical scientists. To a degree, this is not be particularly surprising. Although it cited a number of contemporary scientific studies and was published in a respected journal, the article was largely speculative, acknowledging that more research was required to prove such theories. But viewed in another way, the lack of medical interest, in addition to the paucity of research done to test other theories to explain the rise of allergy and other immune dysfunctions, is depressing, and thus highlights a fundamental problem in how chronic conditions such as these have been explored by at least the mainstream medical community. Specifically, rather than thinking imaginatively or creatively about such diseases, their causes, and what they might denote about our changing relationship with our foods, the environment, or our lifestyles, most clinicians and researchers, especially in the case of food allergy, have expended their energies on defending restrictive dogmas and debating about precise definitions. Worse, this lack of curiosity has flourished not because one theory has been masterful in answering all the questions asked of it but because of the economic and political concerns of allergists—at the expense of patients' health. Rather than contemplating that rising rates of food allergy might be related to changes in Western diets, orthodox allergists continually narrowed the scope of their interest until food allergy was effectively limited to allergies to peanuts and a handful of other foods. Instead of treating patients' accounts at face value, allergists depended on unreliable skin tests and dismissed their symptoms as hypochondriasis if the tests revealed nothing. Likewise, for every Theron Randolph or Albert Rowe meticulously recording the results of elimination diets, there were unscrupulous physicians willing to take advantage of new technologies and immunological theories to sell patients dubious mail-order allergy tests. Unwilling to acknowledge that the link between allergy and mental disturbance might flow in both directions, clinicians either deemed patients to be suffering psychosomatically or, in contrast, failed to recognize that stressful situations could exacerbate an allergic reaction. While there were notable exceptions—A. W. Frankland and Ben Feingold spring to mind—allergists for the most part were polarized by food allergy, resulting in an diminished understanding of what the condition meant, let alone how best to prevent or treat it.

Faced by the epistemological vacuum formed by this stalemate, people who suspect that their chronic health problems are caused by the food that they eat have turned elsewhere, away from allergy. Whether it be the "free-from" aisle at a traditional supermarket or the health-conscious organic alternatives, such as Trader Joe's and Whole Foods Market, the alternative food industry has capitalized on such health concerns, as have a wide range of lay nutritionists, offering dietary advice along with expensive specialty foods.[2] Although there is nothing inherently wrong with people taking ownership over their diets, and although self-medicating using food has been and continues to be central to health practices in countless medical traditions, there remains the risk that many individuals are being exploited, spending too much on hypoallergenic or "free-from" foods that do little to address their specific health problems.[3] Beyond this, however, is the more fundamental problem of the growing nutritional knowledge gap, fueled by growing cynicism about food advice and the food industry. As the food expert Gyorgy Scrinis argues, the politics of nutrition advice during the postwar period resulted in not only unhelpful dietary advice but also ideologically driven schisms about basic nutritional questions: Are all calories created equal? Are there good fats and bad fats? Are some sugars worse for you than others? Should we take vitamins? Are there such things as cancer-fighting foods?[4] Of course the food industry itself has long played and continues to play a tremendous role in influencing the answers to these questions, but with the rise of so many chronic conditions with certain or presumed links to food consumption (obesity, cancer, heart disease, diabetes, and autoimmune diseases, just to name a few), it is also incumbent on national and international health institutions to work harder to resolve such debates in a more constructive and unbiased fashion. The divisions within allergy about food allergy are, in many ways, writ large in the science of food and nutrition more generally.

The seemingly intractable situation in allergy is also reminiscent of another medical field, that of psychiatry, which has similarly suffered from ideological rigidity, internecine debates, and crises of legitimacy. Just as allergy has struggled to explain why some people are allergic and why rates of allergy appear to be increasing, psychiatrists have lurched from one paradigm to the other, each explanation ultimately proving unsatisfactory.[5]

Psychoanalytical theories have vied with genetic, organic, and social hypotheses, with scant appetite for negotiation, compromise, or even the basic recognition that human behavior is complicated and predicated on a wide range of factors.[6] For psychiatry, as with allergy, defining the very subject at hand has been central to these disputes. The rise of peanut allergy has contributed to narrowing the definition of food allergy in a way that suits orthodox allergy, the food industry, and pharmaceutical companies. In addition, the mass-marketing of mental disorder and psychiatric drugs has paradoxically widened the scope of what is considered to be mental illness, so much so that WHO reckons that depression will soon become the biggest threat to the world's health, outpacing both cancer and heart disease. In both cases, however, sophisticated understandings of what mental illness and food allergy actually are, how best to define them, and why they appear to be increasing have proved to be frustratingly elusive. While psychiatrists might at least point hopefully to some strands of DNA or the images from a brain scan, allergists have chosen instead to avoid such issues as much as possible.

There is the argument that pluralistic, nuanced conceptualizations of disease undermine the efficient and inexpensive treatment of patients. Sorting the genetic aspects of a child's hyperactivity from the nutritional, environmental, and psychological aspects is much more difficult than simply prescribing some Ritalin®. Dismissing a patient's symptoms as psychosomatic because those symptoms cannot be linked incontrovertibly to a food allergen by use of a skin test is also much easier than engaging that patient openly and honestly about diet and its possible relationship to chronic health problems. But such approaches do little to add to our deeper understanding of such conditions and, in the long run, are not in the best interest of patients or the potential patients of the future. Research into peanut allergy desensitization is eminently sensible, but surely as much effort should be put into exploring the escalation of such allergies in recent decades, no matter how uncomfortable the answers are. It could well be that, as with psychiatry, the answers are multifaceted, complicated, and troubling, but such is the case with most riddles in medicine. The ultimate goal of medicine is to prevent illness. This is what is truly in the best interest of patients and health-care systems; both psychiatrists and allergists need to renew their efforts to stem the tide of burgeoning mental illness and allergic disease with proactive measures rather than focusing disproportionately on treatment.

There is also, necessarily, a role for history in all of this. In setting out to write this book, I have not attempted to resolve the debates about food allergy or, even more foolishly, explain why allergies to foods such as peanuts are on the increase. This is not what I am trained to do. What I am trained to do as a historian is to analyze why allergists have struggled to answer these questions and to make suggestions, based on the available historical evidence and through the process of looking at the evidence from a wide range of perspectives, about how they might approach such problems differently in the future—a little bit like a management consultant but without the exorbitant salary. If there are any lessons for allergists in this book, they are the same as I have offered to psychiatrists, often for similar reasons. Food allergy, much like mental illness, is a perplexing, alarming, and deeply personal condition, as the observations of insightful physicians dating back to Hippocrates and Galen suggest. And food allergy should be understood as such, not as a neat, precise concept easily defined and described but as an amorphous and complex phenomenon, or set of phenomena, that has and will continue to change over time.[7] It takes creativity, imagination, and open-mindedness to see food allergy in this way, qualities that are not always engendered in either medical education or health-care economies. Nonetheless, if the riddle posed by food allergy is to be solved, it will be attributes such as these that will be most important.

Notes

INTRODUCTION

1. "City Offers Tips," *Edmonton (Alberta) Journal*, August 23, 2009.
2. "Banning Nuts at a Local Stadium?" June 5, 2006, Parenting a Child with a Food Allergy, http://www.childfoodallergy.com/archives/2006/06/banning_nuts_at.html (accessed March 10, 2012).
3. American College of Allergy, Asthma and Immunology, "Food Allergies," http://www.acaai.org/allergist/allergies/Types/food-allergies/Pages/default.aspx (accessed March 7, 2012); National Institute of Allergy and Infectious Diseases, "Report of the Expert Panel on Food Allergy Research," June 30 and July 1, 2003, http://www.niaid.nih.gov/about/organization/dait/documents/june30_2003.pdf (accessed March 1, 2012).
4. American Academy of Allergy, Asthma and Immunology, "Allergy Statistics," http://www.aaaai.org/about-the-aaaai/newsroom/allergy-statistics.aspx#Food_Allergy (accessed March 4, 2012).
5. Amy M. Branum and Susan L. Lukacs, "Food Allergy Among U.S. Children: Trends in Prevalence and Hospitalizations," National Center for Health Statistics Data Brief, no. 10 (2008), http://www.cdc.gov/nchs/data/databriefs/db10.pdf (accessed March 1, 2012).
6. AAAAI, "Allergy Statistics."
7. Quoted in "City Offers Tips." The AC/DC fan's story may seem far-fetched, but near-fatal anaphylaxis triggered by the inhalation of peanuts on airplanes is not unknown. In a recent case, four-year-old Fae Platten became anaphylactic and lost consciousness on a Ryanair flight from the Canary Islands to London when

a passenger sitting four rows away ignored repeated warnings by the cabin crew not to eat peanuts. Fortunately, a paramedic on board was able to inject Fae with adrenaline, and she soon recovered in the hospital. While the offending passenger was banned from flying with Ryanair for two years, Fae is now afraid to fly and has asked her parents never to take her on an airplane again. See "Selfish Flyer Almost Kills Nut Allergy Girl on Plane," *Metro*, August 15, 2014, 7.

8. Quoted in "City Offers Tips."

9. "Give me some peanuts and Cracker Jack. / I don't care if I never get back" ("Take Me Out to the Ball Game" [Jack Norworth and Albert Von Tilzer, 1908]). For more on the history and influence of Cracker Jack, see Andrew F. Smith, *Eating History: 30 Turning Points in the Making of American Cuisine* (New York: Columbia University Press, 2009), 123–30.

10. "Indians Peanut Aware Zone," Major League Baseball, http://mlb.mlb.com/cle/ticketing/super_groups.jsp?group=faan (accessed March 1, 2012).

11. Andrew Ryan, "Cheers from the (No) Peanut Gallery," June 12, 2011, Boston.com, http://articles.boston.com/2011-06-12/lifestyle/29650482_1_peanut-allergy-cracker-jack-fenway-park (accessed March 1, 2012).

12. "NY Lawsuit Says Airline Endangered Child with Peanut Allergy," June 3, 2008, eTN: Global Travel Industry News, http://www.eturbonews.com/2823/ny-lawsuit-says-airline-endangered-child-pean (accessed March 1, 2012).

13. Russ Bynum, "Peanut Ban on Airplanes? FAA Considers Nut Ban on Airlines Because of Allergy," *Huffington Post*, June 12, 2010, http://www.huffingtonpost.com/2010/06/12/peanut-ban-on-airplaines-_n_610247.html (accessed March 1, 2012).

14. Paul Waldie, "Air Canada Told to Provide Nut-Free Zones," *Globe and Mail* (Toronto), January 7, 2010; Dave McGinn, "Air Canada Told to Create Nut-Free Buffer Zones," *Globe and Mail*, October 19, 2010, http://www.theglobeandmail.com/life/the-hot-button/air-canada-told-to-create-nut-free-buffer-zones/article1764118/ (accessed March 1, 2012).

15. Quoted in Waldie, "Air Canada Told to Provide Nut-Free Zones" (emphasis in original).

16. "Edgewater Elementary School Parents Want Student Home Schooled over Peanut Allergy," *Huffington Post*, March 22, 2011, http://www.huffingtonpost.com/2011/03/22/peanut-allergy-edgewater-elementary-school_n_839091.html (accessed March 1, 2012).

17. Walter R. Kessler, "Food Allergy," *Pediatrics* 21 (1958): 523–24.

18. William G. Crook, Walton W. Harrison, and Stanley E. Crawford, "Allergy—The Unanswered Challenge in Pediatric Research, Education and Practice," *Pediatrics* 21 (1958): 649.

19. For some insights into the development of medical facts and the attainment of scientific expertise, see Ludwik Fleck, *Genesis and Development of a Scientific Fact*, trans. Frederick Bradley and Thaddeus J. Trenn (1935; Chicago: University of Chicago Press, 1979); Charles E. Rosenberg, *Explaining Epidemics and Other Stud-*

ies in the History of Medicine (Cambridge: Cambridge University Press, 1992); and Harry Collins and Trevor Pinch, *Dr. Golem: How to Think About Medicine* (Chicago: University of Chicago Press, 2005). Decreasing faith in medicine and the rise of patient consumerism has resulted in patient skepticism about medical knowledge, according to John C. Burnham, "The Decline of the Sick Role," *Social History of Medicine* 25 (2012): 761–76. Perhaps the most striking example of such patient doubt is the controversy in which thousands of parents during the late 1990s and early 2000s declined the uptake of the measles, mumps, and rubella (MMR) vaccine because of fears that it caused autism. Although a rampant measles epidemic occurring in Swansea, Wales, in 2013 is one repercussion of the decline in MMR vaccination, others have linked vaccinations to peanut allergy. See also Collins and Pinch, *Dr. Golem*, 180–204; and Heather Fraser, *The Peanut Allergy Epidemic: What's Causing It and How to Stop It* (New York: Skyhorse, 2011).

20. Steve Sturdy has written about the relationship between medical science and clinical practice, arguing that historians have often exaggerated the gulf between these two ways of looking at medicine, in "Looking for Trouble: Medical Science and Clinical Practice in the Historiography of Modern Medicine," *Social History of Medicine* 24 (2011): 739–59. While this might be true for some fields, it has not been the case in allergy.

21. Matthew Smith, "Psychiatry Limited: Hyperactivity and the Evolution of American Psychiatry," *Social History of Medicine* 21 (2008): 545–46, and *An Alternative History of Hyperactivity: Food Additives and the Feingold Diet* (New Brunswick, N.J.: Rutgers University Press, 2011), 15–35. See also Mark Jackson's description of John Freeman in *Allergy: The History of a Modern Malady* (London: Reaktion, 2006), 90–94.

22. Clemens von Pirquet, "Allergie," *Münchener Medizinische Wochenschrift* 30 (1906): 1457–58.

23. Mark S. Micale and Roy Porter, eds., *Discovering the History of Psychiatry* (Oxford: Oxford University Press, 1994).

24. Warwick Anderson, Myles Jackson, and Barbara Gutmann Rosenkrantz, "Toward an Unnatural History of Immunology," *Journal of the History of Biology* 27 (1994): 575–94; Emily Martin, *Flexible Bodies: Tracking Immunity in American Culture from the Days of Polio to the Age of AIDS* (Boston: Beacon Press, 1994); Alfred I. Tauber, *The Immune Self: Theory or Metaphor?* (Cambridge: Cambridge University Press, 1994); Richard A. Cone and Emily Martin, "Corporeal Flows: The Immune System, Global Economies of Food, and Implications for Health," *Ecologist* 27 (1997): 107–11; Kenton Kroker, "Immunity and Its Other: The Anaphylactic Selves of Charles Richet," *Studies in History and Philosophy of Biological and Biomedical Sciences* 34 (2003): 273–96; Ilana Löwy, "On Guinea Pigs, Dogs and Men: Anaphylaxis and the Study of Biological Individuality, 1902–1939," *Studies in History and Philosophy of Biological and Biomedical Sciences* 34 (2003): 399–423; Thomas Söderqvist, *Science as Autobiography: The Troubled Life of Niels Jerne*, trans. David Mel Paul (New Haven, Conn.: Yale University Press, 2003).

25. Niels Kaj Jerne, "Waiting for the End," *Cold Spring Harbor Symposium on Quantitative Biology* 32 (1967): 591–603.
26. Sheldon G. Cohen, "Preface to the Third Edition," in *Excerpts from Classics in Allergy*, 3rd ed., ed. Sheldon G. Cohen (Bethesda, Md.: National Institutes of Allergy and Infectious Diseases, 2012), vii.
27. Warren T. Vaughan, *Allergy: Strangest of All Maladies* (London: Hutchinson, 1942).
28. Jackson, *Allergy*, 23.
29. Mark Jackson, "'Allergy *con Amore*': Psychosomatic Medicine and the 'Asthmogenic Home' in the Mid-Twentieth Century," in *Health and the Modern Home*, ed. Mark Jackson (New York: Routledge, 2007), 153–74; Carla Keirns, "Better Than Nature: The Changing Treatment of Asthma and Hay Fever in the United States, 1910–1945," *Studies in History and Philosophy of Biological and Biomedical Sciences* 34 (2003): 511–31.
30. Gregg Mitman, "Natural History and the Clinic: The Regional Ecology of Allergy in America," *Studies in History and Philosophy of Biological and Biomedical Sciences* 34 (2003): 491–510, and *Breathing Space: How Allergies Shape Our Lives and Landscapes* (New Haven, Conn.: Yale University Press, 2007).
31. Mitman, *Breathing Space*, 52–129.
32. Jackson, *Allergy*, 103.
33. Mitman, *Breathing Space*, 253.
34. Michelle Murphy, *Sick Building Syndrome and the Problem of Uncertainty: Environmental Politics, Technoscience, and Women Workers* (Durham, N.C.: Duke University Press, 2006), 2.
35. Ibid., 107–9.
36. Ibid., 95–110.
37. Peter Radetsky, *Allergic to the Twentieth Century: The Explosion in Environmental Allergies—From Sick Buildings to Multiple Chemical Sensitivity* (Boston: Little, Brown, 1997); Steve Kroll-Smith and H. Hugh Floyd, *Bodies in Protest: Environmental Illness and the Struggle over Medical Knowledge* (New York: New York University Press, 1997).
38. Jackson, *Allergy*; Mark Jackson, *Asthma: The Biography* (Oxford: Oxford University Press, 2009).
39. For example, Mark Jackson, *The Borderland of Imbecility: Medicine, Society and the Fabrication of the Feeble Mind in Late Victorian and Edwardian England* (Manchester: Manchester University Press, 2000), and *The Age of Stress: Science and the Search for Stability* (Oxford: Oxford University Press, 2013).
40. To give but two examples, compare the progressivist approach of Edward Shorter, *A History of Psychiatry: From the Era of the Asylum to the Age of Prozac* (New York: Wiley, 1997), with the social constructivism of Andrew Scull, *Museums of Madness: The Social Organization of Insanity in Nineteenth-Century England* (London: Allen Lane, 1979).

41. Mark S. Micale, *Approaching Hysteria: Disease and its Interpretations* (Princeton, N.J.: Princeton University Press, 1995).
42. These terms reflect those used by allergists throughout the twentieth century. During the 1960s, the terminology becomes more confusing when many food allergists, such as Theron Randolph, defect from the field of allergy to become clinical ecologists.
43. For perspectives on the relationship between food and health, see Rachel Carson, *Silent Spring* (Boston: Houghton Mifflin, 1962); Joan Jacobs Brumberg, *Fasting Girls: The History of Anorexia Nervosa* (Cambridge, Mass.: Harvard University Press, 1989); Rima D. Apple, *Vitamania: Vitamins in American Culture* (New Brunswick, N.J.: Rutgers University Press, 1996); Cone and Martin, "Corporeal Flows"; Sheldon Krimsky, *Hormonal Chaos: The Scientific and Social Origins of the Environmental Endocrine Hypothesis* (Baltimore: Johns Hopkins University Press, 2000); David F. Smith and Jim Phillips, "Food Policy and Regulation: A Multiplicity of Actors and Experts," in *Food, Science, Policy and Regulation in the Twentieth Century*, ed. David F. Smith and Jim Phillips (London: Routledge, 2000), 1–16; Eric Schlosser, *Fast Food Nation: The Dark Side of the All-American Meal* (New York: Houghton Mifflin, 2001); Marion Nestle, *Food Politics: How the Food Industry Influences Nutrition and Health* (Berkeley: University of California Press, 2002); Warren J. Belasco, *Appetite for Change: How the Counterculture Took on the Food Industry*, 2nd ed. (Ithaca, N.Y.: Cornell University Press, 2007); Sander Gilman, *Fat: A Cultural History of Obesity* (Cambridge: Polity Press, 2008); and Nicholas D. Kristof, "Arsenic in Our Chicken?" *New York Times*, April 4, 2012, http://www.nytimes.com/2012/04/05/opinion/kristof-arsenic-in-our-chicken.html?_r=1&ref=global-home (accessed April 9, 2012).
44. Consider the story of Sweeny Todd, first made popular in the Victorian penny dreadfuls of the 1840s.
45. Smith and Phillips, "Food Policy and Regulation," 1.
46. Charles E. Rosenberg, "Pathologies of Progress: The Idea of Civilization at Risk," *Bulletin of the History of Medicine* 72 (1998): 714–30.

ONE. FOOD ALLERGY BEFORE ALLERGY

1. Clemens von Pirquet, "Allergie," *Münchener Medizinische Wochenschrift* 30 (1906): 1457–58.
2. Ida Macalpine and Richard Hunter, "The 'Insanity' of King George III: A Classic Case of Porphyria," *BMJ* 1 (1966): 65–71; J. W. Paulley, "The Death of Albert Prince Consort: The Case Against Typhoid Fever," *Quarterly Journal of Medicine* 86 (1993): 837–41; Helen Rappaport, *Magnificent Obsession: Victoria, Albert, and the Death that Changed the Monarchy* (New York: St. Martin's Press, 2012).
3. Piers D. Mitchell, "Retrospective Diagnosis and the Use of Historical Texts for Investigating Disease in the Past," *International Journal of Paleopathology* 1 (2011): 81–88.

---

4. David W. Oldbach et al., "A Mysterious Death," *NEJM* 338 (1998): 1764–69; Fernando Orrego and Carlos Quintana, "Darwin's Illness: A Final Diagnosis," *Notes and Records of the Royal Society* 22 (2007): 23–29.

5. Andrew Cunningham, "Identifying Disease in the Past: Cutting the Gordian Knot," *Asclepio* 54 (2002): 13–34; Mark Jackson, "Disease and Diversity in History," *Social History of Medicine* 15 (2002), 323–40; Kevin Siena, "Introduction," in *Sins of the Flesh: Responding to Sexual Disease in Early Modern Europe*, ed. Kevin Siena (Toronto: Centre for Reformation and Renaissance Studies, 2005), 12.

6. Ludwik Fleck, *Genesis and Development of a Scientific Fact*, trans. Frederick Bradley and Thaddeus J. Trenn (1935; Chicago: University of Chicago Press, 1979), 6; Ida Blom, *Medicine, Morality and Political Culture: Legislation and Venereal Disease* (Lund: Nordic Academic Press, 2012), 22.

7. Katherine Ott, *Fevered Lives: Tuberculosis in American Culture Since 1870* (Cambridge, Mass.: Harvard University Press, 1999).

8. Douglas Goldman et al., *Retrospective Diagnoses of Historical Figures as Viewed by Leading Contemporary Psychiatrists* (Bloomfield, N.J.: Schering, 1958), 4, 16.

9. Sami Timimi and Begum Maitra, "ADHD and Globalization," in *Rethinking ADHD: From Brain to Culture*, ed. Sami Timimi and Jonathan Leo (Basingstoke: Palgrave Macmillan, 2009), 203–4.

10. Michael Fitzgerald, *Autism and Creativity: Is There a Link Between Autism in Men and Exceptional Ability?* (New York: Routledge, 2004).

11. Matthew Smith, *Hyperactive: The Controversial History of ADHD: Food Additives and the Feingold Diet* (New Brunswick, N.J.: Rutgers University Press, 2011), 24.

12. Roy Porter and Mark S. Micale, "Introduction: Reflection on Psychiatry and Its Histories," in *Discovering the History of Psychiatry*, ed. Mark S. Micale and Roy Porter (Oxford: Oxford University Press, 1994), 5–6.

13. David Schuster, *Neurasthenic Nation: America's Search for Health, Happiness, and Comfort, 1869–1920* (New Brunswick, N.J.: Rutgers University Press, 2011); Mark S. Micale, *Approaching Hysteria: Disease and its Interpretations* (Princeton, N.J.: Princeton University Press, 1995).

14. Smith, *Hyperactive*, 150–76.

15. Mark Jackson, *Allergy: The History of a Modern Malady* (London: Reaktion, 2006), 10.

16. Ben F. Feingold, *Why Your Child Is Hyperactive* (New York: Random House, 1974), 13; "Dead Poets," an episode in *New Tricks*, BBC, October 8, 2012.

17. Jackson, *Allergy*, 214–15.

18. W. Storm Van Leeuwen, *Allergic Diseases: Diagnosis and Treatment of Asthma, Hay Fever, and Other Allergic Diseases* (Philadelphia: Lippincott, 1925), 10.

19. There are, however, numerous examples of other allergic diseases, including hypersensitivity to insect stings and asthma ("noisy breathing"), from ancient Chinese, Egyptian, and Babylonian sources, according to Sheldon G. Cohen, in *Excerpts from Classics in Allergy*, 3rd ed., ed. Sheldon G. Cohen (Bethesda, Md.: National Institutes of Allergy and Infectious Diseases, 2012), 2–6.

20. Frederic J. Simoons, *Eat Not This Flesh: Food Avoidances in the Old World* (1961; Westport, Conn.: Greenwood Press, 1981), 37–40; 116–17; Peter Farb and George Armelagos, *Consuming Passions: The Anthropology of Eating* (Boston: Houghton Mifflin, 1980), 124–25.

21. Classicists focusing on the history of ancient medicine have argued that classical medicine was more pluralistic than is often portrayed; in other words, there was more to classical medicine than just Hippocrates and Galen. See Philip J. van der Eijk, "Medicine and Health in the Graeco-Roman World," in *The Oxford Handbook of the History of Medicine*, ed. Mark Jackson (Oxford: Oxford University Press, 2012), 21–31. However, since this chapter is partly about how medicine has relied on established theories, such as those offered by Hippocrates and Galen, to explain clinical phenomenon, it is worthwhile to concentrate on them.

22. Vivienne Lo and Penelope Barrett, "Cooking Up Fine Remedies: On the Culinary Aesthetic in a Sixteenth-Century Chinese *Materia Medica*," *Medical History* 49 (2005): 395–422; Warren T. Vaughan, *Practice of Allergy*, 3rd ed. (London: Henry Kimpton, 1954), 271.

23. Elizabeth Craik, "Hippokratic Diaita," in *Food in Antiquity*, ed. John Wilkins, David Harvey, and Mike Dobson (Exeter: University of Exeter Press, 2003), 344–47.

24. Hippocrates, *Ancient Medicine*, Part 20, Perseus Project, http://perseus.uchicago.edu/cgi-bin/philologic/getobject.pl?p.196:29.GreekFeb2011 (accessed September 17, 2014).

25. Ibid.

26. Ibid.

27. Craik, "Hippokratic Diaita," 347.

28. Lucretius, *De Rerum Natura*, trans. Alban Dewes Winspear (New York: Russell, 1956), 162–63. There are many translations of *De Rerum Natura*; some, such as Winspear's, are set in verse, while others are translated in prose.

29. Lucretius, *On the Nature of the Universe*, trans. R. E. Latham, rev. John Godwin (1951; London: Penguin, 1994), 111.

30. Lucretius, *De Rerum Natura*, 163.

31. Alfred I. Tauber, *The Immune Self: Theory or Metaphor?* (Cambridge: Cambridge University Press, 1994), 7, 91–95. According to Tauber, Burnet's original notion of self and non-self was rooted in ecological principles, particularly the idea that stability was desirable in ecosystems, a concept that those in the clinical ecology movement would have found attractive.

32. Frank Macfarlane Burnet, *The Production of Antibodies* (Melbourne: Macmillan, 1941), 126.

33. R. E. Latham, "Introduction," in *On the Nature of the Universe*, by Lucretius, xv.

34. Lucretius, *De Rerum Natura*, 164.

35. Galen, *On the Properties of Foodstuffs*, trans. Owen Powell (Cambridge: Cambridge University Press, 2003), 30–31.

36. Mark Grant, *Galen on Food and Diet* (London: Routledge, 2000), 164.

37. "Is Asparagus Wholesome?" *Lancet* 167 (1906): 1405–6. One fascinating abuse of an idiosyncrasy to strawberries can be found in Sir Thomas More's *History of Richard III*. Knowing his susceptibility to the fruit, Richard III surreptitiously consumed "a messe of strauberies" from the Bishop of Elye, duly broke out into hives, and then blamed it on witchcraft orchestrated by one of his political opponents, Lord Hastings. Hastings was summarily beheaded. See Sir Thomas More, "Richard III: Statesmen, Strawberries, History and Hives," in *Excerpts from Classics in Allergy*, ed. Cohen, 44–45; and *More's History of Richard III*, ed. J. Rawson Lumby (Cambridge: Cambridge University Press, 1883), 46–47.

38. Sami L. Bahna and Douglas Heiner, *Allergies to Milk* (New York: Grune and Stratton, 1980), 1; Arne Høst and Sami L. Bahna, "Cow's Milk Allergy," in *Food Hypersensitivity and Adverse Reactions: A Practical Guide for Diagnosis and Management*, ed. Marianne Frieri and Brett Kettelhut (New York: Dekker, 1999), 99.

39. Vivian Nutton, "Galen and the Traveller's Fare," in *Food in Antiquity*, ed. Wilkins, Harvey, and Dobson, 366–67. Some have also suggested that the practice of the Roman emperor Constantius II (317–361) of avoiding fruit was due to an allergy. See David Rohrbacher, "Why Didn't Constantius II Eat Fruit?" *Classical Quarterly* 55 (2005): 323–26..

40. Nutton, "Galen and the Traveller's Fare," 366 (emphasis in original).

41. Ibid., 367.

42. Ibid.

43. The historian David Gentilcore has noted how the humoral qualities of many fruits and vegetables were questioned by Italians during the Renaissance, in *Pomodoro! A History of the Tomato in Italy* (New York: Columbia University Press, 2010), 27–28.

44. One old adage about fruit that remains popular is "fruit is gold in the morning, silver at noon, and lead at night" (*American Almanac and Repository of Useful Knowledge*, 2nd ed. [Boston: Bowen, 1833], 124; "A Word to the Non-Medical Public," *New York Times*, July 12, 1854).

45. Morton Satin, *Death in the Pot: The Impact of Food Poisoning in History* (New York: Prometheus Books, 2007). For a nineteenth-century account of the pathological effects of diseased meat, see Charles A. Cameron, *A Handy Book on Food and Diet in Health and Disease* (London: Cassell, Petter and Galpin, 1871), 52–53.

46. Occasionally, the word "antipathy" was used as a synonym for "idiosyncrasy," but usually in a looser sense. For instance, the seventeenth-century author Sir Thomas Browne described how he "had no Antipathy, or rather Idio-syncrasy, in Diet, Air, Humour, or any other Thing. I have not wondered at the French for their Dishes of Frogs, Snails, and Toadstools" (*Religio Medici* [1643; London: J. Torbuck, 1736], 152–53). Here, Browne appears to mean "repugnance" rather than a constitutional abnormality; his mentioning of the French and their diet indicates how such antipathies could be common to nations, as well as individuals.

47. While the word "idiosyncrasy" was commonly employed to describe an unusual aspect of a person's health, it was also used to describe an individual's character,

a way of thinking, and, quite often, the peculiarities of particular nations. Writers in the *Times* or the *Economist* often described some of the more frustrating habits of the Irish, Welsh, and French as idiosyncrasies: "We must never forget that the character of the Irishman is singular—full of idiosyncrasies. . . . He will never toil for anything he can dispense with; he will never do anything to-day, which he can possibly put off till to-morrow; and he will never do anything for himself which there is any likelihood of anyone else doing for him" ("Irish Prospects," *Economist*, October 31, 1846, 1417).

48. Avicenna, "Idiosyncrasies of Diet," in *Excerpts from Classics in Allergy*, ed. Cohen, 39.
49. Robert James, *A Medicinal Dictionary; Including Physic, Surgery, Anatomy, Chymistry, and Botany, in all their Branches Relative to Medicine* (London: T. Osborne, 1743), unnumbered page.
50. Ibid. (emphasis in original), referring to *The Whole Works of That Excellent Practical Physician, Dr. Thomas Sydenham*, trans. John Pechey, 9th ed. (London: J. Darby, 1729), 321.
51. James, *Medicinal Dictionary*.
52. Ibid.
53. William Cullen, *Lectures on the Materia Medica* (London: T. Lowndes, 1773), 20.
54. Ibid., 52–53, 148–49.
55. Samuel Ferris, *A Dissertation on Milk* (London: T. Cadell, 1785), 146–47.
56. John Hutchinson, *Pedigree of Disease: Six Lectures on Temperament, Idiosyncrasy and Diathesis* (London: Churchill, 1884), 22.
57. Ibid., 25.
58. Ibid., 35.
59. Ibid., 35–36.
60. J. C. Dodds, "Idiosyncrasy to Eggs," *JAMA* 16 (1891): 827.
61. The first researcher to do so appears to have been the French physiologist François Magendie (1783–1855), who seems to have induced a fatal anaphylaxis in a rabbit by injecting it with albumen, as he reported in *Lectures on the Blood* (Philadelphia: Haswell, Barrington, and Haswell, 1839), 248. See also Ana Maria Saavedra-Delgado, "François Magendie on Anaphylaxis (1839)," *Allergy Proceedings* 12 (1991): 355–56.
62. Rose Terry Cooke, "The Household," *Fort Worth Daily Gazette*, December 6, 1885, 6.
63. Hutchinson, *Pedigree of Disease*, 68. Although the term "idiosyncrasy" would be largely replaced by the word "allergy" in the twentieth century, it does pop up occasionally in the medical literature. For Humphrey Rolleston, "Idiosyncrasy may be defined as an abnormal reaction in an otherwise normal person, which may be either on the one hand greatly exaggerated or on the other hand greatly diminished; more briefly it may be described as an unusual physiological personal equation" (*Idiosyncrasies* [London: Kegan Paul, Trench, Trumpner, 1927], 11).
64. John Fothergill, "Remarks on That Complaint commonly known under the Name of the Sick Head-Ach," in *Medical Observations and Inquiries*, ed. Society of Physi-

cians of London (London: T. Cadell, 1784), 6:103; Edward Liveing, "Observations on Megrim or Sick-Headache," *BMJ* 588 (1872): 364. A number of other historical references to allergies of the nervous system can be found in Frederic Speer, "Historical Development of Allergy of the Nervous System," *Annals of Allergy* 16 (1958): 14–20.

65. Fothergill, "Remarks on That Complaint," 108. Ironically, Fothergill also states that chocolate, associated with migraine for most of the twentieth century, provided a breakfast alternative to butter and toast for those who suffered from sick headache. Gentilcore has noted how the Venetian botanist Pietro Antonio Michiel believed that tomatoes could cause "eye diseases and headaches" reminiscent of those associated with migraine (*Pomodoro!*, 12).

66. Fothergill, "Remarks on That Complaint," 110–14 (emphasis in original).

67. Ibid., 115–17.

68. Stephen Mennell, *All Manners of Food: Eating and Taste in England and France from the Middle Ages to the Present,* 2nd ed. (Urbana: University of Illinois Press, 1996).

69. Ken Albala, *Eating Right in the Renaissance* (Berkeley: University of California Press, 2003), 241–83.

70. George Cheyne, *The English Malady* (London: G. Strahan, 1733), viii.

71. John Sinclair, *The Code of Health and Longevity* (Edinburgh: Constable, 1807), 223.

72. Edward Jukes, *On Indigestion and Costiveness* (London: Effingham Wilson, 1831), 64–65. Given that peas are related to peanuts, Jukes's warning about peas is fascinating: "It is not infrequent for death to ensue in consequence of spasmodic affection of the stomach, induced by eating green peas either not sufficiently cooked, or not broken down by mastication." The "spasmodic affection of the stomach" does not resemble anaphylaxis exactly, but it does indicate the seriousness of some such reactions.

73. Mennell, *All Manners of Food,* 300–301. See also Jane Grigson, who suggests that leeks fell out of fashion in polite society for three hundred years because of their unfortunate effect on the breath and proclivity to cause flatulence, in *Jane Grigson's Vegetable Book* (London: Michael Joseph, 1978).

74. The nineteenth-century physician Edward Liveing commented on the objectivity of physicians who suffered from such headaches, claiming that "the statements of many trustworthy witnesses in this matter [meaning physicians] are of a much more qualified kind, and lend by a very hesitating support to the prevalent notions regarding the influences in question, of which the efficacy has no doubt been enormously overrated" (*On Megrim, Sick-Headache, and Some Allied Disorders* [London: Churchill, 1873], 45).

75. Ibid., 44.

76. Ibid., 229; K. Karbowski, "Samuel Auguste Tissot (1728–1797): His Research on Migraine," *Journal of Neurology* 233 (1986): 123–25.

77. Liveing, *On Megrim,* 6.

78. Ibid., 45, 241.

79. Charles Hinton Fagge and Philip Henry Pye-Smith, *The Principles and Practices of Medicine*, 2nd ed. (London: Churchill, 1888), 787.

80. Ibid., 788–90.

81. Offley Bohun Shore, *Domestic Medicine* (Edinburgh: Nimmo, 1866), 9. See also *Handbook of Domestic Medicine* (London: Bohn, 1855), 254.

82. Mark Jackson, *Asthma: The Biography* (Oxford: Oxford University Press, 2009), 33–55, 63–65; Moses Maimonides, "Treatise on Asthma," in *Excerpts from Classics in Allergy*, ed. Cohen, 54–55; John Floyer, *A Treatise of the Asthma* (London: Richard Wilkin, 1698), 90–99.

83. Jackson, *Asthma*, 33–34. The English physician Thomas Willis (1621–1675) believed that asthma could be triggered by "whatsoever therefore makes the blood to boyl, or raises it into an effervescence, as violent motion of the body or minde, excess of extern cold or heat, the drinking of Wine, Venerey, yea sometimes mere heat of the Bed doth cause asthmatical assaults to such as are predisoposed" (*Pharmaceutice Rationalis: or an Exercitation of the Operations of Medicine in Humane Bodies* [London: T. Dring, C. Harper and J. Leigh, 1679], 83).

84. Floyer, *Treatise of the Asthma*, 95–96.

85. Ibid., 98. More than two hundred years after the publication of Floyer's *Treatise*, a story appeared in a New York newspaper about a young Polish immigrant living in Newark, New Jersey, who had resorted to fasting, when all other attempts to cure her asthma had failed. In this instance, however, divine inspiration, rather than a rebalancing of the humors, was the intended goal of the fast. See "Girl Fasting to Cure Asthma," *New York Tribune*, October 7, 1904.

86. John Millar, *Observations on the Asthma and the Hooping Cough* (London: T. Cadel, 1769), 17, 41, 57, 73, 88; Thomas Withers, *A Treatise on the Asthma* (London: G. G. J. and J. Robinson and W. Richardson, 1786), 52, 101–6; Robert Bree, *A Practical Inquiry into Disordered Respiration* (Birmingham: Swinney and Hawkins, 1800), 144.

87. William Buchan, *Domestic Medicine* (Philadelphia: John Crukshank, Robert Bell, James Bell, 1790), 406–8.

88. Spencer Thomson, *A Dictionary of Domestic Medicine and Household Surgery* (London: Griffin, 1859), 43. Not all of Thomson's contemporaries believed that asthma's treatments were so various. The French scientist and politician François-Vincent Raspail (1794–1878) advocated the "constant inhalation of camphor through the cigarette" (*Domestic Medicine* [London: Weale, 1853], 49, 101). A whole range of cigarettes, burning everything from tobacco and lobelia to potash and stramonium, were recommended for the treatment of asthma between the late nineteenth and early twentieth centuries, as described in Mark Jackson, "'Divine Stramonium': The Rise and Fall of Smoking for Asthma," *Medical History* 54 (2010): 171–94.

89. Alex Sakula, "Henry Hyde Salter (1823–1871): A Biographical Sketch," *Thorax* 40 (1985): 887–88.

90. Henry Hyde Salter, *On Asthma: Its Pathology and Treatment* (London: Churchill, 1860).

91. Henry Hyde Salter, "On the Aetiology of Asthma," *BMJ* 132 (1859): 538.

92. Ibid.

93. Ibid., 539.

94. Ibid.

95. Ibid., 540.

96. Ibid. Salter noted elsewhere that "an observant and thoughtful physician once said to me that he considered dietetic treatment the *only* treatment of asthma" (*On Asthma*, 44 [emphasis in original]).

97. Ibid.

98. Ibid.

99. Henry Hyde Salter, "On Some Points in the Therapeutic and Clinical History of Asthma," *Lancet* 72 (1858): 223–25.

100. Ibid., 472 (emphasis in original).

101. Salter, *On Asthma*, 157.

102. Ibid., 156.

103. Ibid., 47.

104. William John Russell, *Domestic Medicine and Hygiene* (London: Everett. 1878), 262; J. Kost, *Domestic Medicine* (Cincinnati: Melick and Bunn, 1868), 100; Ralph Gooding, *A Manual of Domestic Medicine* (London: Virtue, 1867), 43; Louis Fischer, "Milk Idiosyncrasies in Children," *JAMA* 39 (1902): 247–49. With respect to "particular states of atmosphere," Gooding described how some of his patients would automatically suffer an attack if they slept in a particular room of their house. Other rooms caused no problems whatsoever.

105. Robert Willan described a man being so susceptible to crab that only the smell of crab soup could trigger his rash, in *On Cutaneous Diseases* (Philadelphia: Kimber and Conrad, 1809), 1:306–7. He also described how reactions to lobster and mussels could be fatal and that a colleague of his was "violently affected" by sweet almond, but not blanched almonds. See also William Tilbury Fox, *Atlas of Skin Diseases* (London: Churchill, 1877), 7.

106. Fox, *Atlas of Skin Diseases*, 6.

107. McCall Anderson, "A Lecture on Nettle-Rash," *BMJ* 1197 (1883): 1107–9.

108. Quoted in ibid., 1108.

109. Ibid., 1109.

110. Elsewhere, strawberries were singled out as being a particularly common cause of urticaria, especially when they were consumed in quantity during "strawberry season." See "The Strawberry Season and Its Lessons," *Lancet*, June 20, 1908, 1786.

111. Quoted in Anderson, "Lecture on Nettle-Rash," 1109.

112. Ibid. Anderson did allow that, in some cases, no cause for nettle rash could be found. In such obstinate situations, he recommended a visit to a spa or a change in occupation. Failing that, topical treatments, as simple as vinegar and water, could be used to ease the symptoms. They would not, Anderson cautioned, "cut short the disease."

113. For example, Rudolph L. Baer, "Correspondence," *Journal of Allergy* 27 (1956): 483–84; Louis Webb Hill, "Editorial: Atopic Dermatitis," *Journal of Allergy* 27 (1956): 480–82; and Louis Tuft, "Correspondence," *Journal of Allergy* 27 (1956): 293–94.

114. Stephen Mackenzie, "The Inaugural Address on the Advantages to Be Derived from the Study of Dermatology," *BMJ* 1830 (1896): 195.

115. Ibid., 196.

116. Quoted in W. Allan Jamieson, "A Discussion of Diet in the Etiology and Treatment of Diseases of the Skin," *BMJ* 1822 (1895), 1353.

117. Ibid., 1351.

118. Quoted in ibid., 1353.

119. Quoted in ibid.

120. The historian John Harley Warner has written about the gradual shift during the nineteenth century in the United States from stressing the specific aspects of disease and treatment to emphasizing the universal, in "From Specificity to Universalism in Medical Therapeutics: Transformation in Nineteenth-Century United States," in *Sickness and Health in America: Readings in the History of Medicine and Public Health*, ed. Judith Walzer Leavitt and Ronald S. Numbers, 3rd ed. (Madison: University of Wisconsin Press, 1997), 87–101. In other words, at this time, American physicians regarded disease as a phenomenon inextricably linked with an individual's constitution and predispositions. As such, physicians were compelled to learn a great deal about a patient's history, and treatment, accordingly, was very much individualized. By the 1880s and the development of germ theory and physiology, treatment was much more universal, catering to a particular disease rather than a specific individual. Although this transformation in thinking was undoubtedly beneficial in the treatment of many diseases, it was not necessarily helpful in the treatment of the chronic, intractable conditions associated with food idiosyncrasies.

TWO. ANAPHYLAXIS, ALLERGY, AND THE FOOD FACTOR IN DISEASE

1. Herb Kutchins and Stuart A. Kirk, *Making Us Crazy: DSM: The Psychiatric Bible and the Creation of Mental Disorders* (New York: Free Press, 1997).

2. R. D. Laing, *The Divided Self: An Existential Study in Sanity and Madness* (London: Tavistock, 1960); Angela Woods, *The Sublime Object of Psychiatry Schizophrenia in Clinical and Cultural Theory* (Oxford: Oxford University Press, 2011).

3. Of course, some disorders have also dropped out of *DSM* over the years, the most famous being homosexuality, which was officially considered a mental disorder by the APA until it was removed from *DSM-II* in 1973 (ego-dystonic homosexuality was removed in a revision of *DSM-III* in 1986).

4. Allan Young, *Harmony of Illusions: Inventing Post-Traumatic Stress Disorder* (Princeton, N.J.: Princeton University Press, 1995); Edward Shorter, *A History of Psychiatry: From the Era of the Asylum to the Age of Prozac* (New York: Wiley,

1997); David Healy, *The Antidepressant Era* (Cambridge, Mass.: Harvard University Press, 1997); Matthew Smith, *Hyperactive: The Controversial History of ADHD* (London: Reaktion, 2012).

5. World Health Organization, *Mental Health Atlas* (Geneva: World Health Organization, 2011).

6. Mark J. Tullman, "Overview of the Epidemiology, Diagnosis, and Disease Prevention Associated with Multiple Sclerosis," *American Journal of Managed Care* 19 (2013): S15–20; J. Burisch and P. Munkholm, "Inflammatory Bowel Disease Epidemiology," *Current Opinion in Gastroenterology* 29 (2013): 357–62.

7. Walter R. Kessler, "Food Allergy," *Pediatrics* 21 (1958): 523–25.

8. Ibid.

9. Jonathan Brostoff and Stephen J. Challacombe, "Preface to the Second Edition," in *Food Allergy and Intolerance*, 2nd ed. (London: Saunders, 2002), x.

10. Royal College of Physicians/British Nutrition Foundation, "A Report on Food Intolerance and Food Aversion," *Journal of the Royal College of Physicians* 18 (1984): 83–123.

11. Michael M. Marsh, "Intestinal Pathogenetic Correlates of Clinical Food Allergic Disorders," in *Food Allergy and Intolerance*, ed. Brostoff and Challacombe, 267.

12. Ibid.

13. Since the usage and meaning of the terms "anaphylaxis" and "allergy" fluctuated considerably during the first two decades of the twentieth century, I also use the more generic term "hypersensitivity" to describe when an immune system overreacts to a foreign substance.

14. Mark Jackson, *Allergy: The History of a Modern Malady* (London: Reaktion, 2006), 122.

15. P. G. H. Gell and R. R. A. Coombs, *Clinical Aspects of Immunology* (Oxford: Blackwell, 1963), 317; William E. Fickling and Duncan A. F. Robertson, "Immunologically Mediated Damage of the Gut," in *Food Allergy and Intolerance*, ed. Brostoff and Challacombe, 296–99; Jackson, *Allergy*, 122.

16. Fickling and Robertson, "Immunologically Mediated Damage of the Gut," 296–99; Jackson, *Allergy*, 124.

17. The origins of allergy and anaphylaxis, and specifically ideas about inflammation and "self-destruction," also have their roots in the work of many other investigators, going back decades before these terms were coined, as the historian Ohad Parnes convincingly demonstrates in "'Trouble from Within': Allergy, Autoimmunity, and Pathology in the First Half of the Twentieth Century," *Studies in History and Philosophy of Biological and Biomedical Sciences* 34 (2003): 425–34.

18. Charles Richet was something of a fin-de-siècle renaissance man, having interests in history, poetry, socialism, pacifism, aviation, and spiritualism, or to use his own words, "metapsychical phenomena," which was, among other things, the investigation of "the real nature of things." In the preface to a text on the subject, Richet claimed that science might be able to provide facts about scientific phenomena, such as gravity and conception, but it struggled to provide the under-

lying explanations for them. Writing in 1905, the year of Einstein's *annus mirabilis*, Richet ironically singled out physics as an area that failed to answer such searching "why" questions. Given that Richet is most famous for providing some of the theoretical groundwork for the understanding of allergy, a condition where underlying explanations have also been difficult to pin down, his interest in such questions is especially fascinating. See Charles Richet, "Preface," in *Metapsychical Phenomena*, by J. Maxwell (London: Duckworth, 1905), xv–xxii, and *Traites de métapsychique* (Paris: Librairie Félix Alcan, 1922); and Jacqueline Carroy, "Playing with Signatures: The Young Charles Richet," in *The Mind of Modernism: Medicine, Psychology, and the Cultural Arts in Europe and America, 1880–1940*, ed. Mark S. Micale (Stanford, Calif.: Stanford University Press, 2004), 217–49.

19. For some insights into von Pirquet's death, see Jackson, *Allergy*, 52–53; and Richard Wagner, *Clemens von Pirquet: His Life and Work* (Baltimore: Johns Hopkins University Press, 1968), 184–202.
20. G. Mario Rojido, "One Hundred Years of Anaphylaxis," *Allergología e immunología clínica* 16 (2001): 364–68.
21. Ilana Löwy, "On Guinea Pigs, Dogs and Men: Anaphylaxis and the Study of Biological Individuality, 1902–1939," *Studies in History and Philosophy of Biological and Biomedical Sciences* 34 (2003): 403; Paul Portier and Charles Richet, "De l'action anaphylactique de certains venins," *CR Société Biologie* 54 (1902): 170–72.
22. Löwy, "On Guinea Pigs, Dogs and Men," 403.
23. Ibid.; Charles Richet, "Nobel Prize Lecture," December 11, 1913, http://www.nobelprize.org/nobel_prizes/medicine/laureates/1913/richet-lecture.html (accessed July 8, 2013).
24. Löwy, "On Guinea Pigs, Dogs and Men," 404–5; Stephen R. Boden and A. Wesley Burks, "Anaphylaxis: A History with Emphasis on Food Allergy," *Immunological Reviews* 242 (2011): 247.
25. Löwy, "On Guinea Pigs, Dogs and Men," 418–20.
26. Richet, "Nobel Prize Lecture."
27. Ibid.
28. Löwy, "On Guinea Pigs, Dogs and Men," 401.
29. Charles Richet, "An Address on Ancient Humorism and Modern Humorism," *BMJ* 2596 (1910): 924.
30. Löwy, "On Guinea Pigs, Dogs and Men," 408.
31. Richet, "Nobel Prize Lecture." See also Charles Richet, *L'Anaphylaxie* (Paris: Librairie Félix Alcan, 1912), 124–27.
32. Other contemporary investigators, including the American physiologists Milton J. Rosenau (1869–1946) and John F. Anderson (1873–1958), also used foods to sensitize animals in laboratory investigations, hinting that such studies could lend insight to the work of clinicians: "If man can be sensitized in a similar way by the eating of certain proteid substances, may this not throw light upon those interesting and obscure cases, in which the eating of fish, sea food, and other articles of diet habitually cause sudden and sometimes serious symptoms?" ("A Review of

Anaphylaxis with Especial Reference to Immunity," *Journal of Infectious Diseases* 5 [1908]: 85–105).

33. Richet, "Nobel Prize Lecture." As Parnes has observed, Richet's ideas about humoral individuality resemble the notion of "individual psychology" developed by the Austrian psychiatrist Alfred Adler (1870–1937) and, specifically, his concept of "idiosyncratic neurosis" or "psychical hypersensitivity" ("'Trouble from Within,'" 435–36). Just as Richet was interested in understanding why individuals reacted differently to different foreign substances, Adler wanted "to understand the mechanisms that bring about an endless repertoire of neurotic states," particularly when an individual overreacted disproportionately to fairly innocuous situations.

34. Charles Richet, "Foreword," in *Alimentary Anaphylaxis (Gastro-intestinal Food Allergy)*, by Guy Laroche, Charles Richet Fils, and François Saint-Girons, trans. Mildred P. Rowe and Albert H. Rowe (Berkeley: University of California Press, 1930), 22.

35. See note 18. Richet's interest in the mind–body relationship also helps to explain his attraction to dogs as laboratory animals. The dog's "great intellectual development, the best of man's domesticated animals," made it the necessary "victim of physiological experiments" (Löwy, "On Guinea Pigs, Dogs and Men," 404). Lest one think that Richet callously sacrificed man's best friend to an anaphylactic demise, it should be pointed out that he named all his experimental dogs and could be quite "affected" when they died in the course of research.

36. Michael Worboys, *Spreading Germs: Disease Theories and Medical Practice in Britain, 1865–1900* (Cambridge: Cambridge University Press, 2000).

37. Ibid., 284; Löwy, "On Guinea Pigs, Dogs and Men," 419.

38. Otniel Dror, "The Affect of Experiment: The Turn to Emotions in Anglo-American Experiment," *Isis* 90 (1999): 205–37.

39. Ben F. Feingold et al., "Psychological Studies of Allergic Women: The Relation Between Skin Reactivity and Personality," *Psychosomatic Medicine* 24 (1962): 195–202; Mark Jackson, "'Allergy *con Amore*': Psychosomatic Medicine and the 'Asthmogenic Home' in the Mid-Twentieth Century," in *Health and the Modern Home*, ed. Mark Jackson (New York: Routledge, 2007), 153–74, and *The Age of Stress: Science and the Search for Stability* (Oxford: Oxford University Press, 2013).

40. Jackson, *Allergy*, 29–30; Löwy, "On Guinea Pigs, Dogs and Men," 410. See also Alexandre Besredka, *L'histoire d' une idée* (Paris: Masson, 1921); and Alfred I. Tauber, *The Immune Self: Theory or Metaphor?* (Cambridge: Cambridge University Press, 1994). The Nobel laureate Elie Metchnikoff is also remembered for believing that lactic acid bacteria could reduce the amount of toxic bacteria in the gut and subsequently prolong life, as proclaimed in *The Prolongation of Life: Optimistic Studies*, ed. P. Chalmers Mitchell (New York: Knickerbocker Press, 1908). Practicing what he preached, the Russian drank a glass of sour milk each day.

41. Jackson, *Allergy*, 30–31; Alexandre Besredka, *Anaphylaxis and Anti-Anaphylaxis and Their Experimental Foundations*, ed. S. Roodhouse Gloyne (London: Heinemann, 1919), 1–3.

42. Wagner, *Clemens von Pirquet*, 57.
43. Besredka, *Anaphylaxis and Anti-Anaphylaxis*, 1–2.
44. Arthur Silverstein, *A History of Immunology*, 2nd ed. (London: Elsevier/Academic Press, 2009), 188.
45. Jackson, *Allergy*, 74–76.
46. Alfred T. Schofield, "A Case of Egg Poisoning," *Lancet* 171 (1908): 716.
47. Jackson, *Allergy*, 56–95. See also Gregg Mitman, *Breathing Space: How Allergies Shape Our Lives and Landscapes* (New Haven, Conn.: Yale University Press, 2007), 56–62, and "Natural History and the Clinic: The Regional Ecology of Allergy in America," *Studies in History and Philosophy of Biological and Biomedical Sciences* 34 (2003): 491–503. The immunologist and historian Arthur Silverstein has suggested that the term "desensitization" is actually a "misnomer," since the procedure does not actually reduce the body's sensitivity to allergens but creates "blocking" antibodies, which neutralize the action of the antibodies that would trigger an allergic reaction. See Silverstein, *History of Immunology*, 189.
48. Löwy, "On Guinea Pigs, Dogs and Men" 411; Alexandre Besredka, "Du mécanisme de l'anaphylaxie vis-à-vis sérum de cheval," *Annales de l'Institute Pasteur* 4 (1908): 496–508.
49. Löwy, "On Guinea Pigs, Dogs and Man," 412.
50. For more on von Pirquet, see Jackson, *Allergy*, 10–11, 27–28, 33–44, 52–55.
51. Von Pirquet was also the Silliman lecturer at Yale University during the winter of 1921/1922. See Clemens Pirquet, *An Outline of the Pirquet System of Nutrition* (Philadelphia: Saunders, 1922), 7. Note that for this publication, von Pirquet deleted the "von" in his name, making his surname appear less Germanic.
52. Ibid., 37.
53. Ibid., 37–38.
54. Ibid., 38; Clemens von Pirquet, "Allergie," *Münchener Medizinische Wochenschrift* 30 (1906): 1457–58.
55. Quoted in Wagner, *Clemens von Pirquet*, 64.
56. Jackson, *Allergy*, 38; von Pirquet, "Allergie." Although von Pirquet included hypersensitivity to food as one of the most common clinical manifestations of allergy, he failed to discuss food allergy altogether in his work on developing a more efficient system of childhood nutrition, even though he mentioned other nutritional ailments. Sadly, for von Pirquet, the "Pirquet System of Nutrition" was not well received when it was published in the early 1920s. Instead, it "raised a storm of protest" and was largely "ridiculed," a reception that provides some insight into von Pirquet's unhappiness. Most controversial was von Pirquet's suggestion that the calorie should be replaced by another measure of food value, the "nem." Needless to say, the nem did not have the same success as von Pirquet's previous term. See von Pirquet, *Outline of the Pirquet System*; and Wagner, *Clemens von Pirquet*, 152–62.
57. Jackson, *Allergy*, 40.
58. Ibid. Ironically, Arthur F. Coca and Robert Cooke would further muddy the terminology waters by introducing their own term to the mix in 1923, that of " atopy," a

hereditary predisposition to certain types of allergic reactions, in "On the Classification of the Phenomena of Hypersensitiveness," *Journal of Immunology* 8 (1923):
163–82.

59. For example, eighty-two articles published from 1906 to 1926 with the word "anaphylaxis" in the title can be found on PubMed, compared with sixteen articles
discussing allergy. During the following ten years (1926–1936), thirty articles were
written on anaphylaxis and sixty-seven discussed allergy. When the specific topics of such articles are analyzed, it becomes evident that the use of the term "anaphylaxis" becomes increasingly precise as time goes on. Although not all articles
are listed on PubMed, those that are represented indicate a definite shift in terminology. See www.ncbi.nlm.nih.gov/pubmed.

60. So much so that researchers such as Besredka, Jules Bordet (1870–1961), and Émile
Roux (1853–1933) complained that the use of the term "anaphylaxis" had been ap-
plied "to symptoms that can lay no claim to it" (Roux, quoted in Kenton Kroker,
"Immunity and Its Other: The Anaphylactic Selves of Charles Richet," *Studies in
History and Philosophy of Biological and Biomedical Sciences* 34 [2003]: 285).

61. Jackson, *Allergy*, 78–9.

62. Swelling related to food allergy was not always restricted to the face, throat, and
chest. One fascinating account from 1929 described a woman whose buttocks,
thighs, left arm, and, especially, left foot swelled extraordinarily after she ate
strawberries, in one case, and watermelon, in the other. See H. A. Callis, "Food Allergy: Two Unusual Cases," *Journal of the National Medical Association* 22 (1930):
14–15.

63. J. C. Lindsay, "Food Anaphylaxis," *CMAJ* 16 (1926): 58.

64. Ibid.

65. Warren T. Vaughan, "Minor Allergy: Its Distribution, Clinical Aspects, and Significance," *Journal of Allergy* 5 (1935): 184–96. Vaughan and his distinction between
"fortunate" and "frank" sufferers of allergy are discussed in chapter 3.

66. Callis, "Food Allergy," 15.

67. Warren T. Vaughan, "Allergic Migraine," *JAMA* 88 (1927): 1383–86.

68. A. M. Kennedy, "A Note on Food Allergy," *BMJ* 3729 (1932): 1167–69.

69. Richet, "Nobel Prize Lecture."

70. Parnes, "'Trouble from Within,'" 439–49.

71. Frank Macfarlane Burnet, *The Production of Antibodies* (Melbourne: Macmillan,
1941), 126.

72. Richet, "Address on Ancient Humorism and Modern Humorism," 924.

73. By 1913, Richet had offered an evolutionary explanation for anaphylaxis, arguing
that the phenomenon actually served to benefit the species, rather than the individual. Anaphylaxis "was a mechanism by which the chemical integrity—the pu-
rity—of a species could be maintained against its potential corruption by micro-
bial invaders that threatened to transform its very identity" (Kroker, "Immunity
and Its Other," 274).

74. In addition to Richet's original speculations, some hypothetical evolutionary theories for such reactions have been posited in recent years: N. Bottini et al., "Malaria as a Possible Evolutionary Cause for Allergy," *Allergy* 54 (1999): 188–89; P. N. Le Souëf, J. Goldblatt, and N. R. Lynch, "Evolutionary Adaptation of Inflammatory Immune Responses in Human Beings," *Lancet* 356 (2000): 142–44; J. A. Jenkins, H. Breiteneder, and E. N. Mills, "Evolutionary Distance from Human Homologs Reflects Allergenicity of Animal Food Proteins," *JACI* 120 (2007): 1399–405; A. Daschner, C. Cuéllar, and M. Rodero, "The Anisakis Allergy Debate: Does an Evolutionary Approach Help?" *Trends in Parasitology* 28 (2012): 9–15; and T. A. Platts-Mills, "Allergy in Evolution," *Chemical Immunology and Allergy* 96 (2012): 1–6.

75. Jackson, *Allergy*, 43. Anne Marie Moulin has suggested that von Pirquet's all-encompassing definition did not endure, in *Le dernier langage de la médicine: Histoire de l'immunologie de Pasteur et Sida* (Paris: Presses Universitaires de France, 1991), 391. But in the minds of many food allergists and clinical ecologists, it certainly did.

76. Jackson, *Allergy*, 23. Such thinking was not restricted to food additives, but included the particulates found in polluted air, the chemicals present in modern homes and offices, and pesticides that leached into soil and the water supply. See Michelle Murphy, *Sick Building Syndrome and the Problem of Uncertainty: Environmental Politics, Technoscience, and Women Workers* (Durham, N.C.: Duke University Press, 2006); and Mitman, *Breathing Space*.

77. Jackson, *Allergy*, 23; Charles E. Rosenberg, "Pathologies of Progress: The Idea of Civilization at Risk," *Bulletin of the History of Medicine* 72 (1998): 714–30.

78. Richard Mackarness, *Not All in the Mind: How Unsuspected Food Allergy Can Affect Your Body AND Your Mind* (London: Pan Books, 1976).

79. One recent such example in Ossett, West Yorkshire, involved a black café owner who became annoyed when people entering her premises were surprised to see the color of her skin. She posted a note on her door: "If you are allergic to black people, don't come in" ("Ossett Café Owner 'Warns' Customers She Is Black," BBC News, July 10, 2013, http://www.bbc.co.uk/news/uk-england-leeds-23260860 [accessed July 18, 2013]).

80. "Francis Hare: Noted Physician Passes," *Brisbane Courier*, March 20, 1929.

81. Ibid. See also F. E. Hare, *The Cold-Bath Treatment of Typhoid Fever* (London: Macmillan, 1898).

82. Hare, *Cold-Bath Treatment of Typhoid Fever*, v–ix, 1–5.

83. Parnes, "'Trouble from Within,'" 432–33.

84. Francis Hare, *The Food Factor in Disease* (London: Longmans, Green, 1905), 1:3.

85. Francis Hare, *On Alcoholism: Its Clinical Aspects and Treatment* (London: Churchill, 1912).

86. Theron G. Randolph, *Environmental Medicine: Beginnings and Bibliographies of Clinical Ecology* (Fort Collins, Colo.: Clinical Ecology, 1987), 79–81.

87. Hare, *Cold-Bath Treatment of Typhoid Fever*, vii.

88. Arthur C. Coca, *Familial Nonreaginic Food-Allergy* (Springfield, Ill.: Thomas, 1943); Jackson, *Allergy*, 90–91; Matthew Smith, *An Alternative History of Hyperactivity: Food Additives, and the Feingold Diet* (New Brunswick, N.J.: Rutgers University Press, 2011), 15–35.

89. Hare also admitted later in the book that his theory of hyperpyraemia was based almost exclusively on circumstantial evidence. See Hare, *Food Factor in Disease*, 1:vi, 360–61; and Randolph, *Environmental Medicine*, 84.

90. Such low-carbohydrate, high-protein diets have a long and enduring history, most recently in the form of the Atkins diet (which is more than forty years old) and the South Beach diet.

91. Hare, *Food Factor in Disease*, 1:2.

92. Ibid. (emphasis in original).

93. Ibid., 3.

94. Ibid., 4.

95. Hare, *Food Factor in Disease*, 2:376.

96. Ibid., 213–14.

97. B. Raymond Hoobler, "Some Early Symptoms Suggesting Protein Sensitization in Infancy," *American Journal of Diseases of Children* 12 (1916): 129–35.

98. Randolph, *Environmental Medicine*, viii, 80, 191.

99. Hare, *Food Factor in Disease*, 2:86, 215, 360–64.

100. Ibid., 72, 368, 374.

101. Randolph, *Environmental Medicine*, viii, 89.

102. Hare, *Food Factor in Disease*, 2:407–8.

103. Ibid., 413.

104. Ibid., 430.

105. Ibid., 435, 436–37.

106. Ibid., 393.

107. For a recent endorsement of von Pirquet's definition, see Michelle Jamieson, "Imagining 'Reactivity': Allergy Within the History of Immunology," *Studies in History and Philosophy of Biological and Biomedical Sciences* 41 (2013): 356–66.

108. Wagner, *Clemens von Pirquet*, 56, 63.

109. Ibid., 56, 65.

110. Randolph, *Environmental Medicine*, 81–82.

THREE. STRANGEST OF ALL MALADIES

1. "Book Notices," *JAMA* 113 (1939): 446; Helen Morgan, *You Can't Eat That! A Manual and Recipe Book for Those Who Suffer Either Acutely or Mildly (and Perhaps Unconsciously) from Food Allergy* (New York: Harcourt, Brace, 1939), 3.

2. Morgan, *You Can't Eat That!*, 3; Donna St. George, "Helen Morgan Brooks, 85, a Poet and Teacher for Many Years," *Philadelphia Inquirer*, October 19, 1989, http://articles.philly.com/1989-10-19/news/26115824_1_poetry-collection-poems-family-and-love (accessed August 8, 2013).

3. Morgan, *You Can't Eat That!*, 5, 25.

4. Ibid., 4–6.

5. Ibid., 28.

6. Ibid., 5–6.

7. Ibid., 7.

8. Walter C. Alvarez, "Foreword," in *You Can't Eat That!*, by Helen Morgan, xv.

9. Morgan, *You Can't Eat That!*, 7.

10. Walter C. Alvarez, *Incurable Physician: An Autobiography* (Kingswood: World's Work, 1963), 64, 148. In addition to gastrointestinal troubles, Alvarez believed that his allergy to chicken triggered fatigue, nervous tension, and nightmares.

11. Ibid., 148; Walter C. Alvarez, *How to Help Your Doctor Help You When You Have Food Allergy* (New York: Harper, 1941); "Puzzling Nervous Storms Due to Food Allergy," *Gastroenterology* 7 (1946): 241–52; and "The Production of Food Allergy," *Gastroenterology* 30 (1956): 325–26.

12. Myra May Hass, *Recipes and Menus for Allergics: A Cookbook for the Harassed Housekeeper* (New York: Dodd, Mead, 1939); Warren T. Vaughan, *Allergy: Strangest of All Maladies* (London: Hutchinson, 1942); Albert H. Rowe and Albert H. Rowe Jr., *Food Allergy: Its Manifestations and Control and the Elimination Diets, a Compendium with Important Consideration of Inhalant (Especially Pollen), Drug, and Infectant Allergy* (1931; Springfield, Ill.: Thomas, 1972); Albert H. Rowe, *Clinical Allergy Due to Foods, Inhalants, Contactants, Fungi, Bacteria and Other Causes* (London: Baillière, 1937), and *Elimination Diets and the Patient's Allergies: A Handbook of Allergy* (London: Kimpton, 1941).

13. John Harvey Kellogg's interest in food allergy seems to have flowed neatly from his other nutritionally based health advice and theories, as presented in, for example, "Good Health Question Box," *Evening Public Ledger* (Philadelphia), November 16, 1917. Following a successful career writing health advice books and nationally syndicated medical columns, Leonard Hirshberg was convicted of defrauding investors of approximately $1 million in an investment scam. See "Dr. Hirshberg Gets 4 Years in Prison, " *New York Times*, May 12, 1923; and Leonard Keene Hirshberg, "Beauty, Only Skin Deep, Is Divine Stamp of Health, That Needs Preservation," *Washington Times*, May 24, 1915; "Why You Eat Some Foods with Pleasure and Are Unable to Enjoy Others," *Washington Times*, May 31, 1916; and "Nature Provides Means to Conquer Bacteria and All Their Poisons," *Washington Times*, August 7, 1916. Of course, less sensational health columnists who wrote about food allergy can also be found. See, for example, "Notes and Gleanings," *New York Times*, July 13, 1913; William Brady, "Health Talk: Eczema," *Ogden (Utah) Standard*, March 17, 1917; Uncle Sam, M.D., "Health: Hay Fever, Asthma, Hives, Etc.," *Ogden Standard*, August 10, 1920; and "Causes of Asthma," *Times* (London), January 16, 1929.

14. C. R. Schroeder, "Cow's Milk Protein Hypersensitivity in a Walrus," *Journal of the American Veterinary Medical Association* 83 (1933): 810–15. Food allergy in dogs is discussed in R. Povar, "Food Allergy in Dogs (A Preliminary Report)," *Journal of the American Veterinary Medical Association* 111 (1947): 61–63.

15. Alvarez, *How to Help Your Doctor*, 50; Morgan, *You Can't Eat That!*, 7.

16. Morgan, *You Can't Eat That!*, 7.

17. Ralston Purina helped write some of the recipes in another allergy handbook, this time aimed at general practitioners. See Samuel Feinberg, *Allergy in General Practice* (London: Kimpton, 1934), viii.

18. Ibid., 56–57.

19. Alvarez, *How to Help Your Doctor*, 40.

20. Ibid., 43.

21. Will C. Spain, review of *Food Allergy*, by Herbert J. Rinkel, Theron G. Randolph, and Michael Zeller, *Quarterly Review of Biology* 28 (1953): 97–98.

22. Ibid., 97.

23. Ibid., 98.

24. Another common form of allergy testing was conjunctival testing, which was done by dropping a small amount of allergen into the eye of the patient. This form of testing for allergies is still employed, but is typically restricted to allergies affecting the eyes that cannot be identified using skin tests.

25. Mark Jackson, *Allergy: The History of a Modern Malady* (London: Reaktion, 2006), 42, 46–47.

26. Today, patch tests are also used, in addition to prick-puncture and intradermal tests (traditional scratch tests are not used because they are quite painful and believed to be unreliable). Since skin testing for food allergies remains an inaccurate science, often all three tests are used in diagnosis. See Francis J. Waickman, "Food Allergy/ Sensitivity Diagnosed by Skin Testing," in *Food Allergy and Intolerance*, ed. Jonathan Brostoff and Stephen J. Challacombe, 2nd ed. (London: Saunders, 2002), 831–36.

27. George Frederick Laidlaw, *The Treatment of Hayfever by Rosin-Weed, Ichtyhyol and Faradic Electricity, with a Discussion of the Old Theory of Gout and the New Theory of Anaphylaxis* (New York: Boericke & Runyon, 1917), 119. Some early references to such testing include Oscar M. Schloss, "A Case of Allergy to Common Foods," *American Journal of Diseases of Children* 3 (1912): 341–62; "Eczema and Protein Hypersensitiveness," *JAMA* 67 (1916): 207; Fritz B. Talbot, "Asthma in Children II: Its Relation to Anaphylaxis," *Boston Medical and Surgical Journal* 175 (1916): 191–95, and "The Relation of Food Idiosyncrasies to the Diseases of Childhood," *Boston Medical and Surgical Journal* 179 (1918): 285–88.; and P. Wodehouse, "Preparation of Vegetable Food Proteins for Anaphylactic Tests," *Boston Medical and Surgical Journal* 175 (1916): 195–96.

28. Laidlaw, *Treatment of Hay Fever*, 120 (emphasis in original).

29. Arthur F. Hurst, "An Address on Asthma," *Lancet* 197 (1921): 1113–17.

30. W. Ray Shannon, "Neuropathic Manifestations in Infants and Children as a Result of Anaphylactic Reaction to Foods Contained in Their Dietary," *American Journal of Disease of Children* 24 (1922): 89–94; George Piness and Hyman Miller, "Allergic Manifestations in Infancy and Childhood," *Archives of Pediatrics* 42 (1925): 557–62; Hyman Miller, George Piness, and Willard F. Small, "Allergic Eczema of Infancy

and Childhood: Application of Skin Testing," *California and Western Medicine* 54 (1941): 267–69.

31. Arthur Latham, "An Address on Some Aspects of Bronchial Asthma," *Lancet* 199 (1922): 261–63.

32. John H. Stokes, quoted in Howard Fox and J. Edgar Fisher, "Protein Sensitization in Eczema of Adults," *JAMA* 75 (1920): 910.

33. I was subjected to the full range of allergy skin testing during the early 1980s, when I was about eight years old. It was not pleasant. The result? Mild allergies to dust and mold, left untreated.

34. Warren T. Vaughan, *Practice of Allergy*, 3rd ed. (London: Kimpton, 1954), 276.

35. A. W. Frankland, "Allergy: Immunity Gone Wrong," *Proceedings of the Royal Society of Medicine* 66 (1972): 3. As of 2014, Frankland is still alive and practicing, and was kind enough to be interviewed for this book.

36. A. W. Frankland and R. S. H. Pumfrey, "Acute Allergic Reactions to Foods and Crossreactivity Between Foods," in *Food Allergy and Intolerance*, ed. Brostoff and Challacombe, 416.

37. Waickman, "Food Allergy/Sensitivity," 831, 834.

38. Frederic Speer added that similar confusion and debate had been what spurred Clemens von Pirquet to coin the term "allergy" in the first place, in "What Is Allergy?" *Annals of Allergy* 34 (1975): 49–50.

39. Ibid., 50.

40. G. H. Oriel, *Allergy* (London: Bale and Danielsson, 1932), 55; Feinberg, *Allergy in General Practice*, 112, 275.

41. Rowe and Rowe, *Food Allergy*, vii; quoted in Theron G. Randolph, *Environmental Medicine: Beginnings and Bibliographies of Clinical Ecology* (Fort Collins, Colo.: Clinical Ecology, 1987), 28.

42. Rowe, *Elimination Diets and the Patient's Allergies*. For an example of the often ambivalent manner in which Rowe diets were perceived, see Alice D. Friedman, "Management with the Elimination Diet," in *Introduction to Clinical Allergy*, by Ben F. Feingold (Springfield, Ill: Thomas, 1973), 162–70.

43. Randolph, *Environmental Medicine*, 19.

44. Ibid.

45. Ibid., 20.

46. Spain, review of *Food Allergy*, 98.

47. Herbert J. Rinkel, Theron G. Randolph, and Michael Zeller, *Food Allergy* (Springfield, Ill.: Thomas, 1951), 144–45.

48. Ibid., 146.

49. Vaughan, *Practice of Allergy*, 275.

50. Ibid., 272, 275–76.

51. William B. Sherman, "Presidential Address," *Journal of Allergy* 29 (1958): 274–76; Max Samter, "Presidential Address," *Journal of Allergy* 41 (1960): 88–94.

52. Jackson, *Allergy*, 103.

53. Gregg Mitman, "Natural History and the Clinic: The Regional Ecology of Allergy in America," *Studies in History and Philosophy of Biological and Biomedical Sciences* 34 (2003): 494–510.

54. Jackson, *Allergy*, 127–38.

55. It could be argued that a similar relationship developed between psychiatrists and pharmaceutical companies during the postwar period. For an excellent and provocative account of how ties to the pharmaceutical industrial complex has affected understandings and treatments of asthma, see Gregg Mitman, *Breathing Space: How Allergies Shape Our Lives and Landscapes* (New Haven, Conn.: Yale University Press, 2007).

56. H. J. Gerstenberger and J. H. Davis, "Report of a Case of Anaphylaxis Following an Intradermal Protein Sensitization Test," *JAMA* 76 (1921): 721–23.

57. R. W. Lamson, "So-Called Fatal Anaphylaxis in Man: With Especial Reference to the Diagnosis and Treatment of Clinical Allergies," *JAMA* 93 (1929): 1775–78. Subsequent allergists would also warn about the dangers involved in skin testing. See "News and Notes," *JAMA* 282 (1963): 207; and Feingold, *Introduction to Clinical Allergy*, 148–49.

58. Orville H. Brown, quoted in Alfred H. Rowe, "Gastrointestinal Food Allergy: A Study Based on One Hundred Cases," *Journal of Allergy* 1 (1929–1930): 173.

59. Ibid., 172–77.

60. Alfred H. Rowe, "Food Allergy: Its Manifestations, Diagnosis, and Treatment," *JAMA* 91 (1928): 1623–31, and "Gastrointestinal Food Allergy," 172–77; Randolph, *Environmental Medicine*, 27; Jackson, *Allergy*, 77.

61. Quoted in Randolph, *Environmental Medicine*, 28.

62. For more on the emergence and influence of vitamins, see Rima D. Apple, *Vitamania: Vitamins in American Culture* (New Brunswick, N.J.: Rutgers University Press, 1996).

63. The nutritional adequacies of elimination diets are still discussed, as in Michael M. Marsh, "Elimination Diets as a Diagnostic Tool," in *Food Allergy and Intolerance*, ed. Brostoff and Challacombe, 817–29.

64. "With What We Must Contend," *Annals of Allergy* 19 (1961): 193–95. Nutritional deficiencies were also cited as a criticism of Feingold's food additive–free diet for hyperactivity. See Matthew Smith, *An Alternative History of Hyperactivity: Food Additives, and the Feingold Diet* (New Brunswick, N.J.: Rutgers University Press, 2011), 137.

65. J. H. Baumhauer, "Allergy in Children with Particular Reference to Food Idiosyncrasy; Report of Cases," *Journal of the Medical Association of Alabama* 2 (1932): 195–202; Louis Tuft, *Clinical Allergy* (Philadelphia: Saunders, 1937), 175; Friedman, "Management with the Elimination Diet," 162–70; Richard Mackarness, *Not All in the Mind: How Unsuspected Food Allergy Can Affect Your Body AND Your Mind* (London: Pan Books, 1976), 27.

66. Quoted in Randolph, *Environmental Medicine*, 95.

67. Janet A. Caldwell, "The Manifestations of Food Allergy," *Dallas Medical Journal* 19 (1933): 51–53.
68. Cleveland White, "Acneform Eruptions of the Face: Etiologic Importance of Specific Foods," *JAMA* 103 (1934): 1277–79.
69. Quoted in Rowe, "Gastrointestinal Food Allergy," 176.
70. Quoted in ibid.
71. William G. Crook to Theron G. Randolph and other allergists, undated, Box 7, Folder 20, Theron G. Randolph Papers, 1935–1991, H MS c183, Harvard Medical Library in the Francis A. Countway Library of Medicine, Center for the History of Medicine, Boston.
72. Randolph, *Environmental Medicine*, 79, 110, 114–15.
73. William Waddell Duke, *Allergy, Asthma, Hay Fever, Urticaria, and Allied Manifestations of Reaction* (London: Kimpton, 1925); Rinkel, Randolph, and Zeller, *Food Allergy*, 125; Leandro M. Tocantins, "William Waddell Duke: Notes on the Man and His Work," *Blood* 1 (1946): 455–77.
74. Rinkel, Randolph, and Zeller, *Food Allergy*, 125, 346–47.
75. Bertram J. Sippy, "The Sippy Treatment for Gastric Ulcer," *Journal of the National Medical Association* 16 (1924): 105–7.
76. Rinkel, Randolph, and Zeller, *Food Allergy*, 350–51; Herbert J. Rinkel, "Gastro-Intestinal Allergy: Concerning Mimicry of Peptic Ulcer Syndrome by Symptoms of Food Allergy," *Southern Medical Journal* 27 (1934): 630–33.
77. Ben F. Feingold, "Tonsillectomy in the Allergic Child," *California Medicine* 71 (1949): 341–44, and *Why Your Child Is Hyperactive* (New York: Random House, 1974); Smith, *Alternative History of Hyperactivity*.
78. Vaughan, *Practice of Allergy*, 131–32; Rinkel, Randolph, and Zeller, *Food Allergy*, 379.
79. Rinkel, Randolph, and Zeller, *Food Allergy*, 129.
80. Ibid.
81. Ibid., 351.
82. Ibid., 359–60, 373.
83. Ibid., 125; Warren T. Vaughan, "Food Allergens: Leukopenic Index, Preliminary Report," *Journal of Allergy* (1934): 601, and *Practice of Allergy*, 298.
84. L. P. Gay, "Gastro-Intestinal Allergy IV: The Leucopenic Index as a Method of Diagnosis of Allergy Causing Peptic Ulcer," *JAMA* 106 (1936): 969–76; M. Loveless, R. Dorfman, and L. Downing, "Statistical Evaluation of the Leucopenic Index," *Journal of Allergy* 9 (1938): 321–44; E. Brown and G. P. Wadsworth, "The Leucopenic Index," *Journal of Allergy* 9 (1938): 345–70.
85. [American Association of Immunologists,] "The Founding of *The Journal of Immunology*," http://www.aai.org/about/History/Articles/AAI_History_001.pdf (accessed August 22, 2013).
86. Arthur F. Coca, *The Pulse Test for Allergy* (London: Parrish, 1959), 8–9; Mackarness, *Not All in the Mind*, 62; Mitman, *Breathing Space*, 187–90, 200.

87. Another word that Coca coined was "idioblapsis," used to describe an inherited food allergy that caused an acceleration in the pulse. So, if *Familial Nonreaginic Food-Allergy* was not confusing enough, he could have called his book *Idioblapsis.* Most of Coca's supporters and critics rejected the term as unnecessary and confusing, which is ironic, since Coca himself had criticized von Pirquet's term "allergy" for similar reasons.

88. Arthur F. Coca, *Familial Nonreaginic Food-Allergy* (Springfield, Ill.: Thomas, 1943), 10.

89. Arthur F. Coca first outlined his approach to defining allergy in "Hypersensitiveness," in *Practice of Medicine*, ed. Frederick Tice (Hagerstown, Md.: Prior, 1920), 1:109–99.

90. Randolph, *Environmental Medicine*, 19.

91. L. N. Ettelson and Louis Tuft, "The Value of the Coca Pulse-Acceleration Method in Food Allergy," *Journal of Allergy* 32 (1961): 515.

92. Randolph, *Environmental Medicine*, 92.

93. L. P. Gay, review of *Familial Nonreaginic Food-Allergy*, by Arthur C. Coca, *Quarterly Review of Biology* 21 (1946): 408.

94. Mackarness, *Not All in the Mind*, 62.

95. Theron G. Randolph to Harry G. Clark, August 28, 1951, Box 7, Folder 8, Randolph Papers.

96. Arthur F. Coca to Theron G. Randolph, February 7, 1957, Box 7, Folder 11, Randolph Papers.

97. Spain, review of *Food Allergy*, 98.

98. "Ballad of the Allergists," Box 434, Folder 3, American Academy of Allergy, Asthma and Immunology Records, 1923–2011, University of Wisconsin–Milwaukee Libraries, Archives Department.

99. Rowe, *Elimination Diets*, 33. The notion of the "ideal" food allergy patient persists to this day: "In an ideal scenario patients should be well motivated, keen to take responsibility for their own health, intelligent and with sufficient resources in terms of time and finances. This combination of characteristics is, of course, not usual and in practice it is sometimes those judged to be unable to carry out the diet adequately but who wish to 'give it a go' who have a highly successful outcome" (Gail Pollard, "Practical Application and Hazards of Dietary Management in Food Intolerance," in *Food Allergy and Intolerance*, ed. Brostoff and Challacombe, 908).

100. Bret Ratner, "Diagnosis and Management of the Allergic Child," *JAMA* 96 (1931): 570–75. Ratner carried out his research under the auspices of the Crane Fund for the Study of Allergic Diseases in Children.

101. Vaughan, *Practice of Allergy*, 113.

102. Ibid.

103. Ibid., 136.

104. Ibid., 140.

105. Ibid.

106. Ibid.
107. Some food allergists did provide their patients with hypoallergenic recipes. See Rinkel, Randolph, and Zeller, *Food Allergy*, 115, 294–336.
108. Alfred T. Schofield, "A Case of Egg Poisoning," *Lancet* 171 (1908): 716; Jackson, *Allergy*, 74.
109. Morgan, *You Can't Eat That!*, 7.
110. Harry G. Clark to Theron G. Randolph, March 16, 1950, Box 7, Folder 8, Randolph Papers.
111. Theron G. Randolph, "Allergy as a Causative Factor of Fatigue, Irritability, and Behavior Problems of Children," *Journal of Pediatrics* 31 (1947): 562. See also William Kaufman, "Some Psychosomatic Aspects of Food Allergy," *Psychosomatic Medicine* 16 (1954): 10–40. Randolph's article presents ideas about food allergy and fatigue that would be developed further by Frederic Speer and his "allergic tension fatigue syndrome," as outlined in "Allergic Tension-Fatigue in Children," *Annals of Allergy* 12 (1954): 168–71.
112. A similar relationship can be identified in Michele Murphy, *Sick Building Syndrome and the Problem of Uncertainty: Environmental Politics, Technoscience, and Women Workers* (Durham, N.C.: Duke University Press, 2006).
113. Mackarness, *Not All in the Mind*, 59; Theron G. Randolph, "Biographical Sketch of Herbert J. Rinkel, M.D., Emphasizing His Medical Contributions" (speech presented to the American Society of Opthalmologic and Otolaryngologic Allergy, Las Vegas, Nevada, September 1978), Box 4, Folder 3, Randolph Papers.
114. Mackarness, *Not All in the Mind*, 59; Herbert J. Rinkel, "Role of Food Allergy in Internal Medicine," *Annals of Allergy* 2 (1944): 115–24.
115. Randolph, *Environmental Medicine*, 27.
116. Quoted in ibid., 30.
117. Quoted in ibid., 65.
118. Ibid., 90.
119. Arthur F. Coca to Theron G. Randolph, January 22, 1955, Box 7 Folder 11, Randolph Papers (emphasis in original).
120. Mitman, *Breathing Space*, 188–89. Dust-Seal was the source of a spat between Randolph and Coca, with the former claiming that, far from preventing reactions in patients, the product could cause them. In response, Coca defended the "practically perfect product" and urged Randolph to reconsider the cases in which he believed it caused harm. See Arthur F. Coca to Theron G. Randolph, June 9, 1953, Box 7, Folder 11, Randolph Papers.
121. Theron G. Randolph to Ruth Fox, November 20, 1959, Box 7, Folder 11, Randolph Papers.
122. Guy Laroche, Charles Richet Fils, and François Saint-Girons, *Alimentary Anaphylaxis (Gastro-intestinal Food Allergy)*, trans. Mildred P. Rowe and Albert H. Rowe (Berkeley: University of California Press, 1930), 3; Rinkel, Randolph, and Zeller, *Food Allergy*, 90–112.
123. Coca, *Pulse Test for Allergy*.

124. Coca, *Familial Nonreaginic Food-Allergy*, 11.

125. Warren T. Vaughan, "Minor Allergy: Its Distribution, Clinical Aspects, and Significance," *Journal of Allergy* 5 (1935): 184–96.

126. Ibid., 185.

127. Rinkel, Randolph, and Zeller, *Food Allergy*, 15; Randolph, *Environmental Medicine*, 244–45.

128. Rowe and Rowe, *Food Allergy*, ix, 20.

129. For instance, see Rowe's comments in the following medical articles and newspapers: William C. Voorsanger and Fred Firestone, "Vaccine Therapy in Infectious Bronchitis and Asthma," *California and Western Medicine* 36 (1929): 336–40; Ben F. Feingold, "Treatment of Allergic Disease of the Bronchi," *JAMA* 146 (1951): 319–23; "Most Food Allergies Traceable, Says Doctor," *Los Angeles Examiner*, March 7, 1950; and "May Be Allergic to In-Laws," *Los Angeles Evening Herald-Express*, March 7, 1950.

130. Mackarness, *Not All in the Mind*, 11–13.

131. Francis C. Lowell and Irving W. Schiller, "Editorial: It Is So—It Ain't So," *Journal of Allergy* 25 (1954): 57–59.

132. Horace Baldwin and W. C. Spain, "Editorial," *Journal of Allergy* 20 (1949): 388–90; Ben Z. Rappaport, "President's Address," *Journal of Allergy* 25 (1954): 274–78; Sherman, "Presidential Address," 274–76.

133. Rappaport, "President's Address," 277.

134. Ibid., 275, 278.

135. Leslie N. Gay to B. R. Kirklin, January 20, 1948, Box 432, Folder 1, AAAAI Records.

136. L. N. Gay, review of *Strange Malady*, by Warren T. Vaughan, *Scientific Monthly* 54 (1942): 279–80; review of *Elimination Diets and the Patients' Allergies*, by Albert H. Rowe, *Quarterly Review of Biology* 20 (1945): 183; and review of *Familial Nonreaginic Food-Allergy*.

137. Gay, review of *Elimination Diets*, 183.

138. The respective positions of the AAA and the ACA toward food allergy are clearly indicated in the archives of each association, both located in Wisconsin. Despite ultimately falling out with the ACA, Randolph admitted in the late 1970s that the organization had provided him and his colleagues with opportunities to voice their ideas. See Theron G. Randolph, "Both Allergy and Clinical Ecology Are Needed," *Annals of Allergy* 39 (1977): 215–16.

139. Divisions within medicine based on the desire for more holism or more reductionism in clinical practice were typical of this period, as discussed in Christopher Lawrence and George Weisz, "Medical Holism: The Context," in *Greater Than the Parts: Holism in Biomedicine, 1920–1950*, ed. Christopher Lawrence and George Weisz (New York: Oxford University Press, 1998), 1–22. See also David Cantor, 'The Diseased Body," in *Medicine in the Twentieth Century*, ed. Roger Cooter and John Pickstone (Amsterdam: Harwood Academic, 2000), 347–66.

140. Victor C. Vaughan, "Further Studies of the Protein Poison," *JAMA* 67 (1916): 1559–62; M. Therese Southgate, "The Cover: Victor C. Vaughan," *JAMA* 283 (2000): 848.

FOUR. PANIC? OR THE PANTRY?

1. Ethan Allan Brown, "American Academy of Allergy: The Changing Picture of Allergy," *Journal of Allergy* 28 (1957): 365–66.
2. Ibid., 373.
3. Philip Conford, *Origins of the Organic Movement* (Edinburgh: Floris Books, 2001); Michael Brander, *Eve Balfour: Founder of the Soil Association and Voice of the Organic Movement: A Biography* (Haddington: Glenneil Press, 2003); David Matless, "Bodies Made of Grass Made of Earth Made of Bodies: Organism, Diet, and National Health in Mid-Twentieth-Century England," *Journal of Historical Geography* 27 (2003): 355–76.
4. Rachel Carson, *Silent Spring* (Boston: Houghton Mifflin, 1962).
5. Thirty-eight letters from Beatrice Trim Hunter to Rachel Carson, January 29, 1958–August 10, 1963, Box 23, Beatrice Trum Hunter Collection, Howard Gotlieb Archival Research Center, Boston University.
6. Hunter's contribution to the inspiration of and initial research for *Silent Spring* is made particularly clear in a postcard from Carson to Hunter in which she expresses her gratitude for her "wonderful response to my note of inquiry! I know it represents *hours* of your time. We shall hope to make good use of the wealth of information and reference you have supplied" (Rachel Carson to Beatrice Trum Hunter, February 3, 1958 [emphasis in original]). Given Rachel Carson's domestic and financial difficulties, as well as her cautious, conservative nature—all portrayed in Linda Lear, *Rachel Carson: Witness for Nature* (London: Allen Lane, 1998)—her decision to write such a provocative and divisive book was understandably difficult and was influenced by many factors, including Marjorie Spock's unsuccessful court case. Nevertheless, the influence of her correspondence with Hunter, which occurred earlier, has not yet been documented.
7. Richard A. Merrill, "Food Safety Regulation: Reforming the Delaney Clause," *Annual Review of Public Health* 18 (1997): 313–40; Harvey A. Levenstein, *Fear of Food: A History of Why We Worry About What We Eat* (Chicago: University of Chicago Press, 2012), 111–12.
8. Charles H. Blank, "The Delaney Clause: Technical Naïveté and Scientific Advocacy in the Formulation of Public Health Policies," *California Law Review* 62 (1974): 1088; Harvey A. Levenstein, *Paradox of Plenty: A Social History of Eating in Modern America* (New York: Oxford University Press, 1993), 112.
9. Elizabeth M. Whalen and Frederick J. Stare, *Panic in the Pantry: Food Facts, Fads, and Fallacies* (New York: Athenaeum, 1975).
10. "Frederick Stare," *Economist*, April 18, 2002; D. Mark Hegsted, "Frederick John Stare (1910–2002)," *Journal of Nutrition* 134 (2004): 1007–9. For more on the ACSH and its links to the food, chemical, and pharmaceutical industries, see David Rosner and Gerald Markowitz, "Industry Challenges to the Principle of Prevention in Public Health," *Public Health Reports* 117 (2002): 508–9.
11. Whalen and Stare, *Panic in the Pantry*, v.

12. Ben F. Feingold, "Treatment of Allergic Disease of the Bronchi," *JAMA* 146 (1951): 319–23; Matthew Smith, *An Alternative History of Hyperactivity: Food Additives, and the Feingold Diet* (New Brunswick, N.J.: Rutgers University Press, 2011), 44–45, 96–99, 108–9.

13. Harry G. Clark to Theron G. Randolph, March 6, 1950, Box 7, Folder 8, Theron G. Randolph Papers, 1935–1991, H MS c183, Harvard Medical Library in the Francis A. Countway Library of Medicine, Center for the History of Medicine, Boston.

14. Brown, "American Academy of Allergy," 368.

15. Mark Jackson, "'Allergy *con Amore*': Psychosomatic Medicine and the 'Asthmogenic Home' in the Mid-Twentieth Century," in *Health and the Modern Home*, ed. Mark Jackson (New York: Routledge, 2007), 153–74; Carla Keirns, "Better Than Nature: The Changing Treatment of Asthma and Hay Fever in the United States, 1910–1945," *Studies in History and Philosophy of Biological and Biomedical Sciences* 34 (2003): 511–31.

16. Jackson, "'Allergy *con Amore*,'" 154–55; Henry Hyde Salter, "On the Aetiology of Asthma," *BMJ* 132 (1859): 538.

17. Quoted in Jackson, "'Allergy *con Amore*,'" 156.

18. Ibid., 157–65.

19. T. Wood Clarke, "The Relation of Allergy to Character Problems in Children," *Annals of Allergy* 8 (1950): 21–38.

20. Ibid., 175.

21. Ibid.

22. Ibid.

23. Ibid., 176; T. Wood Clarke, "Neuro-Allergy in Childhood," *New York State Journal of Medicine* 42 (1948): 393–97.

24. Clarke, "Relation of Allergy," 176–77.

25. Ibid., 186

26. Quoted in ibid., 177–78.

27. Quoted in ibid., 178.

28. Ibid., 179.

29. Ibid.

30. Quoted in ibid., 178.

31. Ibid., 185.

32. Ibid.

33. Matthew Smith, "Psychiatry Limited: Hyperactivity and the Evolution of American Psychiatry," *Social History of Medicine* 21 (2008): 541–59.

34. Quoted in Clarke "Relation of Allergy," 177.

35. Quoted in ibid. Similar concerns have been raised recently with respect to peanut allergy.

36. Ibid., 186.

37. Clarke, "Neuroallergy in Childhood," 393.

38. B. Raymond Hoobler, "Some Early Symptoms Suggesting Protein Sensitization in Infancy," *American Journal of Diseases of Children* 12 (1916): 129–35.

39. W. Ray Shannon, "Neuropathic Manifestations in Infants and Children as a Result of Anaphylactic Reaction to Foods Contained in Their Dietary," *American Journal of Disease of Children* 24 (1922): 89–94.

40. Ibid., 90.

41. Alfred T. Schofield, "A Case of Egg Poisoning," *Lancet* 171 (1908): 716; Oscar M. Schloss, "A Case of Allergy to Common Foods," *American Journal of Diseases of Children* 3 (1912): 341–62; William Waddell Duke, *Allergy: Asthma, Hay Fever, Urticaria and Allied Manifestations of Reaction* (London: Kimpton, 1925); George Piness and Hyman Miller, "Allergic Manifestations in Infancy and Childhood," *Archives of Pediatrics* 42 (1925): 557–62; Albert H. Rowe and Albert Rowe Jr., *Food Allergy: Its Manifestations and Control and the Elimination Diets, a Compendium with Important Consideration of Inhalant (Especially Pollen), Drug, and Infectant Allergy* (1931; Springfield, Ill.: Thomas, 1972); Wilmot F. Schneider, "Psychiatric Evaluation of the Hyperkinetic Child," *Journal of Pediatrics* 26 (1945): 559–70; Walter C. Alvarez "Puzzling 'Nervous Storms' Due to Food Allergy," *Gastroenterology* 7 (1946): 241–52; Theron G. Randolph, "Allergy as a Causative Factor of Fatigue, Irritability, and Behavior Problems of Children," *Journal of Pediatrics* 31 (1947): 560–72; Hal M. Davison, "Cerebral Allergy," *Southern Medical Journal* 42 (1949): 712–16.

42. M. W. Laufer and W. E. Denhoff, "Hyperkinetic Behavior Syndrome in Children," *Journal of Pediatrics* 50 (1957): 463–74; M. W. Laufer, W. E. Denhoff, and G. Solomons, "Hyperkinetic Impulse Disorder in Children's Behavior Problems," *Psychosomatic Medicine* 19 (1957): 38–49; Matthew Smith, *Hyperactive: The Controversial History of ADHD* (London: Reaktion, 2012), 46–74.

43. Schneider, "Psychiatric Evaluation," 560, 567.

44. Randolph, "Allergy as a Causative Factor," 560–72.

45. Ibid., 563.

46. Frederic Speer, "Allergic Tension-Fatigue in Children," *Annals of Allergy* 12 (1954): 168–71, and "The Allergic Tension-Fatigue Syndrome," *Pediatric Clinics of North America* 1 (1954): 1029–37.

47. Speer, "Allergic Tension-Fatigue Syndrome," 1029.

48. Alfred A. Strauss and Heinz Werner, "Disorders of Conceptual Thinking in the Brain-Injured Child," *Journal of Nervous and Mental Disease* 96 (1942): 153–72; Paul H. Wender, *Minimal Brain Dysfunction in Children* (New York: Wiley-Interscience, 1971); "Minimal Brain Dysfunction," *Lancet* 302 (1973): 487–88; Rick Mayes and Adam Rafalovich, "Suffer the Restless Children: The Evolution of ADHD and Paediatric Stimulant Use, 1900–1980," *History of Psychiatry* 18 (2007): 435–57; Smith, *Hyperactive*, 20–22; 42–44.

49. Speer, "Allergic Tension-Fatigue Syndrome," 1030.

50. Speer "Allergic Tension-Fatigue in Children," 170.

51. Frederic Speer "The Allergic Tension-Fatigue Syndrome in Children," *International Archives of Allergy and Applied Immunology* 12 (1958): 207–14. For a good comparison, see Paulina F. Kernberg, "The Problem of Organicity in the Child:

Notes on Some Diagnostic Techniques in the Evaluation of Children," *Journal of the American Academy of Child Psychiatry* 8 (1969): 517–41.

52. Frederic Speer, "Historical Development of Allergy of the Nervous System," *Annals of Allergy* 16 (1958): 14–20.

53. Speer listed food dyes as an uncommon cause of such disturbances in 1958, but suggested that milk, chocolate, corn, eggs, and legumes were more commonly at fault, in "Food Allergy in Childhood," *Archives of Pediatrics* 75 (1958): 363–69.

54. Harvey A. Levenstein, *Revolution at the Table: The Transformation of the American Diet* (New York: Oxford University Press, 1988), 39

55. Derek J. Oddy, *From Plain Fare to Fusion Food: The British Diet from the 1890s to the 1990s* (Woodbridge: Boydell Press, 2003), ix, 31.

56. Arthur Kallet and F. J. Schlink, *100,000,000 Guinea Pigs: Dangers in Everyday Foods, Drugs, and Cosmetics* (New York: Vanguard Press, 1933); Laurence B. Glickman, *Buying Power: A History of Consumer Activism in America* (Chicago: University of Chicago Press, 2009), 194–95. Kallet and Schlink were running the consumer activist group Consumer Research when *100,000,000 Guinea Pigs* was published, but their partnership would not last due to political differences. Kallet left Consumer Research in 1936 after Schlink used force to break a strike involving their employees; the following year, Kallet formed a rival consumer watchdog group, the aptly named Consumer Union and Consumer Reports. Kallet, who would be branded as a Communist by the House Un-American Activities Committee in the 1950s, later launched The Medical Letter, a nonprofit foundation that continues to publish the influential *Medical Letter on Drugs and Therapeutics* and *Treatment Guidelines from the Medical Letter*. See Consumer Reports, "Our History," http://www.consumerreports.org/cro/about-us/history/index.htm (accessed September 24, 2013).

57. In addition to their long list of toxic chemicals, Kallet and Schlink warned about the hazards of bran, and Kellogg's All Bran in particular, which they described as "the roughest of roughages," responsible for much indigestion and stomach trouble (*100,000,000 Guinea Pigs*, 3). The medical expert they cited was the gastroenterologist Walter Alvarez, who claimed that "the craze for roughage is worth $300 a month to any good stomach specialist" (20–21).

58. Ibid., 47–60.

59. Levenstein, *Revolution at the Table*, 202.

60. Ernest G. Moore, quoted in Lear, *Rachel Carson*, 413.

61. William S. Gaud, "The Green Revolution: Accomplishments and Apprehensions," (speech presented to the Society for International Development, Washington, D.C., March 8, 1968), http://www.agbioworld.org/biotech-info/topics/borlaug/borlaug-green.html (accessed September 24, 2013).

62. Stephen D. Lockey, "Allergic Reactions Due to Dyes in Foods" (speech presented to the Pennsylvania Allergy Society, Autumn 1948), and "Allergic Reactions Due to FD&C Dyes Used as Coloring and Identifying Agents in Various Medications," *Bulletin* (Lancaster [Pa.] General Hospital), September 1948.

63. Stephen D. Lockey, "Reactions to Hidden Agents in Foods, Beverages and Drugs," *Annals of Allergy* 29 (1971): 461–66; "Sensitizing Properties of Food Additives and Other Commercial Products," *Annals of Allergy* 30 (1972): 638–41; and "Drug Reactions and Sublingual Testing with Certified Food Colors," *Annals of Allergy* 31 (1973): 423–29.

64. Stephen D. Lockey, "Allergic Reactions Due to F. D. and C. Yellow No. 5, Tartrazine, an Aniline Dye Used as a Coloring and Identifying Agent in Various Steroids," *Annals of Allergy* 17 (1959): 719–21. These coal-tar dyes were also the chemical origin of many psychoactive drugs that emerged after the Second World War. See David Healy, *The Antidepressant Era* (Cambridge, Mass: Harvard University Press, 1999).

65. As mentioned in chapter 3, Arthur Coca had also written about allergic reactions to various petrochemical fumes. See Theron G. Randolph, "Allergic Type Reactions to Industrial Solvents and Liquid Fuels"; "Allergic Type Reactions to Mosquito Abatement Fogs and Mists"; "Allergic Type Reactions to Motor Exhaust"; "Allergic Type Reactions to Indoor Utility Gas and Oil Fumes"; "Allergic Type Reactions to Chemical Additives of Foods and Drugs"; "Allergic Type Reactions to Synthetic Drugs and Cosmetics," *Journal of Laboratory and Clinical Medicine* 44 (1954): 910–14, and *Environmental Medicine: Beginnings and Bibliographies of Clinical Ecology* (Fort Collins, Colo.: Clinical Ecology, 1987), viii.

66. Theron G. Randolph to Harry G. Clark, November 1, 1950, Box 7, Folder 8, Randolph Papers; Randolph, *Environmental Medicine*, 76–77.

67. Randolph, *Environmental Medicine*, 32–36.

68. Theron G. Randolph, "Ingredients of Bread: Testimony in the Matter of a Definition and Standard of Identity for Bread and Related Products," docket No. FDC-31(b), Before the Administrator, Federal Security Agency, August 3, 1949, 596–14, 628.

69. Randolph, *Environmental Medicine*, 54.

70. Theron G. Randolph to Harry G. Clark, July 3, 1951, Box 7, Folder 8, Randolph Papers; Randolph, *Environmental Medicine*, 56.

71. The Northwestern School of Medicine has been called the Feinberg School of Medicine since 2002, when Samuel Feinberg's brother, the Chicago banker Reuben Feinberg (1919–2002), donated $75 million to it. Although the article that heralded the donation stated that a chance visit to the hospital after a minor heart attack inspired the donation, clearly there was also a close family connection to the place. See Robert Becker and Meg McSherry Breslin, "Banker Gives $75 Million to NU," *Chicago Tribune*, February 14, 2002, http://articles.chicagotribune.com/2002-02-14/news/0202140008_1_medical-school-nu-bessie-feinberg-foundation (accessed September 25, 2013); Robert Schleimer, "Message from the Division Chief," Northwestern University, Feinberg School of Medicine, http://www.medicine.north western.edu/divisions/allergy-immunology-0 (accessed September 25, 2013); and Samuel Feinberg, *Allergy in General Practice* (London: Kimpton, 1934).

72. Feinberg, *Allergy in General Practice*, 65; Samuel Feinberg, *One Man's Food* (Chicago: Blue Cross Commission, 1953), 2.

73. Samuel M. Feinberg et al., "Reactions to Dextrose," *JAMA* 145 (1951): 666. On the attempts to undermine Randolph's position as president of the Chicago Society of Allergy, see Randolph to Clark, July 3, 1951; Theron G. Randolph to Herbert Rinkel, March 23, 1951, Box 10, Folder 14, both in Randolph Papers. Another letter in the same issue of *JAMA* likened Randolph to the disgraced Soviet biologist Trofim Lysenko (1898–1976): Mary Hewitt Loveless, "Reactions to Dextrose," *JAMA* 145 (1951): 666.

74. Harry G. Clark to Theron G. Randolph, undated, but likely from the early 1950s, Box 7, Folder 8, Randolph Papers.

75. Vilma Kinney, *Theron Grant Randolph, M.D., 1906–1995: A Bibliography: 60 Years of Published Works* (Self-published, 1997), xii.

76. Theron G. Randolph, "Human Ecology and Susceptibility to the Chemical Environment," *Annals of Allergy* 19 (1961): 518–40, 657–77, 779–99, 908–29, and *Human Ecology and Susceptibility to the Chemical Environment* (Springfield, Ill.: Thomas, 1962).

77. Randolph, "Human Ecology," 780 (emphasis in original).

78. Ibid., 782, 791.

79. Theron D. Randolph to Payne Thomas, Mary 18, 1962, Box 2, Folder 13, Randolph Papers.

80. Randolph, "Human Ecology," 915.

81. Ibid., 916 (emphasis in original).

82. Beatrice Trum Hunter, "The Bookhunter," *Herald of Health*, August 12, 1962.

83. Howard W. Mitchell and Byron R. Hubbard to Theron G. Randolph, July 27, 1962, Box 2, Folder 13, Randolph Papers.

84. Randolph, unsurprisingly, did not hesitate to mention this association. See George F. Shambaugh, "Ahead of Their Time," *Archives of Otolaryngology* 79 (1964): 118–19; and Randolph, *Environmental Medicine*, vii.

85. D. Harvey, review of *Human Ecology and Susceptibility to the Chemical Environment*, by Theron G. Randolph, *Nutrition Abstracts and Reviews*, January 1963, 11.

86. Some historians have also chose to ridicule the book, and clinical ecology more generally: Edward Shorter, "Multiple Chemical Sensitivity: Pseudodisease in Historical Perspective," *Scandinavian Journal of Work, Environment, and Health* 23 (1997): 35–42.

87. Theron G. Randolph to Payne Thomas, July 13, 1963, Box 2, Folder 13, Randolph Papers.

88. Randolph, *Environmental Medicine*, 159.

89. Theron D. Randolph, "The Specific Adaptation Syndrome" (manuscript, undated), Box 2, Folder 3, Randolph Papers.

90. For more on Hans Selye, see Mark Jackson, *The Age of Stress: Science and the Search for Stability* (Oxford: Oxford University Press, 2013).

91. Ben F. Feingold, "Allergy to Flea Bites—Clinical and Experimental Observations," *Annals of Allergy* 19 (1961): 1275–89.

92. Ibid., 1282.
93. Ben F. Feingold, *Introduction to Clinical Allergy* (Springfield, Ill.: Thomas, 1973), 157–63.
94. Both Ben F. Feingold, *Why Your Child Is Hyperactive* (New York: Random House, 1974), and its sequel, Ben F. Feingold and Helene S. Feingold, *The Feingold Cookbook for Hyperactive Children* (New York: Random House, 1979), were best sellers, with the latter reaching number four on the *New York Times* best-seller list in 1979. Proceeds from *The Feingold Cookbook* were used to fund the Feingold Association of the United States, which continues to be active. In my history of the Feingold diet, I suggest that, while Feingold's primary goal in writing *Why Your Child Is Hyperactive* was to convince parents, the book was also written with his colleagues in allergy very much in mind. See Smith, *Alternative History of Hyperactivity*, 15–35.
95. Smith, *Alternative History of Hyperactivity*.
96. William J. Crook, "Food Allergy: The Great Masquerader," *Pediatric Clinics of North America* 22 (1975): 227–38; Richard Mackarness, *Not All in the Mind: How Unsuspected Food Allergy Can Affect Your Body AND Your Mind* (London: Pan Books, 1976); Doris J. Rapp, *Allergies and the Hyperactive Child* (New York: Fireside, 1979).
97. William J. Crook, *Can Your Child Write? Is He Hyperactive?* (Jackson, Tenn.: Pedicenter Press, 1975), and *The Yeast Connection: A Medical Breakthrough* (New York: Vintage, 1986).
98. "Misdiagnosed Allergies, Food, and Environment," *Phil Donahue Show*, YouTube, http://www.youtube.com/watch?v=0UUTXTKPusU (accessed September 19, 2014).
99. For information on the Paleo diet, see http://thepaleodiet.com/.
100. Richard Mackarness's opinions about food additives are revealed in the title of another of his books, *Chemical Victims* (London: Pan Books, 1980). See also Richard Mackarness, *Eat Fat and Grow Slim* (Garden City, N.Y.: Doubleday, 1959).
101. For more on the history of hyperactivity, see Smith, *Hyperactive*.
102. Donna McCann et al., "Food Additives and Hyperactive Behaviour in 3-Year-Old and 8/9-Year-Old Children in the Community: A Randomised, Double-Blinded, Placebo-Controlled Trial," *Lancet* 370 (2007): 1560–67; B. Bateman et al., "The Effects of a Double-Blind, Placebo Controlled, Artificial Food Colourings and Benzoate Preservative Challenge on Hyperactivity in a General Population Sample of Preschool Children," *Archives of Disease in Childhood* 89 (2004): 506–11.
103. Smith, *Alternative History of Hyperactivity*, 101.
104. Feingold, *Why Your Child Is Hyperactive*, 156–68. When Feingold, who had published widely in leading medical journals, including *JAMA*, struggled to get journal editors to accept and publish his articles about his hyperactivity hypothesis, he turned to more obscure and more specialist publications, ranging from the *Delaware Medical Journal* and the *American Journal of Nursing* to the *Journal of the American Society for Preventive Dentistry* and the *International Journal of Offender*

Therapy and Comparative Criminology. His last publication was Ben F. Feingold, "The Role of Diet in Behaviour," *Ecology of Disease* 1 (1982): 153–65. Published posthumously, it was accompanied by a warm obituary.

105. Feingold, *Why Your Child Is Hyperactive*, 160.

106. Ibid.

107. Ibid., 162.

108. Ben F. Feingold et al., "Psychological Studies of Allergic Women: The Relation Between Skin Reactivity and Personality," *Psychosomatic Medicine* 24 (1962): 195–202.

109. Ibid., 201.

110. Feingold, "Treatment of Allergic Disease of the Bronchi," 319–23, and *Introduction to Clinical Allergy*, 189–97.

111. Feingold, *Introduction to Clinical Allergy*, 189.

112. Harold A. Abramson "Psychosomatic Aspects of Hay Fever and Asthma Prior to 1900," *Annals of Allergy* 6 (1948): 110. In addition to a historical interest in allergy, Abramson was involved in controversial LSD experiments during the 1950s.

113. Ibid., 110–21.

114. Thomas Morton French and Franz Alexander, *Psychogenic Factors in Bronchial Asthma* (Menasha, Wis.: Banta, 1941).

115. Margaret W. Gerard, "Bronchial Asthma in Children," *Nervous Child* 5 (1946): 327.

116. Ibid., 327–31.

117. Ibid., 329.

118. Ibid.; Leon J. Saul, "The Relations to the Mother as Seen in Cases of Allergy," *Nervous Child* 5 (1946): 332–38.

119. Albert H. Rowe, Albert Rowe Jr., and E. James Young, "Bronchial Asthma Due to Food Allergy Alone in Ninety-Five Patients," *Allergy Abstracts* 24 (1959): 1158.

120. Saul, "Relations to the Mother as Seen in Cases of Allergy," 334.

121. Felix Deutsch and Raymond Nadell, "Psychological Aspects of Dermatology with Special Consideration of Allergic Phenomena," *Nervous Child* 5 (1946): 355.

122. Ibid.

123. Ibid., 344.

124. Jackson, *Allergy*, 89.

125. Harold A. Abramson, "The Present Status of Allergy," *Nervous Child* 7 (1948): 99.

126. L. P. Gay, review of *Elimination Diets and the Patients' Allergies*, by Albert H. Rowe, *Quarterly Review of Biology* 20 (1945): 183.

127. L. P. Gay, review of *Strange Malady*, by Warren T. Vaughn, *Scientific Monthly* 54 (1942): 279–80.

128. Henry G. Clark to Theron G. Randolph, March 16, 1950, Box 7, Folder 8, Randolph Papers. Randolph did offer to present his research to psychiatrists, but most of his overtures went unrewarded.

129. John H. Mitchell et al., "Personality Factors in Allergic Disorder," *Journal of Allergy* 18 (1947): 337–40.

130. See the case of Joanna in Mackarness, *Not All in the Mind*.
131. Randolph, *Environmental Medicine*, viii.
132. J. S. Lebovidge et al., "Assessment of Psychological Distress Among Children and Adolescents with Food Allergy," *JACI* 124 (2009): 1282–88; A. J. Cummings et al., "Management of Nut Allergy Influences Quality of Life and Anxiety in Children and Their Mothers," *Pediatric Allergy and Immunology* 21 (2010): 586–94; K. M. Roy and M. C. Roberts, "Peanut Allergy in Children: Relationships to Health-Related Quality of Life, Anxiety, and Parental Stress," *Clinical Pediatrics* 50 (2011): 1045–51.
133. Feingold, *Introduction to Clinical Allergy*, 189–95.
134. Some new research in this area can be found in Christiane Liezmann, Burghard Klapp, and Eva M. J. Peters, "Stress, Atopy, and Allergy," *Dermatoendocrinology* 3 (2011): 37–40.
135. Hans Selye, *The Stress of Life* (London: Longman, Green, 1957); Russell Viner, "Putting Stress in Life: Hans Selye and the Making of Stress Theory," *Social Studies of Science* 29 (1999): 391–410; Jackson, *Age of Stress*.
136. Mackarness, *Not All in the Mind*, 42. Not all food allergists subscribed to Selye's theories. Coca, for instance, found Selye's ideas to be "imaginative" but also believed that he misused the term "adaptation" by focusing too much on the effects of adaptation rather what caused the need for it. See Arthur F. Coca to Theron G. Randolph, February 7, 1957, Box 7, Folder 11, Randolph Papers.
137. Randolph, "Human Ecology and Susceptibility to the Chemical Environment," 520–21.
138. Smith, "Psychiatry Limited."

FIVE. AN IMMUNOLOGICAL EXPLOSION?

1. Susan Donaldson James, "Weird Food Allergy Stresses Mom, Baffles Doctors," ABC News, April 1, 2013, http://abcnews.go.com/Health/weird-food-allergy-stresses-moms-baffles-doctors/story?id=18843611#.UVsgSo6K420 (accessed October 8, 2013).
2. Warren T. Vaughan, "Minor Allergy: Its Distribution, Clinical Aspects, and Significance," *Journal of Allergy* 5 (1935): 184–96.
3. Frederic Speer, "Is Allergy Extinct?" *Annals of Allergy* 2 (1967): 47–48.
4. For example, Speer argued that the "thrust" of the AAA and the ACA was "divided and not always coordinated" (ibid., 47).
5. Kimishige Ishizaka, Teruko Ishizaka, and M. Hornbrook, "Physicochemical Properties of Reaginic Antibody IV. Presence of a Unique Immunoglobulin as a Carrier of Reaginic Activity," *Journal of Immunology* 97 (1966): 75–85. For more details about why Denver was an appropriate place for IgE to be discovered, see Gregg Mitman, *Breathing Space: How Allergies Shape Our Lives and Landscapes* (New Haven, Conn.: Yale University Press, 2007), 89–129, 194, 236–37.

6. S. G. Johansson and H. Bennich, "Immunological Studies of an Atypical (Myeloma) Immunoglobulin," *Immunology* 13 (1967): 381–89; Gunnar Johansson, Hans Bennich, and Leif Wide, "Expanding the Scope of IgE, RAST," in *Excerpts from Classics in Allergy*, 3rd ed., ed. Sheldon G. Cohen (Bethesda, Md.: National Institutes of Allergy and Infectious Diseases, 2012), 314.

7. J. D. Gryboski, "Gastrointestinal Milk Allergy in Infants," *Pediatrics* 40 (1967): 354–62; H. Moria et al., "Gastrointestinal Food Allergy in Infants," *Allergology International* 62 (2013): 297–307.

8. William B. Sherman, "President's Address," *Journal of Allergy* 29 (1958): 275; T. Berg, H. Bennich, and S. G. Johansson, "In Vitro Diagnosis of Atopic Allergy. I. A Comparison of Provocation Tests and the Radioallergosorbent Test," *International Archives of Allergy and Applied Immunology* 40 (1971): 770–78; William T. Knicker, quoted in Mark Jackson, *Allergy: The History of a Modern Malady* (London: Reaktion, 2006), 126.

9. D. R. and Z. H. Haddad, "Diagnosis of IgE-Mediated Reactions to Food Antigens by Radioimmunoassay," *JACI* 54 (1974): 165–73. For a more recent use of the phrase, see S. L. Taylor and S. L. Hefle, "Food as Allergens," in *Food Allergy and Intolerance*, ed. Jonathan Brostoff and Stephen J. Challacombe, 2nd ed. (London: Saunders, 2002), 403–12.

10. P. G. H. Gell and R. R. A. Coombs, eds., *Clinical Aspects of Immunology* (Oxford: Blackwell, 1963).

11. W. R. Brown, B. K. Borthistle, and S. T. Chen, "Immunoglobulin E (IgE) and IgE-Containing Cells in Human Gastrointestinal Fluids and Tissues," *Clinical and Experimental Immunology* 20 (1975): 227–37; Johansson and Bennich, "Immunological Studies"; D. M. Ure, "Negative Association Between Allergy and Cancer," *Scottish Medical Journal* 14 (1969): 51–54; Michelle C. Turner, "Epidemiology: Allergy History, IgE, and Cancer," *Cancer Immunology, Immunotherapy* 62 (2012): 1493–510.

12. Jackson, *Allergy*, 125.

13. Harold M. Schmeck, "Doctors Seek Keys to Defenses of the Body," *New York Times*, December 29, 1972.

14. John W. Yunginger and Gerald J. Gleich, "The Impact of the Discovery of IgE on the Practice of Allergy," *Pediatric Clinics of North America* 22 (1975): 12.

15. Kenton Kroker, Pauline M. H. Mazumdar, and Jennifer Keelen, "Editor's Introduction," in *Crafting Immunity: Working Histories of Clinical Immunology*, ed. Kenton Kroker, Pauline M. H. Mazumdar, and Jennifer Keelen (Aldershot: Ashgate, 2008), 1; Ilana Löwy, *Between Bench and Bedside: Science, Healing, and Interleukin-2 in a Cancer Ward* (Cambridge, Mass.: Harvard University Press, 1996).

16. Mark Jackson, "'A Private Line to Medicine': The Clinical and Laboratory Contours of Allergy in the Early Twentieth Century," in *Crafting Immunity*, ed. Kroker, Mazumdar, and Keelen, 55–76.

17. Lucia Fisher-Pap, quoted in ibid., 56.

18. Ibid., 67–68.

19. Ibid., 67.

20. Prior to the certification of allergy as a specialty unto itself, it had been a subspecialty of both internal medicine (1936) and pediatrics (1944). Attempts to achieve board certification were often hampered by divisions between the AAA and the ACA, as well as the fact that other medical practitioners, particularly otolaryngologists, practiced allergy. See Horace S. Baldwin and W. C. Spain, "Editorial," *Journal of Allergy* 20 (1949): 388–90; Merle W. Moore, "More Stress on Education in Allergy," *Journal of Allergy* 31 (1959): 42–45; "The Underprivileged Child: Where Are We in Pediatric Allergy?" *Journal of Allergy* 19 (1961): 1196–97; and William G. Crook, Walton W. Harrison, and Stanley E. Crawford, "Allergy—The Unanswered Challenge in Pediatric Research, Education, and Practice," *Pediatrics* 21 (1958): 649–54.

21. Jerome Glaser, "Gastrointestinal Allergy in Infancy and Childhood," *Journal of the Medical Association of Georgia* 45 (1956): 514–18.

22. Ben Z. Rappaport, "President's Address," *Journal of Allergy* 25 (1954): 274–78.

23. Orval R. Withers, "The Allergist as a Clinician," *Journal of Allergy* 29 (1958): 278.

24. Max Samter, "On the Impossible," *Journal of Allergy* 31 (1960): 91.

25. One of Samter's research findings was that sensitivity to aspirin was nonallergic and, instead, an example of a pharmacological intolerance. He is known today for "Samter's Triad," a condition combining aspirin sensitivity, asthma, and nasal polyps. See Max Samter and R. F. Beers Jr., "Concerning the Nature of Intolerance to Aspirin," *Journal of Allergy* 40 (1967): 281–93.

26. Walter R. Kessler, "Food Allergy," *Pediatrics* 21 (1958): 523–25.

27. Ibid., 523.

28. Edward L. Pratt, "Food Allergy and Food Intolerance in Relation to the Development of Good Eating Habits," *Pediatrics* 21 (1958): 642–48.

29. Elliot F. Ellis, "Foreword," *Pediatric Clinics of North America* 22 (1975): 1.

30. Debra Jan Bibel, *Milestones in Immunology: A Historical Exploration* (Madison, Wis.: Science Tech, 1988), 57.

31. Jackson, *Allergy*, 47.

32. Arthur Silverstein, *A History of Immunology*, 2nd ed. (London: Elsevier/Academic Press, 2009), 180–87.

33. Milton J. Rosenau and John F. Anderson, *Studies upon Hypersusceptibility and Immunity* (Washington, D.C.: Government Printing Office, 1906); Victor C. Vaughan, "The Protein Poison and Its Relation to Disease," *JAMA* 61 (1913): 1761–64.

34. Carl Prausnitz, whose mother was English, later adopted her maiden name, Giles, when he left Nazi Germany for the Isle of Wight in 1935. Thus he is sometimes referred to as Carl Prausnitz-Giles or Carl Giles. See A. W. Frankland, "Carl Prausnitz: A Personal Memoir," *JACI* 114 (2004): 700–705.

35. Silverstein, *History of Immunology*, 183.

36. William Waddell Duke, *Allergy, Asthma, Hay Fever, Urticaria, and Allied Manifestations of Reaction* (London: Kimpton, 1925), 128; Albert H. Rowe and Albert Rowe

Jr., *Food Allergy: Its Manifestations and Control and the Elimination Diets, a Compendium with Important Consideration of Inhalant (Especially Pollen), Drug, and Infectant Allergy* (1931; Springfield, Ill.: Thomas, 1972).

37. Such tests fell out of favor when it emerged that certain blood-borne diseases, including hepatitis, could be transferred along with the sera. See Sheldon G. Cohen and Myrna Zelaya-Quesada, "Prausnitz and Küstner Phenomenon: The P-K Reaction," *JACI* 114 (2004): 705–10.

38. Frankland, "Carl Prausnitz," 702.

39. Arthur F. Coca and Ella F. Grove, "Studies in Hypersensitiveness XIII: A Study of the Atopic Reagins," *Journal of Immunology* 10 (1925): 445–64.

40. Silverstein, *History of Immunology*, 135.

41. Callen Black, "A Brief History of the Discovery of Immunoglobulins and the Origin of the Modern Immunoglobulin Nomenclature," *Immunology and Cell Biology* 75 (1997): 65–68.

42. Joseph F. Heremans, M. T. Heremans, and H. E. Schultze, "Isolation and Description of a Few Properties of ɣ2A-Globulin of Human Serum," *Clinica Chimica Acta* 4 (1959): 96–102; Thomas B. Tomasi Jr. et al., "Characteristics of an Immune System Common to Certain External Secretions," *Journal of Experimental Medicine* 121 (1965): 101–24; Thomas B. Tomasi, "The Discovery of Secretory IgA and the Mucosal Immune System," *Immunology Today* 13 (1992): 416–18; Bibel, *Milestones in Immunology*, 107; Silverstein, *History of Immunology*, 187.

43. Ishizaka, Ishizaka, and Hornbrook, "Physicochemical Properties of Reaginic Antibody," 75–85; Johansson and Bennich, "Immunological Studies," 381–89.

44. IgE was secretive partly because it is found in such low quantities in normal human serum. See H. Alice Orgel, "Genetic and Developmental Aspects of IgE," *Pediatric Clinics of North America* 22 (1975): 17–32.

45. Bibel, *Milestones in Immunology*, 107.

46. Ibid.

47. "Reagin and IgE," *Lancet* 291, no. 7552 (1968): 1131–32.

48. Bibel, *Milestones in Immunology*, 44.

49. R. S. Hogarth-Scott, S. G. Johansson, and H. Bennich, "Antibodies to *Toxocara* in the Sera of Visceral Larva Migrans Patients: The Significance of Raised Levels of IgE," *Clinical and Experimental Immunology* 5 (1969): 619–25; M. Ogawa et al., "Clinical Aspects of IgE Myeloma," *NEJM* 281 (1969): 1217–20; K. Ishizaka, H. Tomioka, and T. Ishizaka, "Mechanism of Passive Sensitization. I. Presence of IgE and IgG Molecules on Human Leukocytes," *Journal of Immunology* 105 (1970): 1459–67; K. Nilsson et al., "Established Immunoglobulin Producing Myeloma (IgE) and Lymphoblastoid (IgG) Cell Lines from an IgE Myeloma Patient," *Clinical and Experimental Immunology* 7 (1970): 477–89.

50. W. D. Mackay, "The Incidence of Allergic Disorders and Cancer," *British Journal of Cancer* 20 (1966): 434–37.

51. E. G. Martin, "Predisposing Factors and Diagnosis of Rectal Cancer: A Discussion of Allergy," *Annals of Surgery* 102 (1935): 56–61; J. Logan and D. Saker, "The Inci-

dence of Allergic Disorders in Cancer," *New Zealand Medical Journal* 52 (1953): 210–12; E. W. Fisherman, "Does the Allergic Diathesis Influence Malignancy?" *JACI* 31 (1960): 74–78; Mackay, "Incidence of Allergic Disorders"; Turner, "Epidemiology," 1493–510.

52. Manuel L. Penichet and Erika Jensen-Jarolim, eds., *Cancer and IgE: Introducing the Concept of AllergoOncology* (Totowa, N.J.: Humana Press, 2010).

53. B. M. Ogilvie, "Reagin-Like Antibodies in Animals Immune to Helminth Parasites," *Nature* 204 (1964): 91–92; Hogarth-Scott, Johansson, and Bennich, "Antibodies to *Toxocara*," 619–25; E. B. Rosenberg, S. H. Polmar, and G. E. Whalen, "Increased Circulating IgE in Trichinosis," *Annals of Internal Medicine* 75 (1971): 575–78.

54. R. G. Bell, "IgE, Allergies and Helminth Parasites: A New Perspective on an Old Conundrum," *Immunology and Cell Biology* 74 (1996): 337–45.

55. B. P. Bielory, T. Mainardi, and M. Rottem, "Evolutionary Immune Response to Conserved Domains in Parasites and Aeroallergens," *Allergy and Asthma Proceedings* 34 (2013): 93–102.

56. C. M. Fitzsimmons and D. W. Dunne, "Survival of the Fittest: Allergology or Parasitology?" *Trends in Parasitology* 25 (2009): 447–51; D. E. Elliott and J. V. Weinstock, "Where Are We on Worms?" *Current Opinion in Gastroenterology* 28 (2012): 551–56.

57. J. W. Gerrard, C. A. Geddes, et al., "Serum IgE Levels in White and Métis Communities in Saskatchewan," *Annals of Allergy* 37 (1976): 91–100.

58. N. R. Lynch, M. C. Di Prisco-Fuenmayor, and J. M. Soto, "Diagnosis of Atopic Conditions in the Tropics," *Annals of Allergy* 51 (1983): 547–51. Another article, which appeared to discuss IgE levels in conditions other than allergy, actually delved more into techniques for measuring it rather than what its presence actually meant: Douglas C. Heiner and Bram Rose, "Elevated Levels of Gamma-E (IgE) in Conditions Other Than Classic Allergy," *Journal of Allergy* 45 (1970): 30–42.

59. For instance, E. E. Jarrett and D. C. Stewart, "Potentiation of Rat Reaginic (IgE) Antibody by Helminth Infection," *Immunology* 23 (1972): 749–55; Biroum-Noerjasin, "Serum IgE Concentrations in Relation to Anti-Helminthic Treatment in a Javanese Population with Hookworm," *Clinical and Experimental Immunology* 13 (1973): 454–51; M. L. Ghosh, "Eosinophilia, Increased IgE Toxocariasis in Children," *Indian Journal of Pediatrics* 41 (1974): 11–14.

60. Ben F. Feingold mentioned that IgE must have a function in healthy individuals, but that it had not yet been demonstrated, in *Introduction to Clinical Allergy* (Springfield, Ill.: Thomas, 1973). 16. Given Feingold's breadth of immunological knowledge, it is surprising that he would not have mentioned the connections with helminths and cancer. The omission, whether due to ignorance or apathy, is likely representative of how other allergists understood the potentially broader role of IgE in healthy humans.

61. John W. Yunginger and Gerald J. Gleich, "The Impact of the Discovery of IgE on the Practice of Allergy," *Pediatric Clinics of North America* 22 (1975): 3–15; Leif Wide, "Clinical Significance of Measurement of Reaginic (IgE) Antibody by RAST," *Clini-*

cal Allergy 3 (1973): 583–95; Johansson, Bennich, and Wide, "Expanding the Scope of IgE, RAST," 314.

62. *In vivo* (within the living) tests are conducted on living organisms; *in vitro* (within the glass) tests are done in test tubes or under similar laboratory conditions. Since skin tests were conducted on patients, they were *in vivo* procedures.

63. Although total IgE tests have also been used in certain circumstances, a recent paper published by the American Academy of Allergy, Asthma and Immunology, outlining practice parameters on diagnosis, stated that they were only of "modest value" ("Allergy Diagnostic Testing: An Updated Practice Parameter," *Annals of Allergy, Asthma and Immunology* 100 [2008]: S10).

64. Yunginger and Gleich, "Impact of the Discovery of IgE," 8.

65. Ibid., 9–11.

66. Ibid., 12.

67. The pharmaceutical potential of IgE has also been discussed in Jackson, *Allergy*, 126; and Mitman, *Breathing Space*, 236–37.

68. Yunginger and Gleich, "Impact of the Discovery of IgE," 9.

69. William T. Knicker, "Is the Choice of Allergy Skin Testing Versus *In Vitro* Determination of Specific IgE No Longer a Scientific Issue?" *Annals of Allergy* 62 (1989): 373.

70. Ibid., 373–74.

71. The AAA changed its name to the AAAI in 1982, in part to emphasize the immunological nature of allergy. It then became the American Academy of Allergy, Asthma and Immunology (AAAAI) in 1995. I have attempted to use the abbreviation that would have been used during the time period described.

72. American Academy of Allergy and Immunology, "Position Statement of the Practice Standards Committee, Skin Testing and Radioallergosorbent Testing (RAST) for Diagnosis of Specific Allergens Responsible for IgE-Mediated Diseases," *JACI* 72 (1983): 515–17.

73. Knicker, "Choice of Allergy Skin Testing," 374.

74. RAST is still used, but it remains less sensitive than skin testing. The costs of such tests also continue to pose a challenge to both allergists and patients. Moreover, most allergy associations stress that any test must be interpreted in conjunction with a comprehensive account of the patient's history. See AAAAI, "Allergy Diagnostic Testing," S1-S148.

75. Susan J. Thorpe et al., "The Third International Standard for Serum IgE," World Health Organization, http://www.who.int/biologicals/BS_2220_Candidate_Preparation.pdf (accessed October 22, 2013).

76. Jackson, *Allergy*, 126.

77. J. W. Gerrard, D. C. Heiner, et al., "Immunoglobulin Levels in Smokers and Non-Smokers," *Annals of Allergy* 44 (1980): 261–63; B. Burrows et al, "The Relation of Serum Immunoglobulin E and Cigarette Smoking," *Annals of Allergy* 44 (1980): 523–25; R. Hällgren and L. Lundin, "Increased Total Serum IgE in Alcoholics," *Acta Medica Scandinavica* 213 (1983): 99–103.

78. Heiner and Rose, "Elevated Levels of Gamma-E (IgE)."

79. A. A. Sugarman, D. L. Southern, and J. F. Curran, "A Study of Antibody Levels in Alcoholic, Depressive, and Schizophrenic Patients," *Annals of Allergy* 48 (1982): 166–71.

80. Deborah A. Meyers and David G. Marsh, "Report on a National Institute of Allergy and Infectious Diseases–Sponsored Workshop on the Genetics of Total Immunoglobulin E Levels in Humans," *JACI* 67 (1981): 167–70.

81. A. W. Frankland, "Allergy: Immunity Gone Wrong," *Proceedings of the Royal Society of Medicine* 66 (1972): 1.

82. Ibid.

83. A. W. Frankland, "Some Observations on the RAST Test," *Annals of Allergy* 33 (1974): 105–6.

84. Frankland, "Allergy," 1.

85. John C. Selner to Leonard Bernstein, August 17, 1972, Box 361, Folder 9, American Academy of Allergy, Asthma and Immunology Records, 1923–2011, University of Wisconsin–Milwaukee Libraries, Archives Department.

86. Ibid. Although Selner was originally sympathetic to some of clinical ecology's tenets, he eventually determined, in collaboration with psychologist Herman Staudenmeyer, that the origin of many MCS sufferers' symptoms was childhood sexual abuse. See Peter Radetsky, *Allergic to the Twentieth Century: The Explosion in Environmental Allergies—From Sick Buildings to Multiple Chemical Sensitivity* (Boston: Little, Brown, 1997), 122–27.

87. William G. Crook, "Food Allergy: The Great Masquerader," *Pediatric Clinics of North America* 22 (1975): 227–38.

88. Crook's two camps of physicians resemble the dichotomy provided by Frederic Speer, "What Is Allergy?" *Annals of Allergy* 34 (1975): 49–50.

89. Crook, "Food Allergy," 235.

90. James E. Strain, "Biographical Sketches of the First Editorial Board and Those Who Have Edited *Pediatrics*," *Pediatrics* 102 (1998): 191–93; Charles D. May, "Food Allergy: A Commentary," *Pediatric Clinics of North America* 22 (1975): 217–20.

91. May, "Food Allergy: Commentary," 217–19; Charles D. May, "Food Allergy: Lessons from the Past," *JACI* 69 (1982): 255–59, and "Food Sensitivities: Facts and Fancies," *Nutrition Reviews* 42 (1984): 72–78; "Dr. Charles D. May, 84; Debunked Myth That Linked Asthma Food Allergies," *Boston Globe*, June 18, 1992.

92. May, "Food Allergy: Commentary," 219.

93. Wayne A. Lake, review of *Clinical Ecology*, by Lawrence D. Dickey, *Annals of Allergy* 37 (1976): 444.

94. William G. Crook, "To the Editor," *Annals of Allergy* 38 (1977): 285.

95. Theron G. Randolph, "Both Allergy and Clinical Ecology Are Needed," *Annals of Allergy* 39 (1977): 215–16.

96. Theron G. Randolph, *Environmental Medicine: Beginnings and Bibliographies of Clinical Ecology* (Fort Collins, Colo.: Clinical Ecology, 1987), 220.

97. Theron G. Randolph and R. W. Moss, *Allergies: Your Hidden Enemy* (Winnipeg: Turnstone Press, 1980), 11.

98. The AAAAI was even hesitant to have papers presented on food allergy at its annual conference, as letters in its archive indicate. See Box 361, Folder 9, AAAAI Records.

99. Minutes of the New Board of Regents of the American College of Allergists, April 8, 1981, Box 20, Folder 8, American College of Allergy, Asthma and Immunology Records, 1928–[ongoing], University of Wisconsin–Parkside Libraries, Archives Department.

100. Advisory Board of Allergy to American Boards for Medical Specialties and of Internal Medicine and Pediatrics [letter], undated, Box 432 Folder 1, AAAAI Records.

101. Ibid.

102. Randolph, "Allergy and Clinical Ecology," 215–16.

103. Randolph, *Environmental Medicine*, 214.

104. While it is difficult to estimate what Randolph charged, a similar unit in Dallas during the 1990s charged an outpatient $5,500 for lab work, skin testing, and office visits over a two-week period. Doris Rapp charged her patients $1,200 for three days' worth of testing. Blue Cross was unwilling to pay any of these costs incurred by one of Rapp's patients until the patient threatened legal action, according to Radetsky, *Allergic to the Twentieth Century*, 109–10.

105. Ibid. By the end of the year, financial problems would also result in the closure of ninety-nine-year-old Henrotin Hospital, which had been most famous for its expertise in treating gunshot injuries, as reported in Ron Kotulak, "Henrotin Hospital Closing Set," *Chicago Tribune*, October 2, 1986.

106. Douglas C. Heiner, "Sublingual Testing in the Diagnosis of Food Allergy," *Western Journal of Medicine* 121 (1974): 152; Food Allergy Committee of the American College of Allergists, "Final Report of the Food Allergy Committee of the American College of Allergists on the Clinical Evaluation of Sublingual Provocative Testing Method for Diagnosis of Food Allergy," *Annals of Allergy* 33 (1974): 164–66.

107. Oscar L. Frick to Roger Hirsch and Jordan Fink, December 29, 1977, Box 122, Folder 9, AAAAI Records; T. E. Van Metre Jr. et al., "A Controlled Study of the Effectiveness of the Rinkel Method of Immunotherapy for Ragweed Pollen Hay Fever," *JACI* 65 (1980): 288–97. A much more recent study, however, indicated that such sublingual desensitization might in fact be more effective than subcutaneous injections: D. D. Skoner et al., "Sublingual Immunotherapy in Patients with Allergic Rhinoconjunctivitis Caused by Ragweed Pollen," *JACI* 125 (2010): 660–66.

108. For more on changes in American attitudes to food during the 1960s, see Harvey A. Levenstein, *Paradox of Plenty: A Social History of Eating in Modern America* (New York: Oxford University Press, 1993); Warren J. Belasco, *Appetite for Change: How the Counterculture Took on the Food Industry*, 2nd ed. (Ithaca, N.Y.: Cornell University Press, 2007); and Matthew Smith, *An Alternative History of Hyperactivity: Food Additives, and the Feingold Diet* (New Brunswick, N.J.: Rutgers University Press, 2011), 68–86.

109. New York Metabolic Group, "The Foods You Love May Not Love You" [advertisement], *New York Times*, June 27, 1984, Box 361, Folder 1, AAAAI Records.

110. Rotary diversified diets, originally devised by Herbert Rinkel, were controversial regimens prescribed to patients based on the clinical ecological theory that food allergy was addictive; in other words, people were pathologically driven to eat foods to which they were allergic. In order to prevent this, patients were told to diversify their diet as much as possible and avoid eating the same food repeatedly. Extremely hypersensitive people had to undertake extreme measures to ensure this diversity, including eating exotic foods, such as kangaroo, elephant, and lion meat. The apparent eccentricity of such diets, however effective they may have been, did little for the reputation of clinical ecologists. Beatrice Trum Hunter, interview with author, December 8, 2007.

111. New York Metabolic Group, "Foods You Love May Not Love You."

112. National Allergy Clinics, "All Cytotoxic Labs Are Not Created Equal" [advertisement], *Wall Street Journal*, undated, Box 361, Folder 1, AAAAI Records (emphasis in original).

113. One advertisement for Dr. James Braly's Optimum Health Labs indicated that it charged $580 for a "Comprehensive Allergy and Nutrition Program." Individual services ranged from $9.50 for a "blood chemical test" to $395 for a "Food Immune Complex Assay" (Box 115, Folder 12, AAAAI Records).

114. Raymond G. Slavin to Donald McNeil, October 20, 1983; Raymond G. Slavin to Mike Whitney, July 15, 1983, both in Box 361, Folder 1, AAAAI Records. With respect to the *Women's Wear Daily* article, Slavin told McNeil that he "hadn't read anything in a long time that gives our position as succinctly. . . . When you see something like this in a reputable magazine it gives one a bit of hope about the future." McNeil replied to Slavin that "the story is but one of a continuing application of nails of truth to the coffin lid of clinical ecology" (Donald McNeil to Raymond G. Slavin, November 7, 1983, Box 361, Folder 1, AAAAI Records).

115. Macy I. Levin to Jordan N. Fink, December 5, 1984, Box 171, Folder 13, AAAAI Records.

116. Yehuda Barsel, "Identify and Treat Children's Allergies Early," *Jewish Times*, July 19, 1984, Box 361, Folder 1, AAAAI Records.

117. *Daily Register* (Shrewsbury, N.J.), July 6, 1982, A4.

118. "Disciplinary Actions: April 1, 1984 to September 30, 1984, Physicians and Surgeons," May 23, 1984, Box 361, Folder 1, AAAAI Records.

119. AAAAI, form letter, Box 361, Folder 1, AAAAI Records.

120. Quoted in Jeanie Wilson, "New Hope for the Allergic," *Town and Country*, August 1984, Box 361, Folder 1, AAAAI Records.

121. Helen Krause to Raymond G. Slavin, August 23, 1984; Jerome G. Goldstein to Raymond G. Slavin, August 24, 1983, both in Box 361, Folder 1, AAAAI Records. The AAO continues to be quite broadminded when it comes to food allergy. See American Academy of Otolaryngology–Head and Neck Surgery, "Fact Sheet: Pediatric Food Allergies," http://www.entnet.org/HealthInformation/pediatricFood Allergies.cfm (accessed October 28, 2012)

122. AAAAI correspondence, Box 122, Folder 8; Box 137, Folder 2; Box 361, Folders 9–11, AAAAI Records.

123. Donald McNeil to Grace Powers Monaco, December 1, 1983, Box 361, Folder 7, AAAAI Records.

124. Carol Barr, *International Allergy Workbook* (Captain Cook, Hawaii: Barr, 1986), Box 115, Folder 11, AAAAI Records.

125. Carol Barr to American Academy of Allergy and Immunology, undated, Box 115, Folder 11, AAAAI Records (emphasis in original).

126. Thomas E. Stenzel, International Food Information Council, to Donald McNeil, November 13, 1986, Box 221, Folder 11, AAAAI Records; "Allergies" [advertising supplement], *Time*, May 9, 1988. By 1991, the AAAI had reached its goal of earning more than $1 million in sponsorships from pharmaceutical companies, which went toward courses, fellowships, lectures, awards, and research, as well as catering, entertainment, and gaming at meetings. Although there were guidelines on such relationships, some allergists were not comfortable with them. See American Academy of Allergy and Immunology, "Policies Related to Support from Pharmaceutical Industries," memorandum, August 1991; and Jordan N. Fink to American Academy of Allergy and Immunology Executive Committee Members, memorandum, February 11, 1991, both in Box 253, Folder 6, AAAAI Records.

127. *William Rea, et al. v. American Academy of Allergies and Immunologies* [sic], Civil Action No. CA3-84-0219-R, United States District Court, Northern District of Texas, Dallas Division, 1984, Box 366, Folder 3, AAAAI Records.

128. Ibid. The court also determined that the number of clinical ecologists represented by the suit (3,000) and, by extension, the number of patients was unrealistic.

129. Ibid.

130. John E Salvaggio to Timothy J. Sullivan, February 12, 1986, Box 361, Folder 7, AAAAI Records.

131. Randolph, *Environmental Medicine*, 289; Jackson, *Allergy*, 201–3.

132. Anthony S. Fauci, "The Revolution in the Approach to Allergic and Immunologic Diseases," *Annals of Allergy* 55 (1985): 632–33.

SIX. THE PROBLEM WITH PEANUTS

1. Jean Mayer, "Better Labeling Laws Are Needed," *Pittsburgh Post-Gazette*, June 5, 1972, 12.

2. Quoted in ibid (emphasis in original).

3. Ibid.

4. Despite working with Frederick Stare, Mayer's approach to the issue of food additives and health was quite nuanced, as exemplified by his writing about the Feingold diet. See Matthew Smith, *An Alternative History of Hyperactivity: Food Additives, and the Feingold Diet* (New Brunswick, N.J.: Rutgers University Press, 2011), 82, 99–105. Some of Nader's and Hunter's work on food additives and labeling

can be found in James S. Turner, *The Chemical Feast: The Ralph Nader Study Group Report on Food Protection and the Food and Drug Administration* (New York: Grossman, 1970); and Beatrice Trum Hunter, *Beatrice Trum Hunter's Additives Book* (New Canaan, Conn.: Keats, 1972), and *The Mirage of Safety: Food Additives and Federal Policy* (Brattleboro, Vt.: Greene, 1975).

5. Mayer, "Better Labeling Laws Are Needed." Rosenthal lamented that the labeling requirements for pet food were more rigorous than that for human food, as reported in "Coalition Asks More Specific Ingredient Labeling for Food," *Daily Herald*, December 13, 1973.

6. In 1966, the Fair Packaging and Labeling Act had been passed, but this had more to do with ensuring that the volume of contents in any commodity, including foods, was accurately measured so that consumers could enough information to choose between products. The next major labeling legislation affecting food was the Nutrition Labeling and Education Act, which required the nutritional contents of most foods to be identified, but many food experts remain skeptical about its effectiveness. See Michele Simon, *Appetite for Profit: How the Food Industry Undermines Our Health and How to Fight Back* (New York: Nation Books, 2006); and Marion Nestle, *Food Politics: How the Food Industry Influences Nutrition and Health* (Berkeley: University of California Press, 2002).

7. Joseph H. Fries, "Peanuts: Allergic and Other Untoward Reactions," *Annals of Allergy* 48 (1982): 220–26.

8. Charles A. Hannigan to American Academy of Allergy, December 22, 1978, Box 137, Folder 2, American Academy of Allergy, Asthma and Immunology Records, 1923–2011, University of Wisconsin–Milwaukee Libraries, Archives Department. The Hollister-Stier Ana-kit was recalled in 1999 and 2009 due to ineffectiveness.

9. S. L. Taylor et al., "Peanut Oil Is Not Allergenic to Peanut-Sensitive Individuals," *JACI* 68 (1981): 372–75.

10. Gerald M. Sapers to American Academy of Allergy, March 14, 1972, Box 137, Folder 2, AAAAI Records.

11. Charles D. May, "Food Allergy: A Commentary," *Pediatric Clinics of North America* 22 (1975): 217–20, a rejoinder to William G. Crook, "Food Allergy: The Great Masquerader," *Pediatric Clinics of North America* 22 (1975): 227–38.

12. Charles D. May to Martin D. Valentine, August 21, 1978, Box 137, Folder 2; Charles D. May to Roberta Buckley, August 22, 1979, Box 443, Folder 10, both in AAAAI Records.

13. Some of these other foods will be discussed later in this chapter, but included in their number were milk, egg, wheat, seafood, soya, nuts, and wheat.

14. Andrew F. Smith, *Peanuts: The Illustrious History of the Goober Pea* (Champaign: University of Illinois Press, 2002), 6.

15. B. W. Higman, *How Food Made History* (Oxford: Wiley-Blackwell, 2012), 41.

16. Jon Krampner, *Creamy and Crunchy: An Informal History of Peanut Butter, the All-American Food* (New York: Columbia University Press, 2013), 4.

17. Smith, *Peanuts*, 20–21. The musicians who have recorded or performed versions of "Eating Goober Peas" include Burl Ives, Johnny Cash, the Kingston Trio, and Elton John.

18. Krampner, *Creamy and Crunchy*, 14–16.

19. Kara Newman, *The Secret Financial Life of Food: From Commodities Markets to Supermarkets* (New York: Columbia University Press, 2013), 141.

20. One of the first places Americans had peanut butter was at the Louisiana Purchase Exposition, or St. Louis World's Fair, in 1904, along with equally all-American hot dogs, hamburgers, and ice-cream cones, according to Krampner, *Creamy and Crunchy*, 26–38.

21. Smith, *Peanuts*, 35.

22. Krampner, *Creamy and Crunchy*, 44–45.

23. Smith, *Peanuts*, 126–29.

24. Krampner, *Creamy and Crunchy*, 57.

25. Apart from Canada, the Netherlands, Australia, Haiti, and a small number of other countries that have their own peanut butter traditions, most peanut butter consumed outside the United States is eaten by American ex-pats. Interestingly, the oldest peanut butter brand is not American but Australian, first produced in 1898 by Edward Halsey, a Seventh-Day Adventist who had worked with John Harvey Kellogg. See ibid., 125, 127–92.

26. Ibid., 163.

27. Ibid., 166–71.

28. R. N. Adsule, K. M. Lawande, and S. S. Kadam, "Peanuts," in *Handbook of World Food Legumes*, ed. D. K. Salunkhe and S. S. Kadam (Boca Raton, Fla.: CRC Press, 1989), 2:193–214; National Peanut Council of America, *Peanuts: The Inside Story* (Alexandria, Va.: National Peanut Council of America, 1993).

29. Peanuts also have many nonfood applications, being used in paints, polishes, textiles, insecticides, fertilizers, creams, shampoos, soaps, oils, and vaccines, some of which have been implicated in the emergence of peanut allergy. The African American scientist George Washington Carver (1864–1943) is said to have invented more than a hundred uses for the peanut, though these claims have been contested. See George Washington Carver, *How to Grow the Peanut and 105 Ways of Preparing It for Human Consumption*, 7th ed. (Tuskegee, Ala.: Tuskegee Institute Press, 1940); and Krampner, *Creamy and Crunchy*, 39–43.

30. Adsule, Lawande, and Kadam, "Peanuts," 193; Krampner, *Creamy and Crunchy*, 210–19.

31. Suzanne White Junod, "The Rise and Fall of Federal Food Standards in the United States: The Case of the Peanut Butter and Jelly Sandwich," in *The Food and Drug Administration*, ed. Meredith A. Hickman (Hauppauge, N.Y.: Nova Science, 2003), 35–48.

32. Krampner, *Creamy and Crunchy*, 63–68, 175–79, 199–209.

33. Eleven proteins found in peanuts have been found to be allergenic. See J. E. Knoll et al., "TILLING for Allergen Reduction and Improvement of Quality Traits in Peanut (Arachis Hypogaea L.)," *BMC Plant Biology* 11 (2011): 81–99.
34. S. F. Kemp and R. F. Lockey, "Peanut Anaphylaxis from Food Cross-Contamination," *JAMA* 275 (1996): 1636–37.
35. M. U. Keating et al., "Immunoassay of Peanut Allergens in Food-Processing Materials and Finished Foods," *JACI* 86 (1990): 41–44.
36. A. W. Frankland and R. S. H. Pumphrey, "Acute Allergic Reactions to Foods and Crossreactivity Between Foods," in *Food Allergy and Intolerance*, ed. Jonathan Brostoff and Stephen J. Challacombe, 2nd ed. (London: Saunders, 2002), 413–23.
37. Ibid., 416.
38. Joseph H. Fries, "Food Faddism—the Dilemma of Diet," *Annals of Allergy* 39 (1977): 288–89, and "Chocolate: A Review of Published Reports of Allergic and Other Deleterious Effects, Real or Presumed," *Annals of Allergy* 41 (1978): 195–207.
39. Joseph H. Fries, "Studies on the Allergenicity of the Soy Bean," *Annals of Allergy* 29 (1971): 1–7, and "Food Allergy—Current Concerns," *Annals of Allergy* 46 (1981): 260–63.
40. Fries, "Peanuts," 220.
41. Ibid.
42. Bret Ratner, quoted in Fries, "Peanuts," 226.
43. The number of American peanut farmers dropped by 50 percent, due to land costs, conglomeration of agribusinesses, and foreign competition, according to Smith, *Peanuts*, 121.
44. The Danish political drama *Borgen* recently had a plotline in which a character suffered an allergic reaction to penicillin after eating pork contaminated with antibiotics.
45. Harold M. Schmeck Jr., "Doctors Seek Keys to Body's Defenses," *New York Times*, December 29, 1972.
46. Ben F. Feingold, *Introduction to Clinical Allergy* (Springfield, Ill: Thomas, 1973), 149.
47. D. Barnett, B. A. Baldo, and M. E. Howden, "Multiplicity of Allergens in Peanuts," *JACI* 58 (1983): 61–68; A. S. Kemp et al., "Skin Test, RAST, and Clinical Reactions to Peanut Allergens in Children," *Clinical Allergy* 1 (1985): 73–78; J. W. Gerrard and L. Perelmutter, "IgE-Mediated Allergy to Peanut, Cow's-Milk, and Egg in Children with Special Reference to Maternal Diet," *Annals of Allergy* 56 (1986): 351–54.
48. Susan Evans, Danna Skea, and Jerry Dolovich, "Fatal Reaction to Peanut Antigen in Almond Icing," *CMAJ* 139 (1988): 231–32.
49. J. Michael White, "Fatal Food Allergy," *CMAJ* 139 (1988): 8. A more recent piece of Ontario legislation tackling anaphylactic food allergy is "Sabrina's Law" (2005), which requires schools to establish prevention and contingency plans for allergic students. See Legislative Assembly of Ontario, 38:1 Bill 3, Sabrina's Law (2005), http://www.ontla.on.ca/web/bills/bills_detail.do?locale=en&BillID=135&isCurrent=false&ParlSessionID=38:1 (accessed August 8, 2014).

50. J. W. Yunginger et al., "Fatal Food-Induced Anaphylaxis," *JAMA* 260 (1988): 1450–52.
51. Ibid., 1451.
52. Guy A. Settipane, "Anaphylactic Deaths in Asthmatic Patients," *Allergy Proceedings* 10 (1989): 271–74; Hugh A. Sampson, Louis Mendelson, and James A. Rosen, "Fatal and Near-Fatal Anaphylactic Reactions to Food in Children and Adolescents," *NEJM* 327 (1992): 380–84.
53. Sampson, Mendelson, and Rosen, "Fatal and Near-Fatal Anaphylactic Reactions," 383.
54. Ibid., 384.
55. Timothy J. Sullivan to William A. Pierson, March 20, 1991, Box 668, Folder 7, AAAAI Records.
56. Ibid.
57. The AAAAI was nudged into action in other ways as well. A 1994 letter in the AAAAI archive from a law office, for instance, encouraged it to investigate peanut allergy more thoroughly following the death of a woman who unknowingly ate peanuts contained in pesto served at a restaurant in New Hampshire. Although the letter made no mention of litigation, the looming possibility of legal action in cases of accidental anaphylaxis also spurred orthodox allergists to consider food allergies more seriously. See Richard C. Bardi to Donald L. McNeil, February 24, 1994, Box 668, Folder 7, AAAAI Records.
58. Quoted in William R. Greer, "Warnings on Food Allergies," *New York Times*, March 29, 1986.
59. As quotations from previous chapters demonstrate, food allergists and clinical ecologists were not hesitant to provide vibrant, often impassioned descriptions of the tribulations faced by their patients. Orthodox allergists, particularly by the 1980s, were less willing to do so and tended to present their "data" in the dry, detached manner adopted by many other medical disciplines. This shift from colorful case studies to terse, economical reviews is also marked in psychiatry during the same period, as literature dominated by psychoanalysts was replaced by that of biological psychiatrists. See Matthew Smith, "Psychiatry Limited: Hyperactivity and the Evolution of American Psychiatry," *Social History of Medicine* 21 (2008): 541–59.
60. Here I focus on FAN; Mark Jackson has discussed the AC in *Allergy: The History of a Modern Malady* (London: Reaktion, 2006).
61. Anne Muñoz-Furlong's other daughter developed an anaphylactic allergy to seafood in her early thirties. Anne Muñoz-Furlong, interview with author, October 9, 2010.
62. Jackson, *Allergy*, 146, 190–91; Muñoz-Furlong interview; for information on David Reading, see Anaphylaxis Campaign: Supporting People with Severe Allergies, http://www.anaphylaxis.org.uk/about-us/our-vice-president (accessed September 22, 2014).
63. Muñoz-Furlong interview.

64. Ibid. Parents' struggles with attaining helpful advice are well documented in Rima D. Apple, *Perfect Motherhood: Science and Childrearing in America* (New Brunswick, N.J.: Rutgers University Press, 2006).

65. In my previous work on food additives and hyperactivity, many parents interviewed described struggling to find support from friends and family. This is one of the reasons they turned instead to support groups, as discussed in Smith, *Alternative History of Hyperactivity*, 131–52.

66. Muñoz-Furlong interview.

67. "How to Read a Label for a Peanut-Free Diet," Box 216, Folder 1, AAAAI Records.

68. Muñoz-Furlong interview.

69. Anne Muñoz-Furlong, "Final Report," August 6, 1996, Box 216, Folder 1, AAAAI Records.

70. Anne Muñoz-Furlong and A. Wesley Burks, *Food Allergy and Atopic Dermatitis* (Fairfax, Va.: Food Allergy Network, 1992); Anne Muñoz-Furlong and Robert S. Zeiger, *Off to School with Food Allergies* (Fairfax, Va.: Food Allergy Network, 1992).

71. Harvey A. Levenstein, *Paradox of Plenty: A Social History of Eating in Modern America* (New York: Oxford University Press, 1993), 112; Smith, *Alternative History of Hyperactivity*, 70.

72. Related Industries Committee, correspondence, Box 253, Folder 6, AAAAI Records.

73. Jordan N. Fink to John A. Anderson, June 19, 1990, Box 253, Folder 6, AAAAI Records. An earlier letter by Fink suggested that the AAAAI "solicit" companies outside the United States as well.

74. Andrew Purvis, "Just What the Patient Ordered," *Time*, May 28, 1990, 42.

75. Lisa A. Bero, Alison Galbraith, and Drummond Rennie, "The Publication of Sponsored Symposiums in Medical Journals," *NEJM* 327 (1992): 1135–40.

76. Jordan N. Fink to American Academy of Allergy and Immunology Executive Committee Members, memorandum, February 11, 1991, Box 253, Folder 6, AAAAI Records. To give an example of what such funding provided, a 1994 letter from AAAI to potential sponsors cited that for $85,000, companies could host their Sunday evening symposia; the Wednesday afternoon symposia was a bargain at $60,000. See AAAI, form letter, 1994, Box 253, Folder 7, AAAAI Records.

77. Jackson, *Allergy*, 103–47; Gregg Mitman, *Breathing Space: How Allergies Shape Our Lives and Landscapes* (New Haven, Conn.: Yale University Press, 2007), 206–50.

78. "Adrenaline Epipens for Anaphylactic Shock to 'Expire,'" BBC News, December 10, 2009, http://news.bbc.co.uk/1/hi/health/8404536.stm (accessed November 21, 2013).

79. "President Signs Epinephrine Incentive Bill," News 4 San Antonio, November 14, 2013, http://news4sanantonio.com/news/features/top-stories/stories/president-signs-epinephrine-incentive-bill-5724.shtml (accessed November 21, 2013).

80. AAAI to IFIC, July 1, 1992, Box 221, Folder 12, AAAAI Records.

81. International Food Information Council Foundation, Food Insight: Your Nutrition and Food Safely Resource, http://www.foodinsight.org/Content/6/FINAL_Understanding-Food-Allergy_5-22-07.pdf.

82. Muñoz-Furlong interview.

83. Elliot F. Ellis to Joseph J. Lotharius, May 30, 1986, Box 366, Folder 6, AAAAI Records.

84. National Restaurant Association, *What You Need to Know About Allergies* (Washington, D.C.: National Restaurant Association, undated), Box 514, Folder 1, AAAAI Records.

85. Food allergy awareness is now part of the curriculum in many cooking schools, according to Giorgio Locatelli, interview with author, October 15, 2010.

86. Ian Mosby, "'That Won-Ton Soup Headache': The Chinese Restaurant Syndrome, MSG, and the Making of American Food, 1968–1980," *Social History of Medicine* 22 (2009): 133–51.

87. Food Allergy and Anaphylaxis Network, "Sarah Weaver, Allergic to Peanuts," Box 116, Folder 2, AAAAI Records.

88. Muñoz-Furlong interview.

89. Scott H. Sicherer et al., "A Voluntary Registry for Peanut and Tree Nut Allergy: Characteristics of the First 5149 Registrants," *JACI* 108 (2001): 128–32.

90. S. Allan Bock, Anne Muñoz-Furlong, and Hugh A. Sampson, "Fatalities Due to Anaphylactic Reactions Due to Foods," *JACI* 107 (2001): 191–93.

91. Gwen Smith and Karen Eck, "Teen Food Allergy Deaths: Lessons from Tragedy," *Allergic Living*, Summer 2006, http://allergicliving.com/index.php/2010/07/02/food-allergy-teen-tragedies (accessed November 26, 2013). See also Clive Seale, *Media and Health* (London: Sage, 2002).

92. Donald M. Arnold at al., "Passive Transfer of Peanut Hypersensitivity from Fresh Frozen Plasma," *Archives of Internal Medicine* 167 (2010): 853–54.

93. Smith, *Peanuts*, 124.

94. Airlines were among the first to institute a peanut ban, possibly given their early action on smoking and the risk of inhalant peanut allergy.

95. Nsikan Akpan, "Goldendoodle Sniffs Out Peanuts to Protect Seven-Year-Old Girl, Meghan Weingarth, from a Deadly Nut Allergy," *Medical Daily*, August 9, 2013, http://www.medicaldaily.com/goldendoodle-sniffs-out-peanuts-protect-7-year-old-girl-meghan-weingarth-deadly-nut-allergy-250095 (accessed November 26, 2013).

96. Eyal Shemesh et al., "Child and Parental Reports of Bullying in a Consecutive Sample of Children with Food Allergy," *Pediatrics* 131 (2013): e10–e17.

97. "Teenage Bully Pushes the Limit at Lunch," news.com.au, June 14, 2006, http://www.childfoodallergy.com/archives/2006/06/teenage_bully_p.html (accessed November 26, 2013).

98. Peter Jackson, "The Peanut Detectives," BBC News, February 24, 2009, November 2, 2013, http://news.bbc.co.uk/1/hi/uk/7868115.stm (accessed November 2, 2013).

99. Ibid.

100. Nicholas A. Christakis, "This Allergies Hysteria Is Just Nuts," *BMJ* 337 (2008): 1384.

101. Ibid. Other social scientists have described such reactions using softer language, such as "moral regulation" as opposed to "moral panic," explaining the phenom-

enon as part of Ulrich Beck's argument that the Western world increasingly con-
ceptualizes itself as a "risk society," which is filled with hidden environmental
threats that fuel uncertainty and promote a "risk management culture" (*World
Risk Society* [Malden, Mass.: Polity Press, 1999]). See also Trevor Rous and Alan
Hunt, "Governing Peanuts: The Regulation of the Social Bodies of Children and
the Risks of Food Allergies," *Social Science and Medicine* 58 (2004): 825–36.

102. Muñoz-Furlong interview.

103. Krampner *Creamy and Crunchy*; Smith, *Peanuts*, 133.

104. Frankland and Pumphrey, "Acute Allergic Reactions," 419.

105. Centers for Disease Control and Prevention, *Asthma Facts* (Atlanta: U.S. Department of Health and Human Services, Centers for Disease Control and Prevention,
2013), http://www.cdc.gov/asthma/pdfs/asthma_facts_program_grantees.pdf
(accessed November 27, 2013).

106. Mitman, *Breathing Space*.

107. Smith, *Alternative History of Hyperactivity*.

108. Michael C. Young, Anne Muñoz-Furlong, and Scott H. Sicherer, "Management of
Food Allergies in Schools: A Perspective for Allergists," *JACI* 124 (2009): 175–82.

109. Among the strategies outlined by FARE to tackle the question in the future were
using animal models more effectively, creating a food allergy biorepository, and
encouraging more scientists to study the problem, as outlined in *A Vision and Plan
for Food Allergy Research* (McLean, Va.: FARE, 2013), http://www.foodallergy.org/
document.doc?id=250 (accessed November 27, 2013).

110. Dry roasting, which uses higher temperatures, apparently increases the allergenic property (Ara h 1) of peanut proteins, whereas frying or boiling peanuts
seems to reduce the allergenicity of peanuts. A case study found that

> the protein fractions of . . . peanuts were altered to a similar degree by frying or boil-
> ing. Compared with roasted peanuts, the relative amount of Ara h 1 was reduced in
> the fried and boiled preparations, resulting in a significant reduction of IgE-binding
> intensity. In addition, there was significantly less IgE binding to Ara h 2 and Ara h 3 in
> fried and boiled peanuts compared with that in roasted peanuts. (K. Beyer, E. Morrow,
> X.-M. Li, L. Bardina, G. A. Bannon, A. W. Burks, and H. A. Sampson, "Effects of Cooking
> Methods on Peanut Allerginicity," *JACI* 107 [2001]: 1077)

111. W. Ray Shannon, "Demonstration of Food Proteins in Human Breast Milk by
Anaphylactic Experiments in Guinea Pigs," *American Journal of Diseases of Childhood* 22 (1921): 223–31.

112. Food Standards Agency, "Peanuts During Pregnancy, Breastfeeding and Early
Childhood," August 24, 2009, http://www.food.gov.uk/policy-advice/allergyintol/
peanutspregnancy#.UpXxmdK-0yo (accessed November 27, 2013).

113. A. DesRoches et al., "Peanut Allergy: Is Maternal Transmission of Antigens
During Pregnancy and Breastfeeding a Risk Factor?" *Journal of Investigative Allergology and Clinical Immunology* 20 (2010): 289–94.

114. Ekaterina Maslova et al., "Peanut and Tree Nut Consumption During Pregnancy and Allergic Disease in Children—Should Mothers Decrease Their Intake? Longitudinal Evidence from the Danish National Birth Cohort," *JACI* 130 (2012): 724–32.

115. Gideon Lack et al., "Factors Associated with the Development of Peanut Allergy in Childhood," *NEJM* 348 (2003): 977–85.

116. Joanne M. Duncan and Malcolm R. Sears, "Breastfeeding and Allergies: Time for a Change in Paradigm?" *Current Opinion in Allergy and Clinical Immunology* 8 (2008): 398–405.

117. D. Strachan, "Hay Fever, Hygiene and Household Size," *BMJ* 299 (1989): 1259–60.

118. Charles E. Rosenberg, "Pathologies of Progress: The Idea of Civilization at Risk," *Bulletin of the History of Medicine* 72 (1998): 714–30.

119. Heather Fraser, *The Peanut Allergy Epidemic: What's Causing It and How to Stop It* (New York: Skyhorse, 2011).

120. Ibid., 92–94.

121. Ibid., 100–101.

122. The death of Michael Gryzbinski in 1972, discussed at the beginning of this chapter, is the only example I have come across.

123. Fraser, *Peanut Allergy Epidemic*, 107.

124. Ibid., 122–29.

125. Chloe Silverman, *Understanding Autism: Parents, Doctors, and the Understanding of a Disorder* (Princeton, N.J.: Princeton University Press, 2013), 197–228; Emily Underwood, "Gut Microbes Linked to Autism-Like Symptoms in Mice," *Science Now*, December 5, 2013, http://news.sciencemag.org/biology/2013/12/gut-microbes-linked-autismlike-symptoms-mice (accessed December 11, 2013).

126. There are fewer than a handful of exceptions, and most concern peanut oil found in topical medications, some ironically for eczema, rather than vaccines. See J. Ring and M. Möhrenschlager, "Allergy to Peanut Oil—Clinically Relevant?" *Journal of the European Academy of Dermatology and Venereology* 21 (2007): 452–55; and Viktoria Dixon, Shaymau Habeeb, and Raman Lakshman, "Did You Know This Medicine Has Peanut Butter in It, Doctor?" *Archives of Disease in Childhood* 92 (2007): 654.

127. Phil Liebermann, "Is Peanut Antigen in Vaccines," American Academy of Allergy, Asthma and Immunology, Ask the Expert, http://www.aaaai.org/ask-the-expert/peanut-antigen-in-vaccines.aspx (accessed November 28, 2013).

128. A. T. Clark et al., "Successful Oral Tolerance Induction in Severe Peanut Allergy," *Allergy* 64 (2009): 1218–20.

129. Aziz Shiekh, "Oral Immunotherapy for Peanut Allergy," *BMJ* 341 (2010): 264; American Academy of Allergy, Asthma and Immunology, "Swish or Swallow: Comparing Oral and Sublingual Immunotherapy for Peanut Allergy," March 26, 2013, http://www.aaaai.org/global/latest-research-summaries/Current-JACI-Research/oral-sublingual-immunotherapy-peanut-allergy.aspx (accessed December 2, 2013); Hugh A. Sampson, "Peanut Oral Immunotherapy: Is It Ready for Clinical Practice?" *JACI: In Practice* 1 (2013): 15–21.

CONCLUSION

1. Richard A. Cone and Emily Martin, "Corporeal Flows: The Immune System, Global Economies of Food, and Implications for Health," *Ecologist* 27 (1997): 107–11.
2. Michael Mikulak argues that large organic food multinationals are particularly guilty of exploiting individuals' efforts to purchase environmentally friendly and healthy food products that, in reality, do little to address the food crisis facing the planet, in *The Politics of the Pantry: Stories, Food, and Social Change* (Montreal: McGill-Queen's University Press, 2013).
3. Nancy N. Chen, *Food, Medicine, and the Quest for Good Health* (New York: Columbia University Press, 2009).
4. Gyorgy Scrinis, *Nutritionism: The Science and Politics of Dietary Advice* (New York: Columbia University Press, 2013).
5. Thomas Kuhn, *The Structure of Scientific Revolutions* (Chicago: University of Chicago Press, 1962).
6. Matthew Smith, "Psychiatry Limited: Hyperactivity and the Evolution of American Psychiatry," *Social History of Medicine* 21 (2008): 541–59.
7. Mark Jackson, *Allergy: The History of a Modern Malady* (London: Reaktion, 2006), 216–20.

Bibliography

ARCHIVAL SOURCES

American Academy of Allergy, Asthma and Immunology Records, 1923–2011. University of Wisconsin–Milwaukee Libraries, Archives Department.

American College of Allergy, Asthma and Immunology Records, 1928–[ongoing]. University of Wisconsin–Parkside Libraries, Archives Department.

Beatrice Trum Hunter Collection, Howard Gotlieb Archival Research Center, Boston University.

Theron G. Randolph Papers, 1935–1991, H MS c183. Harvard Medical Library in the Francis A. Countway Library of Medicine, Center for the History of Medicine, Boston.

PUBLISHED SOURCES

Abramson, Harold A. "The Present Status of Allergy." *Nervous Child* 7 (1948): 86–101.

——. "Psychosomatic Aspects of Hay Fever and Asthma Prior to 1900." *Annals of Allergy* 6 (1948): 110–21.

"Adrenaline Epipens for Anaphylactic Shock to 'Expire.'" BBC News, December 10, 2009. http://news.bbc.co.uk/1/hi/health/8404536.stm. Accessed November 21, 2013.

Adsule, R. N., K. M. Lawande, and S. S. Kadam. "Peanuts." In *Handbook of World Food Legumes*, edited by D. K. Salunkhe and S. S. Kadam, 2:193–214. Boca Raton, Fla.: CRC Press, 1989.

Akpan, Nsikan. "Goldendoodle Sniffs Out Peanuts to Protect Seven-Year-Old Girl, Meghan Weingarth, from a Deadly Nut Allergy." *Medical Daily*, August 9, 2013.

http://www.medicaldaily.com/goldendoodle-sniffs-out-peanuts-protect-7-year-old-girl-meghan-weingarth-deadly-nut-allergy-250095. Accessed November 26, 2013.

Albala, Ken. *Eating Right in the Renaissance*. Berkeley: University of California Press, 2003.

Alvarez, Walter C. "Foreword." In *You Can't Eat That! A Manual and Recipe Book for Those Who Suffer Either Acutely or Mildly (And Perhaps Unconsciously) from Food Allergy*, by Helen Morgan. New York: Harcourt, Brace, 1939.

——. *Incurable Physician: An Autobiography*. Kingswood: World's Work, 1963.

——. "The Production of Food Allergy." *Gastroenterology* 30 (1956): 325–26.

——. "Puzzling Nervous Storms Due to Food Allergy." *Gastroenterology* 7 (1946): 241–52.

American Academy of Allergy, Asthma and Immunology. "Allergy Diagnostic Testing: An Updated Practice Parameter." *Annals of Allergy Asthma, and Immunology* 100 (2008): S10.

——. "Allergy Statistics." http://www.aaaai.org/about-the-aaaai/newsroom/allergy -statistics.aspx#Food_Allergy. Accessed March 4, 2012.

——. "Swish or Swallow: Comparing Oral and Sublingual Immunotherapy for Peanut Allergy." March 26, 2013. http://www.aaaai.org/global/latest-research-summaries /Current-JACI-Research/oral-sublingual-immunotherapy-peanut-allergy.aspx. Accessed December 2, 2013.

American Academy of Allergy and Immunology. "Position Statement of the Practice Standards Committee, The American Academy of Allergy and Immunology: Skin Testing and Radioallergosorbent Testing (RAST) for Diagnosis of Specific Allergens Responsible for IgE-Mediated Diseases." *JACI* 72 (1983): 515–17.

American Academy of Otolaryngology–Head and Neck Surgery. "Fact Sheet: Pediatric Food Allergies." http://www.entnet.org/HealthInformation/pediatricFood Allergies.cfm. Accessed October 28, 2013.

American Almanac and Repository of Useful Knowledge. 2nd ed. Boston: Bowen, 1833.

[American Association of Immunologists.] "The Founding of *The Journal of Immunology*." http://www.aai.org/about/History/Articles/AAI_History_001.pdf. Accessed August 22, 2013.

American College of Allergy, Asthma and Immunology. "Food Allergies." http://www .acaai.org/allergist/allergies/Types/food-allergies/Pages/default.aspx. Accessed March 7, 2012.

Anderson, McCall. "A Lecture on Nettle Rash." *BMJ* 1197 (1883): 1107–9.

Anderson, Warwick, Myles Jackson, and Barbara Gutmann Rosenkrantz. "Toward an Unnatural History of Immunology." *Journal of the History of Biology* 27 (1994): 575–94.

Apple, Rima D. *Perfect Motherhood: Science and Childrearing in America*. New Brunswick, N.J.: Rutgers University Press, 2006.

——. *Vitamania: Vitamins in American Culture*. New Brunswick, N.J.: Rutgers University Press, 1996.

Arnold, Donald M., Morris A. Blajchman, Julie DiTomasso, Myron Kulczycki, and Paul K. Keith. "Passive Transfer of Peanut Hypersensitivity from Fresh Frozen Plasma." *Archives of Internal Medicine* 167 (2010): 853–54.

Baer, Rudolph L. "Correspondence." *Journal of Allergy* 27 (1956): 483–84.

Bahna, Sami L., and Douglas C. Heiner. *Allergies to Milk*. New York: Grune and Stratton, 1980.

Baldwin, Horace S., and W. C. Spain. "Editorial." *Journal of Allergy* 20 (1949): 388–90.

"Banning Nuts at a Local Stadium?" June 5, 2006. Parenting a Child with a Food Allergy. http://www.childfoodallergy.com/archives/2006/06/banning_nuts_at.html. Accessed March 10, 2012.

Barnett, D., B. A. Baldo, and M. E. Howden. "Multiplicity of Allergens in Peanuts." *JACI* 58 (1983): 61–68.

Bateman, B., J. O. Warner, E. Hutchinson, T. Dean, P. Rowlandson, C. Grant, J. Grundy, C. Fitzgerald, and J. Stephenson. "The Effects of a Double-Blind, Placebo Controlled, Artificial Food Colourings and Benzoate Preservative Challenge on Hyperactivity in a General Population Sample of Preschool Children." *Archives of Disease in Childhood* 89 (2004): 506–11.

Baumhauer, J. H. "Allergy in Children with Particular Reference to Food Idiosyncrasy; Report of Cases." *Journal of the Medical Association of Alabama* 2 (1932): 195–202.

Beck, Ulrich. *World Risk Society*. Malden, Mass.: Polity Press, 1999.

Becker, Robert, and Meg McSherry Breslin. "Banker Gives $75 Million to NU." *Chicago Tribune*, February 14, 2002. http://articles.chicagotribune.com/2002-02-14/news/0202140008_1_medical-school-nu-bessie-feinberg-foundation. Accessed September 25, 2013.

Belasco, Warren J. *Appetite for Change: How the Counterculture Took on the Food Industry*. 2nd ed. Ithaca, N.Y.: Cornell University Press, 2007.

Bell, R. G. "IgE, Allergies and Helminth Parasites: A New Perspective on an Old Conundrum." *Immunology and Cell Biology* 74 (1996): 337–45.

Berg, T., H. Bennich, and S. G. Johansson. "In Vitro Diagnosis of Atopic Allergy. I. A Comparison of Provocation Tests and the Radioallergosorbent Test." *International Archives of Allergy and Applied Immunology* 40 (1971): 770–78.

Bero, Lisa A., Alison Galbraith, and Drummond Rennie. "The Publication of Sponsored Symposiums in Medical Journals." *NEJM* 327 (1992): 1135–40.

Besredka, Alexandre. *Anaphylaxis and Anti-Anaphylaxis and Their Experimental Foundations*. Edited by S. Roodhouse Gloyne. London: Heinemann, 1919.

——. "Du mécanisme de l'anaphylaxie vis-à-vis sérum de cheval." *Annales de l'Institute Pasteur* 4 (1908): 496–508.

——. *L'histoire d' une idée*. Paris: Masson, 1921.

Beyer, K., E. Morrow, X.-M. Li, L. Bardina, G. A. Bannon, A. W. Burks, and H. A. Sampson. "Effects of Cooking Methods on Peanut Allerginicity." *JACI* 107, no. 6 (2001): 1077–81.

Bibel, Debra Jan. *Milestones in Immunology: A Historical Exploration*. Madison, Wis.: Science Tech, 1988.

Bielory, B. P., T. Mainardi, and M. Rottem. "Evolutionary Immune Response to Conserved Domains in Parasites and Aeroallergens." *Allergy and Asthma Proceedings* 34 (2013): 93–102.

Biroum-Noerjasin. "Serum IgE Concentrations in Relation to Anti-Helminthic Treatment in a Javanese Population with Hookworm." *Clinical and Experimental Immunology* 13 (1973): 454–51.

Black, Callen. "A Brief History of the Discovery of Immunoglobulins and the Origin of the Modern Immunoglobulin Nomenclature." *Immunology and Cell Biology* 75 (1997): 65–68.

Blank, Charles H. "The Delaney Clause: Technical Naïveté and Scientific Advocacy in the Formulation of Public Health Policies." *California Law Review* 62 (1974): 1084–120.

Blom, Ida. *Medicine, Morality and Political Culture: Legislation and Venereal Disease.* Lund: Nordic Academic Press, 2012.

Bock, S. Allan, Anne Muñoz-Furlong, and Hugh A. Sampson. "Fatalities Due to Anaphylactic Reactions Due to Foods." *JACI* 107 (2001): 191–93.

Boden, Stephen R., and A. Wesley Burks. "Anaphylaxis: A History with Emphasis on Food Allergy." *Immunological Reviews* 242 (2011): 247–57.

"Book Notices." *JAMA* 113 (1939): 446.

Bottini, N., M. P. Ronchetti, F. Gloria-Bottini, and L. Fontana. "Malaria as a Possible Evolutionary Cause for Allergy." *Allergy* 54 (1999): 188–89.

Brady, William. "Health Talk: Eczema." *Ogden (Utah) Standard*, March 17, 1917.

Brander, Michael. *Eve Balfour: Founder of the Soil Association and Voice of the Organic Movement: A Biography.* Haddington: Glenneil Press, 2003.

Branum, Amy M., and Susan L. Lukacs. "Food Allergy Among U.S. Children: Trends in Prevalence and Hospitalizations." National Center for Health Statistics Data Brief, no. 10 (2008). http://www.cdc.gov/nchs/data/databriefs/db10.pdf. Accessed March 1, 2012.

Bree, Robert. *A Practical Inquiry into Disordered Respiration.* Birmingham: Swinney and Hawkins, 1800.

Brostoff, Jonathan, and Stephen J. Challacombe, eds. *Food Allergy and Intolerance.* 2nd ed. London: Saunders, 2002.

Brown, E. A., and G. P. Wadsworth. "The Leucopenic Index." *Journal of Allergy* 9 (1938): 345–70.

Brown, Ethan Allan. "American Academy of Allergy: The Changing Picture of Allergy." *Journal of Allergy* 28 (1957): 365–66.

Brown, W. R., B. K. Borthistle, and S. T. Chen. "Immunoglobulin E (IgE) and IgE-Containing Cells in Human Gastrointestinal Fluids and Tissues." *Clinical and Experimental Immunology* 20 (1975): 227–37.

Browne, Thomas. *Religio Medici.* 1643. London: J. Torbuck, 1736.

Brumberg, Joan Jacobs. *Fasting Girls: The History of Anorexia Nervosa.* Cambridge, Mass.: Harvard University Press, 1989.

Buchan, William. *Domestic Medicine.* Philadelphia: John Crukshank, Robert Bell, James Bell, 1790.

Burisch, J., and P. Munkholm. "Inflammatory Bowel Disease Epidemiology." *Current Opinion in Gastroenterology* 29 (2013): 357–62.

Burnet, Frank Macfarlane. *The Production of Antibodies.* Melbourne: Macmillan, 1941.

Burnham, John C. "The Decline of the Sick Role." *Social History of Medicine* 25 (2012): 761–76.

Burrows, B., M. Halonen, R. A. Barbee, and M. Lebowitz. "The Relation of Serum Immunoglobulin E and Cigarette Smoking." *American Review of Respiratory Disease* 124 (1981): 523–25.

Bynum, Russ. "Peanut Ban on Airplanes? FAA Considers Nut Ban on Airlines Because of Allergy." *Huffington Post*, June 12, 2010. http://www.huffingtonpost .com/2010/06/12/peanut-ban-on-airplaines-_n_610247.html. Accessed March 1, 2012.

Caldwell, Janet A. "The Manifestations of Food Allergy." *Dallas Medical Journal* 19 (1933): 51–53.

Callis, H. A. "Food Allergy: Two Unusual Cases." *Journal of the National Medical Association* 22 (1930): 14–15.

Cameron, Charles A. *A Handy Book on Food and Diet in Health and Disease.* London: Cassell, Petter and Galpin, 1871.

Cantor, David. "The Diseased Body." In *Medicine in the Twentieth Century*, edited by Roger Cooter and John Pickstone, 347–66. Amsterdam: Harwood Academic, 2000.

Carroy, Jacqueline. "Playing with Signatures: The Young Charles Richet." In *The Mind of Modernism: Medicine, Psychology, and the Cultural Arts in Europe and America, 1880–1940*, edited by Mark S. Micale, 217–49. Stanford, Calif.: Stanford University Press, 2004.

Carson, Rachel. *Silent Spring.* Boston: Houghton Mifflin, 1962.

Carver, George Washington. *How to Grow the Peanut and 105 Ways of Preparing It for Human Consumption.* 7th ed. Tuskegee, Ala.: Tuskegee Institute Press, 1940.

"Causes of Asthma." *Times* (London), January 16, 1929.

Centers for Disease Control and Prevention. *Asthma Facts.* Atlanta: U.S. Department of Health and Human Services, Centers for Disease Control and Prevention, 2013. http://www.cdc.gov/asthma/pdfs/asthma_facts_program_grantees.pdf. Accessed November 27, 2013.

Chen, Nancy N. *Food, Medicine, and the Quest for Good Health.* New York: Columbia University Press, 2009.

Cheyne, George. *The English Malady.* London: G. Strahan, 1733.

Christakis, Nicholas A. "This Allergies Hysteria Is Just Nuts." *BMJ* 337 (2008): 1384.

"City Offers Tips." *Edmonton (Alberta) Journal*, August 23, 2009.

Clark, A. T., S. Islam, Y. King, J. Deighton, K. Anagnostou, and P. W. Ewan. "Successful Oral Tolerance Induction in Severe Peanut Allergy." *Allergy* 64 (2009): 1218–20.

Clarke, T. Wood. "Neuro-Allergy in Childhood." *New York State Journal of Medicine* 42 (1948): 393–97.

——. "The Relation of Allergy to Character Problems in Children." *Annals of Allergy* 8 (1950): 21–38.

"Coalition Asks More Specific Ingredient Labeling for Food." *Daily Herald*, December 13, 1973.

Coca, Arthur F. *Familial Nonreaginic Food-Allergy*. Springfield, Ill.: Thomas, 1943.

——. "Hypersensitiveness." In *Practice of Medicine*, edited by Frederick Tice, 1:109–99. Hagerstown, Md.: Prior, 1920.

——. *The Pulse Test for Allergy*. London: Parrish, 1959.

Coca, Arthur F., and Robert Cooke. "On the Classification of the Phenomena of Hypersensitiveness." *Journal of Immunology* 8 (1923): 163–82.

Coca, Arthur F., and Ella F. Grove. "Studies in Hypersensitiveness 13: A Study of the Atopic Reagins." *Journal of Immunology* 10 (1925): 445–64.

Cohen, Sheldon G., ed. *Excerpts from Classics in Allergy*. 3rd ed. Bethesda, Md.: National Institutes of Allergy and Infectious Diseases, 2012.

Cohen, Sheldon G., and Myrna Zelaya-Quesada. "Prausnitz and Küstner Phenomenon: The P-K Reaction." *JACI* 114 (2004): 705–10.

Collins, Harry, and Trevor Pinch. *Dr. Golem: How to Think About Medicine*. Chicago: University of Chicago Press, 2005.

Cone, Richard A., and Emily Martin. "Corporeal Flows: The Immune System, Global Economies of Food, and Implications for Health." *Ecologist* 27 (1997): 107–11.

Conford, Philip. *Origins of the Organic Movement*. Edinburgh: Floris Books, 2001.

Consumer Reports. "Our History." http://www.consumerreports.org/cro/about-us/history/index.htm. Accessed September 24, 2013.

Cooke, Rose Terry. "The Household." *Fort Worth Daily Gazette*, December 6, 1885.

Craik, Elizabeth. "Hippokratic Diaita." In *Food in Antiquity*, edited by John Wilkins, David Harvey, and Mike Dobson, 343–50. Exeter: University of Exeter Press, 2003.

Crook, William G. *Can Your Child Write? Is He Hyperactive?* Jackson, Tenn.: Pedicenter Press, 1975.

——. "Food Allergy: The Great Masquerader." *Pediatric Clinics of North America* 22 (1975): 227–38.

——. "To the Editor." *Annals of Allergy* 38 (1977): 285.

——. *The Yeast Connection: A Medical Breakthrough*. New York: Vintage, 1986.

Crook, William G., Walton W. Harrison, and Stanley E. Crawford. "Allergy—The Unanswered Challenge in Pediatric Research, Education, and Practice." *Pediatrics* 21 (1958): 649–54.

Cullen, William. *Lectures on the Materia Medica*. London: T. Lowndes, 1773.

Cummings, A. J., R. C. Knibb, M. Erlewynn-Lajeunesse, R. M. King, G. Roberts, and J. S. Lucas. "Management of Nut Allergy Influences Quality of Life and Anxiety in Children and Their Mothers." *Pediatric Allergy and Immunology* 21 (2010): 586–94.

Cunningham, Andrew. "Identifying Disease in the Past: Cutting the Gordian Knot." *Asclepio* 54 (2002): 13–34.

Daschner, A., C. Cuéllar, and M. Rodero. "The Anisakis Allergy Debate: Does an Evolutionary Approach Help?" *Trends in Parasitology* 28 (2012): 9–15.

Davison, Hal M. "Cerebral Allergy." *Southern Medical Journal* 42 (1949): 712–16.

DesRoches, A., C. Infante-Rivard, L. Paradis, J. Paradis, and E. Haddad. "Peanut Allergy: Is Maternal Transmission of Antigens During Pregnancy and Breastfeeding a Risk Factor?" *Journal of Investigative Allergology and Clinical Immunology* 20 (2010): 289–94.

Deutsch, Felix, and Raymond Nadell. "Psychological Aspects of Dermatology with Special Consideration of Allergic Phenomena." *Nervous Child* 5 (1946): 339–64.

Dixon, Viktoria, Shaymau Habeeb, and Raman Lakshman. "Did You Know This Medicine Has Peanut Butter in It, Doctor?" *Archives of Disease in Childhood* 92 (2007): 654.

Dodds, J. C. "Idiosyncrasy to Eggs." *JAMA* 16 (1891): 827.

"Dr. Charles D. May, 84; Debunked Myth That Linked Asthma to Food Allergies." *Boston Globe*, June 18, 1992.

"Dr. Hirshberg Gets 4 Years in Prison." *New York Times*, May 12, 1923.

Dror, Otniel. "The Affect of Experiment: The Turn to Emotions in Anglo-American Experiment." *Isis* 90 (1999): 205–37.

Duke, William Waddell. *Allergy, Asthma, Hay Fever, Urticaria, and Allied Manifestations of Reaction*. London: Kimpton, 1925.

Duncan, Joanne M., and Malcom R. Sears. "Breastfeeding and Allergies: Time for a Change in Paradigm?" *Current Opinion in Allergy and Clinical Immunology* 8 (2008): 398–405.

"Eczema and Protein Hypersensitiveness." *JAMA* 67 (1916): 207.

"Edgewater Elementary School Parents Want Student Home Schooled over Peanut Allergy." *Huffington Post*, March 22, 2011. http://www.huffingtonpost.com/2011/03/22/peanut-allergy-edgewater-elementary-school_n_839091.html. Accessed March 1, 2012.

Eijk, Philip J. van der. "Medicine and Health in the Graeco-Roman World." In *The Oxford Handbook of the History of Medicine*, edited by Mark Jackson, 21–39. Oxford: Oxford University Press, 2012.

Elliott, D. E., and J. V. Weinstock. "Where Are We on Worms?" *Current Opinion in Gastroenterology* 28 (2012): 551–56.

Ellis, Elliot F. "Foreword." *Pediatric Clinics of North America* 22 (1975): 1–2.

Ellis, Sydney. Review of *Human Ecology and Susceptibility to the Chemical Environment*, by Theron G. Randolph. *Archives of Environmental Health* 6 (1963): 814.

Ettelson, L. N., and Louis Tuft. "The Value of the Coca Pulse-Acceleration Method in Food Allergy." *Journal of Allergy* 32 (1961): 514–24.

Evans, Susan, Danna Skea, and Jerry Dolovich. "Fatal Reaction to Peanut Antigen in Almond Icing." *CMAJ* 139 (1988): 231–32.

Fagge, Charles Hinton, and Philip Henry Pye-Smith. *The Principles and Practices of Medicine*. 2nd ed. London: Churchill, 1888.

Farb, Peter, and George Armelagos. *Consuming Passions: The Anthropology of Eating.* Boston: Houghton Mifflin, 1980.

Fauci, Anthony S. "The Revolution in the Approach to Allergic and Immunologic Diseases." *Annals of Allergy* 55 (1985): 632–33.

Feinberg, Samuel. *Allergy in General Practice.* London: Kimpton, 1934.

——. *One Man's Food.* Chicago: Blue Cross Commission, 1953.

Feinberg, Samuel M., Harry L. Huber, J. Harvey Black, and Karl D. Figley. "Reactions to Dextrose." *JAMA* 145 (1951): 666.

Feingold, Ben F. "Allergy to Flea Bites—Clinical and Experimental Observations." *Annals of Allergy* 19 (1961): 1275–89.

——. *Introduction to Clinical Allergy.* Springfield, Ill: Thomas, 1973.

——. "The Role of Diet in Behaviour." *Ecology of Disease* 1 (1982): 153–65.

——. "Tonsillectomy in the Allergic Child." *California Medicine* 71 (1949): 341–44.

——. "Treatment of Allergic Disease of the Bronchi." *JAMA* 146 (1951): 319–23.

——. *Why Your Child Is Hyperactive.* New York: Random House, 1974.

Feingold, Ben F., and Helene S. Feingold. *The Feingold Cookbook for Hyperactive Children.* New York: Random House, 1979.

Feingold, Ben F., Frank J. Gorman, Margaret Thaler Singer, and Kurt Schlesinger. "Psychological Studies of Allergic Women: The Relation Between Skin Reactivity and Personality." *Psychosomatic Medicine* 24 (1962): 195–202.

Ferris, Samuel. *A Dissertation on Milk.* London: T. Cadell, 1785.

Fickling, William E., and Duncan A. F. Robertson. "Immunologically Mediated Damage of the Gut." In *Food Allergy and Intolerance*, edited by Jonathan Brostoff and Stephen J. Challacombe, 293–301. 2nd ed. London: Saunders, 2002.

Fischer, Louis. "Milk Idiosyncrasies in Children." *JAMA* 39 (1902): 247–49.

Fisherman, E. W. "Does the Allergic Diathesis Influence Malignancy?" *JACI* 31 (1960): 74–78.

Fitzgerald, Michael. *Autism and Creativity: Is There a Link Between Autism in Men and Exceptional Ability?* New York: Routledge, 2004.

Fitzsimmons, C. M., and D. W. Dunne. "Survival of the Fittest: Allergology or Parasitology?" *Trends in Parasitology* 25 (2009): 447–51.

Fleck, Ludwik. *Genesis and Development of a Scientific Fact.* Translated by Frederick Bradley and Thaddeus J. Trenn. 1935. Chicago: University of Chicago Press, 1979.

Floyer, John. *A Treatise of the Asthma.* London: R. Wilkin, 1698.

Food Allergy Committee of the American College of Allergists. "Final Report of the Food Allergy Committee of the American College of Allergists on the Clinical Evaluation of Sublingual Provocative Testing Method for Diagnosis of Food Allergy." *Annals of Allergy* 33 (1974): 164–66.

Food Allergy Research and Education. *A Vision and Plan for Food Allergy Research.* McLean, Va.: FARE, 2013. http://www.foodallergy.org/document.doc?id=250. Accessed November 27, 2013.

Food Standards Agency. "Peanuts During Pregnancy, Breastfeeding and Early Childhood." August 24, 2009. http://www.food.gov.uk/policy-advice/allergyintol/peanuts pregnancy#.UpXxmdK-0yo. Accessed November 27, 2013.

Fothergill, John. "Remarks on That Complaint commonly known under the Name of the Sick Head-Ach." In *Medical Observations and Inquiries*, edited by the Society of Physicians of London, 6:103–34. London: T. Cadell, 1784.

Fox, Howard, and J. Edgar Fisher. "Protein Sensitization in Eczema of Adults." *JAMA* 75 (1920): 910.

Fox, William Tilbury. *Atlas of Skin Diseases*. London: Churchill, 1877.

"Francis Hare: Noted Physician Passes." *Brisbane Courier*, March 20, 1929.

Frankland, A. W. "Allergy: Immunity Gone Wrong." *Proceedings of the Royal Society of Medicine* 66 (1972): 1–4.

——. "Carl Prausnitz: A Personal Memoir." *JACI* 114 (2004): 700–705.

——. "Some Observations on the RAST Test." *Annals of Allergy* 33 (1974): 105–6.

Frankland, A. W., and R. S. H. Pumfrey. "Acute Allergic Reactions to Foods and Crossreactivity Between Foods." In *Food Allergy and Intolerance*, edited by Jonathan Brostoff and Stephen J. Challacombe, 413–23. 2nd ed. London: Saunders, 2002.

Fraser, Heather. *The Peanut Allergy Epidemic: What's Causing It and How to Stop It*. New York: Skyhorse, 2011.

"Frederick Stare." *Economist*, April 18, 2002.

French, Thomas Morton, and Franz Alexander. *Psychogenic Factors in Bronchial Asthma*. Menasha, Wis.: Banta, 1941.

Friedman, Alice D. "Management with the Elimination Diet." In *Introduction to Clinical Allergy*, by Ben F. Feingold, 162–70. Springfield, Ill: Thomas, 1973.

Fries, Joseph H. "Chocolate: A Review of Published Reports of Allergic and Other Deleterious Effects, Real or Presumed." *Annals of Allergy* 41 (1978): 195–207.

——. "Food Allergy—Current Concerns." *Annals of Allergy* 46 (1981): 260–63.

——. "Food Faddism—The Dilemma of Diet." *Annals of Allergy* 39 (1977): 288–89.

——. "Peanuts: Allergic and Other Untoward Reactions." *Annals of Allergy* 48 (1982): 220–26.

——. "Studies on the Allergenicity of the Soy Bean." *Annals of Allergy* 29 (1971): 1–7.

Galen. *On the Properties of Foodstuffs*. Translated by Owen Powell. Cambridge: Cambridge University Press, 2003.

Gaud, William S. "The Green Revolution: Accomplishments and Apprehensions." Speech presented to the Society for International Development, Washington, D.C., March 8, 1968. http://www.agbioworld.org/biotech-info/topics/borlaug/borlaug -green.html. Accessed September 24, 2013.

Gay, L. P. "Gastro-Intestinal Allergy IV: The Leucopenic Index as a Method of Diagnosis of Allergy Causing Peptic Ulcer." *JAMA* 106 (1936): 969–76.

——. Review of *Elimination Diets and the Patients' Allergies*, by Albert H. Rowe. *Quarterly Review of Biology* 20 (1945): 183.

——. Review of *Familial Nonreaginic Food-Allergy*, by Arthur F. Coca. *Quarterly Review of Biology* 21 (1946): 408.

——. Review of *Strange Malady*, by Warren T. Vaughn. *Scientific Monthly* 54 (1942): 279–80.

Gell, P. G. H., and R. R. A. Coombs, eds. *Clinical Aspects of Immunology*. Oxford: Blackwell, 1963.

Gentilcore, David. *Pomodoro! A History of the Tomato in Italy*. New York: Columbia University Press, 2010.

Gerard, Margaret W. "Bronchial Asthma in Children." *Nervous Child* 5 (1946): 327–31.

Gerrard, J. W., C. A. Geddes, P. L. Reggin, C. D. Gerrard, and S. Horne. "Serum IgE Levels in White and Métis Communities in Saskachewan." *Annals of Allergy* 37 (1976): 91–100.

Gerrard, J. W., D. C. Heiner, C. G. Co, J. Mink, A. Meyers, and J. A. Dosman. "Immunoglobulin Levels in Smokers and Non-Smokers." *Annals of Allergy* 44 (1980): 261–63.

Gerrard, J. W., and L. Perelmutter. "IgE-Mediated Allergy to Peanut, Cow's-Milk, and Egg in Children with Special Reference to Maternal Diet." *Annals of Allergy* 56 (1986): 351–54.

Gerstenberger, H. J., and J. H. Davis. "Report of a Case of Anaphylaxis Following an Intradermal Protein Sensitization Test." *JAMA* 76 (1921): 721–23.

Ghosh, M. L. "Eosinophilia, Increased IgE Toxocariasis in Children." *Indian Journal of Pediatrics* 41 (1974): 11–14.

Gilman, Sander. *Fat: A Cultural History of Obesity*. Cambridge: Polity, 2008.

"Girl Fasting to Cure Asthma." *New York Tribune*, October 7, 1904.

Glaser, Jerome. "Gastrointestinal Allergy in Infancy and Childhood." *Journal of the Medical Association of Georgia* 45 (1956): 514–18.

Glickman, Laurence B. *Buying Power: A History of Consumer Activism in America*. Chicago: University of Chicago Press, 2009.

Goldman, Douglas, Nathan S. Kline, Veronica M. Pennington, and Burtrum C. Schiele. *Retrospective Diagnoses of Historical Figures as Viewed by Leading Contemporary Psychiatrists*. Bloomfield, N.J.: Schering, 1958.

Gooding, Ralph. *A Manual of Domestic Medicine*. London: Virtue, 1867.

Grant, Mark. *Galen on Food and Diet*. London: Routledge, 2000.

Greer, William R. "Warnings on Food Allergies." *New York Times*, March 29, 1986.

Grigson, Jane. *Jane Grigson's Vegetable Book*. London: Michael Joseph, 1978.

Gryboski, J. D. "Gastrointestinal Milk Allergy in Infants." *Pediatrics* 40 (1967): 354–62.

Hällgren, R., and L. Lundin. "Increased Total Serum IgE in Alcoholics." *Acta Medica Scandinavica* 213 (1983): 99–103.

Handbook of Domestic Medicine. London: Bohn, 1855.

Hare, F. E. *The Cold-Bath Treatment of Typhoid Fever*. London: Macmillan, 1898.

Hare, Francis. *The Food Factor in Disease: Being an Investigation into the Humoral Causation, Meaning, Mechanism, and Rational Treatment, Preventive and Curative, of the Paroxysmal Neuroses (Migraine, Asthma, Angina Pectoris, Epilepsy, Etc.), Bilious Attacks, Gout, Catarrhal and Other Affections, High Blood-Pressure, Circulatory, Renal and Other Degenerations*. 2 vols. London: Longmans, Green, 1905.

——. *On Alcoholism: Its Clinical Aspects and Treatment*. London: Churchill, 1912.

Harvey, D. Review of *Human Ecology and Susceptibility to the Chemical Environment*, by Theron G. Randolph. *Nutrition Abstracts and Reviews*, January 1963, 11.

Hass, Myra May. *Recipes and Menus for Allergics: A Cookbook for the Harassed Housekeeper*. New York: Dodd, Mead, 1939.

Healy, David. *The Antidepressant Era.* Cambridge, Mass.: Harvard University Press, 1997.

Hegsted, D. Mark. "Frederick John Stare (1910–2002)." *Journal of Nutrition* 134 (2004): 1007–9.

Heiner, Douglas C. "Sublingual Testing in the Diagnosis of Food Allergy." *Western Journal of Medicine* 121 (1974): 152.

Heiner, Douglas C., and Bram Rose. "Elevated Levels of Gamma-E (IgE) in Conditions Other Than Classic Allergy." *Journal of Allergy* 45 (1970): 30–42.

Heremans, Joseph F., M. T. Heremans, and H. E. Schultze. "Isolation and Description of a Few Properties of ɤ2A-Globulin of Human Serum." *Clinica Chimica Acta* 4 (1959): 96–102.

Higman, B. W. *How Food Made History.* Oxford: Wiley-Blackwell, 2012.

Hill, Louis Webb. "Editorial: Atopic Dermatitis." *Journal of Allergy* 27 (1956): 480–82.

Hippocrates. *Ancient Medicine.* Part 20. Perseus Project. http://perseus.uchicago.edu/cgi-bin/philologic/getobject.pl?p.196:29.GreekFeb2011. Accessed September 17, 2014.

Hirshberg, Leonard Keene. "Beauty, Only Skin Deep, Is Divine Stamp of Health, That Needs Preservation." *Washington Times,* May 24, 1915.

———. "Nature Provides Means to Conquer Bacteria and All Their Poisons." *Washington Times,* August 7, 1916.

———. "Why You Eat Some Foods with Pleasure and Are Unable to Enjoy Others." *Washington Times,* May 31, 1916.

Hoffman, D. R., and Z. H. Haddad. "Diagnosis of IgE-Mediated Reactions to Food Antigens by Radioimmunoassay." *JACI* 54 (1974): 165–73.

Hogarth-Scott, R. S., S. G. Johansson, and H. Bennich. "Antibodies to *Toxocara* in the Sera of Visceral Larva Migrans Patients: The Significance of Raised Levels of IgE." *Clinical and Experimental Immunology* 5 (1969): 619–25.

Hoobler, B. Raymond. "Some Early Symptoms Suggesting Protein Sensitization in Infancy." *American Journal of Diseases of Children* 12 (1916): 129–35.

Høst, Arne, and Sami L. Bahna. "Cow's Milk Allergy." In *Food Hypersensitivity and Adverse Reactions: A Practical Guide for Diagnosis and Management,* edited by Marianne Frieri and Brett Kettelhut, 99–112. New York: Dekker, 1999.

Hunter, Beatrice Trum. *Beatrice Trum Hunter's Additives Book.* New Canaan, Conn.: Keats, 1972.

———. "The Bookhunter." *Herald of Health,* August 12, 1962.

———. *The Mirage of Safety: Food Additives and Federal Policy.* Brattleboro, Vt.: Greene, 1975.

Hurst, Arthur F. "An Address on Asthma." *Lancet* 197 (1921): 1113–17.

Hutchinson, John. *Pedigree of Disease: Six Lectures on Temperament, Idiosyncrasy and Diathesis.* London: Churchill, 1884.

"Irish Prospects." *Economist,* October 31, 1846.

"Is Asparagus Wholesome?" *Lancet* 167 (1906): 1405–6.

Ishizaka, K., H. Tomioka, and T. Ishizaka. "Mechanism of Passive Sensitization. I. Presence of IgE and IgG Molecules on Human Leukocytes." *Journal of Immunology* 105 (1970): 1459–67.

Ishizaka, Kimishige, Teruko Ishizaka, and M. Hornbrook. "Physicochemical Properties of Reaginic Antibody IV. Presence of a Unique Immunoglobulin as a Carrier of Reaginic Activity." *Journal of Immunology* 97 (1966): 75–85.

Jackson, Mark. *The Age of Stress: Science and the Search for Stability.* Oxford: Oxford University Press, 2013.

——. *Allergy: The History of a Modern Malady.* London: Reaktion, 2006.

——. "'Allergy *con Amore*': Psychosomatic Medicine and the 'Asthmogenic Home' in the Mid-Twentieth Century." In *Health and the Modern Home*, edited by Mark Jackson, 153–74. New York: Routledge, 2007.

——. *Asthma: The Biography.* Oxford: Oxford University Press, 2009.

——. *The Borderland of Imbecility: Medicine, Society and the Fabrication of the Feeble Mind in Late Victorian and Edwardian England.* Manchester: Manchester University Press, 2000.

——. "Disease and Diversity in History." *Social History of Medicine* 15 (2002), 323–40.

——. "'Divine Stramonium': The Rise and Fall of Smoking for Asthma." *Medical History* 54 (2010): 171–94.

——. "'A Private Line to Medicine': The Clinical and Laboratory Contours of Allergy in the Early Twentieth Century." In *Crafting Immunity: Working Histories of Clinical Immunology*, edited by Kenton Kroker, Pauline M. H. Mazumdar, and Jennifer Keelen, 55–76. Aldershot: Ashgate, 2008.

Jackson, Peter. "The Peanut Detectives." BBC News, February 24, 2009. http://news .bbc.co.uk/1/hi/uk/7868115.stm. Accessed November 2, 2013.

James, Robert. *A Medicinal Dictionary; Including Physic, Surgery, Anatomy, Chymistry, and Botany, in all their Branches Relative to Medicine.* London: T. Osborne, 1743.

James, Susan Donaldson. "Weird Food Allergy Stresses Mom, Baffles Doctors." ABC News, April 1, 2013. http://abcnews.go.com/Health/weird-food-allergy-stresses-moms-baffles-doctors/story?id=18843611#.UVsgSo6K420. Accessed October 8, 2013.

Jamieson, Michelle. "Imagining 'Reactivity': Allergy Within the History of Immunology." *Studies in History and Philosophy of Biological and Biomedical Sciences* 41 (2013): 356–66.

Jamieson, W. Allan. "A Discussion of Diet in the Etiology and Treatment of Diseases of the Skin." *BMJ* 1822 (1895): 1351–56.

Jarrett, E. E., and D. C. Stewart. "Potentiation of Rat Reaginic (IgE) Antibody by Helminth Infection." *Immunology* 23 (1972): 749–55.

Jenkins, J. A., H. Breiteneder, and E. N. Mills. "Evolutionary Distance from Human Homologs Reflects Allergenicity of Animal Food Proteins." *JACI* 120 (2007): 1399–405.

Jerne, Niels Kaj. "Waiting for the End." *Cold Spring Harbor Symposium on Quantitative Biology* 32 (1967): 591–603.

Johansson, S. G., and H. Bennich. "Immunological Studies of an Atypical (Myeloma) Immunoglobulin." *Immunology* 13 (1967): 381–89.

Jukes, Edward. *On Digestion and Costiveness*. London: Effingham Wilson, 1831.

Junod, Suzanne White. "The Rise and Fall of Federal Food Standards in the United States: The Case of the Peanut Butter and Jelly Sandwich." In *The Food and Drug Administration*, edited by Meredith A. Hickman, 35–48. Hauppauge, N.Y.: Nova Science, 2003.

Kallet, Arthur, and F. J. Schlink. *100,000,000 Guinea Pigs: Dangers in Everyday Foods, Drugs, and Cosmetics*. New York: Vanguard, 1933.

Karbowski, K. "Samuel Auguste Tissot (1728–1797): His Research on Migraine." *Journal of Neurology* 233 (1986): 123–25.

Kaufman, William. "Some Psychosomatic Aspects of Food Allergy." *Psychosomatic Medicine* 16 (1954): 10–40.

Keating, M. U., R. T. Jones, N. J. Worley, C. A. Shively, and J. W. Yunginger. "Immunoassay of Peanut Allergens in Food-Processing Materials and Finished Foods." *JACI* 86 (1990): 41–44.

Keirns, Carla. "Better Than Nature: The Changing Treatment of Asthma and Hay Fever in the United States, 1910–1945." *Studies in History and Philosophy of Biological and Biomedical Sciences* 34 (2003): 511–31.

Kellogg, John Harvey. "Good Health Question Box." *Evening Public Ledger* (Philadelphia), November 16, 1917, December 31, 1917.

Kemp, A. S., C. M. Mellis, D. Barnett, E. Sharota, and J. Simpson. "Skin Test, RAST, and Clinical Reactions to Peanut Allergens in Children." *Clinical Allergy* 1 (1985): 73–78.

Kemp, S. F., and R. F. Lockey. "Peanut Anaphylaxis from Food Cross-Contamination." *JAMA* 275 (1996): 1636–37.

Kennedy, A. M. " A Note on Food Allergy." *BMJ* 3729 (1932): 1167–69.

Kernberg, Paulina F. "The Problem of Organicity in the Child: Notes on Some Diagnostic Techniques in the Evaluation of Children." *Journal of the American Academy of Child Psychiatry* 8 (1969): 517–41.

Kessler, Walter R. "Food Allergy." *Pediatrics* 21 (1958): 523–25.

Kinney, Vilma. *Theron Grant Randolph, M.D., 1906–1995: A Bibliography: 60 Years of Published Works*. Self-published, 1997.

Knicker, William T. "Is the Choice of Allergy Skin Testing Versus *In Vitro* Determination of Specific IgE No Longer a Scientific Issue?" *Annals of Allergy* 62 (1989): 373–74.

Knoll, J. E., M. L. Ramos, Y. Zeng, C. C. Holybrook, M. Chow, S. Chen, S. Maleki, A. Bhattacharya, and P. Ozias-Akins. "TILLING for Allergen Reduction and Improvement of Quality Traits in Peanut (Arachis Hypogaea L.)." *BMC Plant Biology* 11 (2011): 81–99.

Kost, J. *Domestic Medicine*. Cincinnati: Melick and Bunn, 1868.

Kotulak, Ron. "Henrotin Hospital Closing Set." *Chicago Tribune*, October 2, 1986.

Krampner, Jon. *Creamy and Crunchy: An Informal History of Peanut Butter, the All-American Food*. New York: Columbia University Press, 2013.

Krimsky, Sheldon. *Hormonal Chaos: The Scientific and Social Origins of the Environmental Endocrine Hypothesis*. Baltimore: Johns Hopkins University Press, 2000.

Kristof, Nicholas D. "Arsenic in Our Chicken?" *New York Times*, April 4, 2012. http://
www.nytimes.com/2012/04/05/opinion/kristof-arsenic-in-our-chicken.html?_
r=1&ref=global-home. Accessed April 9, 2012.

Kroker, Kenton. "Immunity and Its Other: The Anaphylactic Selves of Charles Richet."
Studies in History and Philosophy of Biological and Biomedical Sciences 34 (2003):
273–96.

Kroker, Kenton, Pauline M. H. Mazumdar, and Jennifer Keelen. "Editor's Introduction."
In *Crafting Immunity: Working Histories of Clinical Immunology*, edited by Kenton
Kroker, Pauline M. H. Mazumdar, and Jennifer Keelen, 1–16. Aldershot: Ashgate, 2008.

Kroll-Smith, Steve, and H. Hugh Floyd. *Bodies in Protest: Environmental Illness and
the Struggle over Medical Knowledge*. New York: New York University Press, 1997.

Kuhn, Thomas. *The Structure of Scientific Revolutions*. Chicago: University of Chicago
Press, 1962.

Kutchins, Herb, and Stuart A. Kirk. *Making Us Crazy: DSM: The Psychiatric Bible and
the Creation of Mental Disorders*. New York: Free Press, 1997.

Lack, Gideon, Deborah Fox, Kate Northstone, and Jean Golding. "Factors Associated
with the Development of Peanut Allergy in Childhood." *NEJM* 348 (2003): 977–85.

Laidlaw, George Frederick. *The Treatment of Hayfever by Rosin-Weed, Ichtyhyol and
Faradic Electricity, with a Discussion of the Old Theory of Gout and the New Theory
of Anaphylaxis*. New York: Boericke & Runyon, 1917.

Laing, R. D. *The Divided Self: An Existential Study in Sanity and Madness*. London: Tavistock, 1960.

Lake, Wayne A. Review of *Clinical Ecology*, by Lawrence D. Dickey. *Annals of Allergy* 37
(1976): 444.

Lamson, R. W. "So-Called Fatal Anaphylaxis in Man: With Especial Reference to the
Diagnosis and Treatment of Clinical Allergies." *JAMA* 93 (1929): 1775–78.

Laroche, Guy, Charles Richet Fils, and François Saint-Girons. *Alimentary Anaphylaxis
(Gastro-intestinal Food Allergy)*. Translated by Mildred P. Rowe and Albert H. Rowe.
Berkeley: University of California Press, 1930.

Latham, Arthur. "An Address on Some Aspects of Bronchial Asthma." *Lancet* 199
(1922): 261–63.

Laufer, M. W., and W. E. Denhoff, "Hyperkinetic Behavior Syndrome in Children." *Journal of Pediatrics* 50 (1957): 463–74.

Laufer, M., W. E. Denhoff, and G. Solomons. "Hyperkinetic Impulse Disorder in Children's Behavior Problems." *Psychosomatic Medicine* 19 (1957): 38–49.

Lawrence, Christopher, and George Weisz. "Medical Holism: The Context." In *Greater
Than the Parts: Holism in Biomedicine, 1920–1950*, edited by Christopher Lawrence
and George Weisz, 1–22. New York: Oxford University Press, 1998.

Lear, Linda. *Rachel Carson: Witness for Nature*. London: Allen Lane, 1998.

Lebovidge, J. S., H. Strauch, L. A. Kalish, and L. C. Schneider. "Assessment of Psychological Distress Among Children and Adolescents with Food Allergy." *JACI* 124 (2009):
1282–88.

Le Souëf, P. N., J. Goldblatt, and N. R. Lynch. "Evolutionary Adaptation of Inflammatory Immune Responses in Human Beings." *Lancet* 356 (2000): 142–44.

Levenstein, Harvey A. *Fear of Food: A History of Why We Worry About What We Eat.* Chicago: University of Chicago Press, 2012.

——. *Paradox of Plenty: A Social History of Eating in Modern America.* New York: Oxford University Press, 1993.

——. *Revolution at the Table: The Transformation of the American Diet.* New York: Oxford University Press, 1988.

Liebermann, Phil. "Is Peanut Antigen in Vaccines?" American Academy of Allergy, Asthma and Immunology, Ask the Expert. http://www.aaaai.org/ask-the-expert/peanut-antigen-in-vaccines.aspx. Accessed November 28, 2013.

Liezmann, Christiane, Burghard Klapp, and Eva M. J. Peters. "Stress, Atopy and Allergy." *Dermatoendocrinology* 3 (2011): 37–40.

Lindsay, J. C. "Food Anaphylaxis." *CMAJ* 16 (1926): 58.

Liveing, Edward. "Observations on Megrim or Sick-Headache." *BMJ* 588 (1872): 364–66.

——. *On Megrim, Sick-Headache, and Some Allied Disorders.* London: Churchill, 1873.

Lo, Vivienne, and Penelope Barrett. "Cooking Up Fine Remedies: On the Culinary Aesthetic in a Sixteenth-Century Chinese *Materia Medica*." *Medical History* 49 (2005): 395–422.

Lockey, Stephen D. "Allergic Reactions Due to Dyes in Foods." Speech presented to the Pennsylvania Allergy Society, Autumn 1948.

——. "Allergic Reactions Due to FD&C Dyes Used as Coloring and Identifying Agents in Various Medications." *Bulletin* (Lancaster [Pa.] General Hospital), September 1948.

——. "Allergic Reactions Due to FD. and C. Yellow No. 5, Tartrazine, an Aniline Dye Used as a Coloring and Identifying Agent in Various Steroids." *Annals of Allergy* 17 (1959): 719–21.

——. "Drug Reactions and Sublingual Testing with Certified Food Colors." *Annals of Allergy* 31 (1973): 423–29.

——. "Reactions to Hidden Agents in Foods, Beverages and Drugs." *Annals of Allergy* 29 (1971): 461–66.

——. "Sensitizing Properties of Food Additives and Other Commercial Products." *Annals of Allergy* 30 (1972): 638–41.

Logan, J., and D. Saker. "The Incidence of Allergic Disorders in Cancer." *New Zealand Medical Journal* 52 (1953): 210–12.

Loveless, M., R. Dorfman, and L. Downing. "Statistical Evaluation of the Leucopenic Index." *Journal of Allergy* 9 (1938): 321–44.

Loveless, Mary Hewitt. "Reactions to Dextrose." *JAMA* 145 (1951): 666.

Lowell, Francis C., and Irving W. Schiller. "Editorial: It Is So—It Ain't So." *Journal of Allergy* 25 (1954): 57–59.

Löwy, Ilana. *Between Bench and Bedside: Science, Healing, and Interleukin-2 in a Cancer Ward.* Cambridge, Mass.: Harvard University Press, 1996.

——. "On Guinea Pigs, Dogs and Men: Anaphylaxis and the Study of Biological Individuality, 1902–1939." *Studies in History and Philosophy of Biological and Biomedical Sciences* 34 (2003): 399–423.

Lucretius. *De Rerum Natura.* Translated by Alban Dewes Winspear. New York: Russell, 1956.

——. *On the Nature of the Universe.* Translated by R. E. Latham. Revised by John Godwin. 1951. London: Penguin, 1994.

Lynch, N. R., M. C. Di Prisco-Fuenmayor, and J. M. Soto. "Diagnosis of Atopic Conditions in the Tropics." *Annals of Allergy* 51 (1983): 547–51.

Macalpine, Ida, and Richard Hunter. "The 'Insanity' of King George III: A Classic Case of Porphyria." *BMJ* 1 (1966): 65–71.

Mackarness, Richard. *Chemical Victims.* London: Pan Books, 1980.

——. *Eat Fat and Grow Slim.* Garden City, N.Y.: Doubleday, 1959.

——. *Not All in the Mind: How Unsuspected Food Allergy Can Affect Your Body AND Your Mind.* London: Pan Books, 1976.

Mackay, W. D. "The Incidence of Allergic Disorders and Cancer." *British Journal of Cancer* 20 (1966): 434–37.

Mackenzie, Stephen. "The Inaugural Address on the Advantages to Be Derived from the Study of Dermatology." *BMJ* 1830 (1896): 193–97.

Magendie, François. *Lectures on the Blood.* Philadelphia: Haswell, Barrington, and Haswell, 1839.

Marsh, Michael M. "Elimination Diets as a Diagnostic Tool." In *Food Allergy and Intolerance*, edited by Jonathan Brostoff and Stephen J. Challacombe, 817–29. 2nd ed. London: Saunders, 2002.

——. "Intestinal Pathogenetic Correlates of Clinical Food Allergic Disorders." In *Food Allergy and Intolerance*, edited by Jonathan Brostoff and Stephen J. Challacombe, 267–75. 2nd ed. London: Saunders, 2002.

Martin, E. G. "Predisposing Factors and Diagnosis of Rectal Cancer: A Discussion of Allergy." *Annals of Surgery* 102 (1935): 56–61.

Martin, Emily. *Flexible Bodies: Tracking Immunity in American Culture from the Days of Polio to the Age of AIDS.* Boston: Beacon Press, 1994.

Maslova, Ekaterina, Charlotta Granström, Susanne Hansen, Sesilje B. Petersen, Marin Strøm, Walter C. Willet, and Sjurdur F. Olsen. "Peanut and Tree Nut Consumption During Pregnancy and Allergic Disease in Children—Should Mothers Decrease Their Intake? Longitudinal Evidence from the Danish National Birth Cohort." *JACI* 130 (2012): 724–32.

Matless, David. "Bodies Made of Grass Made of Earth Made of Bodies: Organism, Diet, and National Health in Mid-Twentieth-Century England." *Journal of Historical Geography* 27 (2003): 355–76.

May, Charles D. "Food Allergy: A Commentary." *Pediatric Clinics of North America* 22 (1975): 217–20.

——. "Food Allergy: Lessons from the Past." *JACI* 69 (1982): 255–59.

——. "Food Sensitivities: Facts and Fancies." *Nutrition Reviews* 42 (1984): 72–78.

"May Be Allergic to In-Laws." *Los Angeles Evening Herald-Express*, March 7, 1950.

Mayer, Jean. "Better Labeling Laws Are Needed." *Pittsburgh Post-Gazette*, June 5, 1972.

Mayes, Rick, and Adam Rafalovich. "Suffer the Restless Children: The Evolution of ADHD and Paediatric Stimulant Use, 1900–1980." *History of Psychiatry* 18 (2007): 435–57.

McCann, Donna, Angelina Barrett, Alison Cooper, Debbie Crumpler, Lindy Dalen, Kate Grimshaw, Elizabeth Kitchin, Kris Lok, Lucy Porteous, Emily Prince, Edmund Sonuga-Barke, John O. Warner, and Jim Stevenson. "Food Additives and Hyperactive Behaviour in 3-Year-Old and 8/9-Year-Old Children in the Community: A Randomised, Double-Blinded, Placebo-Controlled Trial." *Lancet* 370 (2007): 1560–67.

McGinn, Dave. "Air Canada Told to Create Nut-Free Buffer Zones." *Globe and Mail* (Toronto), October 19, 2010. http://www.theglobeandmail.com/life/the-hot-button/air-canada-told-to-create-nut-free-buffer-zones/article1764118/. Accessed March 1, 2012.

Mennell, Stephen. *All Manners of Food: Eating and Taste in England and France from the Middle Ages to the Present.* 2nd ed. Urbana: University of Illinois Press, 1996.

Merrill, Richard A. "Food Safety Regulation: Reforming the Delaney Clause." *Annual Review of Public Health* 18 (1997): 313–40.

Metchnikoff, Elie. *The Prolongation of Life: Optimistic Studies.* Edited by P. Chalmers Mitchell. New York: Knickerbocker Press, 1908.

Meyers, Deborah A., and David G. Marsh. "Report on a National Institute of Allergy and Infectious Diseases–Sponsored Workshop on the Genetics of Total Immunoglobulin E Levels in Humans." *JACI* 67 (1981): 167–70.

Micale, Mark S. *Approaching Hysteria: Disease and Its Interpretations.* Princeton, N.J.: Princeton University Press, 1995.

Micale, Mark S., and Roy Porter, eds. *Discovering the History of Psychiatry.* Oxford: Oxford University Press, 1994.

Mikulak, Michael. *The Politics of the Pantry: Stories, Food, and Social Change.* Montreal: McGill-Queen's University Press, 2013.

Millar, John. *Observations on the Asthma and the Hooping Cough.* London: T. Cadel, 1769.

Miller, Hyman, George Piness, and Willard F. Small. "Allergic Eczema of Infancy and Childhood: Application of Skin Testing." *California and Western Medicine* 54 (1941): 267–69.

"Minimal Brain Dysfunction." *Lancet* 302 (1973): 487–88.

Mitchell, John H., Charles A. Curran, William F. Mitchell, Iola Sivon, and Ruth Myers. "Personality Factors in Allergic Disorder." *Journal of Allergy* 18 (1947): 337–40.

Mitchell, Piers D. "Retrospective Diagnosis and the Use of Historical Texts for Investigating Disease in the Past." *International Journal of Paleopathology* 1 (2011): 81–88.

Mitman, Gregg. *Breathing Space: How Allergies Shape Our Lives and Landscapes.* New Haven, Conn.: Yale University Press, 2007.

——. "Natural History and the Clinic: The Regional Ecology of Allergy in America." *Studies in History and Philosophy of Biological and Biomedical Sciences* 34 (2003): 491–510.

Moore, Merle W. "More Stress on Education in Allergy." *Journal of Allergy* 31 (1959): 42–45.

Morgan, Helen. *You Can't Eat That! A Manual and Recipe Book for Those Who Suffer Either Acutely or Mildly (And Perhaps Unconsciously) from Food Allergy.* New York: Harcourt, Brace, 1939.

Moria, H., I. Nomura, A. Matsuda, H. Saito, and K. Matsumoto. "Gastrointestinal Food Allergy in Infants." *Allergology International* 62 (2013): 297–307.

Mosby, Ian. "'That Won-Ton Soup Headache': The Chinese Restaurant Syndrome, MSG, and the Making of American Food, 1968–1980." *Social History of Medicine* 22 (2009): 133–51.

"Most Food Allergies Traceable, Says Doctor." *Los Angeles Examiner*, March 7, 1950.

Moulin, Anne Marie. *Le dernier langage de la médecine: Histoire de l'immunologie de Pasteur et Sida.* Paris: Presses Universitaires de France, 1991.

Muñoz-Furlong, Anne, and A. Wesley Burks. *Food Allergy and Atopic Dermatitis.* Fairfax, Va.: Food Allergy Network, 1992.

Muñoz-Furlong, Anne, and Robert S. Zeiger. *Off to School with Food Allergies.* Fairfax, Va.: Food Allergy Network, 1992.

Murphy, Michelle. *Sick Building Syndrome and the Problem of Uncertainty: Environmental Politics, Technoscience, and Women Workers.* Durham, N.C.: Duke University Press, 2006.

National Institute of Allergy and Infectious Diseases (NIAID). "Report of the Expert Panel on Food Allergy Research." June 30 and July 1, 2003. http://www.niaid.nih.gov/about/organization/dait/documents/june30_2003.pdf. Accessed March 1, 2012.

National Peanut Council of America. *Peanuts: The Inside Story.* Alexandria, Va.: National Peanut Council of America, 1993.

Nestle, Marion. *Food Politics: How the Food Industry Influences Nutrition and Health.* Berkeley: University of California Press, 2002.

Newman, Kara. *The Secret Financial Life of Food: From Commodities Markets to Supermarkets.* New York: Columbia University Press, 2013.

"News and Notes." *JAMA* 282 (1963): 207.

Nilsson, K., H. Bennich, S. G. Johansson, and J. Pontén. "Established Immunoglobulin Producing Myeloma (IgE) and Lymphoblastoid (IgG) Cell Lines from an IgE Myeloma Patient." *Clinical and Experimental Immunology* 7 (1970): 477–89.

"Notes and Gleanings." *New York Times*, July 13, 1913.

Nutton, Vivian. "Galen and the Traveller's Fare." In *Food in Antiquity*, edited by John Wilkins, David Harvey, and Mike Dobson, 359–70. Exeter: University of Exeter Press, 2003.

"NY Lawsuit Says Airline Endangered Child with Peanut Allergy." June 3, 2008. eTN: Global Travel Industry News. http://www.eturbonews.com/2823/ny-lawsuit-says -airline-endangered-child-pean. Accessed March 1, 2012.

Oddy, Derek J. *From Plain Fare to Fusion Food: The British Diet from the 1890s to the 1990s*. Woodbridge: Boydell Press, 2003.

Ogawa, M., S. Kochwa, C. Smith, K. Ishizaka, and O. R. McIntyre. "Clinical Aspects of IgE Myeloma." *NEJM* 281 (1969): 1217–20.

Ogilvie, B. M. "Reagin-Like Antibodies in Animals Immune to Helminth Parasites." *Nature* 204 (1964): 91–92.

Oldbach, David W., Robert E. Richard, Eugene N. Borza, and R. Michael Benitez. "A Mysterious Death." *NEJM* 338 (1998): 1764–69.

Orgel, H. Alice. "Genetic and Developmental Aspects of IgE." *Pediatric Clinics of North America* 22 (1975): 17–32.

Oriel, G. H. *Allergy*. London: Bale and Danielsson, 1932.

Orrego, Fernando, and Carlos Quintana. "Darwin's Illness: A Final Diagnosis." *Notes and Records of the Royal Society* 22 (2007): 23–29.

"Ossett Café Owner 'Warns' Customers She Is Black." BBC News, July 10, 2013. http://www.bbc.co.uk/news/uk-england-leeds-23260860. Accessed July 18, 2013.

Ott, Katherine. *Fevered Lives: Tuberculosis in American Culture Since 1870*. Cambridge, Mass.: Harvard University Press, 1999.

Parnes, Ohad. "'Trouble from Within': Allergy, Autoimmunity, and Pathology in the First Half of the Twentieth Century." *Studies in History and Philosophy of Biological and Biomedical Sciences* 34 (2003): 425–54.

Paulley, J. W. "The Death of Albert Prince Consort: The Case Against Typhoid Fever." *Quarterly Journal of Medicine* 86 (1993): 837–41.

Penichet, Manuel L., and Erika Jensen-Jarolim, eds. *Cancer and IgE: Introducing the Concept of AllergoOncology*. Totowa, N.J.: Humana Press, 2010.

Piness, George, and Hyman Miller. "Allergic Manifestations in Infancy and Childhood." *Archives of Pediatrics* 42 (1925): 557–62.

Pirquet, Clemens von. "Allergie." *Münchener Medizinische Wochenschrift* 30 (1906): 1457–58.

——. *An Outline of the Pirquet System of Nutrition*. Philadelphia: Saunders, 1922.

Platts-Mills, T. A. "Allergy in Evolution." *Chemical Immunology and Allergy* 96 (2012): 1–6.

Pollard, Gail. "Practical Application and Hazards of Dietary Management in Food Intolerance." In *Food Allergy and Intolerance*, edited by Jonathan Brostoff and Stephen J. Challacombe, 907–19. 2nd ed. London: Saunders, 2002.

Portier, Paul, and Charles Richet. "De l'action anaphylactique de certains venins." *CR Société Biologie* 54 (1902): 170–72.

Povar, R. "Food Allergy in Dogs (A Preliminary Report)." *Journal of the American Veterinary Medical Association* 111 (1947): 61–63.

Pratt, Edward L. "Food Allergy and Food Intolerance in Relation to the Development of Good Eating Habits." *Pediatrics* 21 (1958): 642–48.

"President Signs Epinephrine Incentive Bill." News 4 San Antonio, November 14, 2013. http://news4sanantonio.com/news/features/top-stories/stories/president-signs-epinephrine-incentive-bill-5724.shtml. Accessed November 21, 2013.

Purvis, Andrew. "Just What the Patient Ordered." *Time*, May 28, 1990.

Radetsky, Peter. *Allergic to the Twentieth Century: The Explosion in Environmental Allergies—From Sick Buildings to Multiple Chemical Sensitivity*. Boston: Little, Brown, 1997.

Randolph, Theron G. "Allergic Type Reactions to Industrial Solvents and Liquid Fuels;" "Allergic Type Reactions to Mosquito Abatement Fogs and Mists"; "Allergic Type Reactions to Motor Exhaust"; "Allergic Type Reactions to Indoor Utility Gas and Oil Fumes"; "Allergic Type Reactions to Chemical Additives of Foods and Drugs"; "Allergic Type Reactions to Synthetic Drugs and Cosmetics." *Journal of Laboratory and Clinical Medicine* 44 (1954): 910–14.

——. "Allergy as a Causative Factor of Fatigue, Irritability, and Behavior Problems of Children." *Journal of Pediatrics* 31 (1947): 560–72.

——. "Both Allergy and Clinical Ecology Are Needed." *Annals of Allergy* 39 (1977): 215–16.

——. *Environmental Medicine: Beginnings and Bibliographies of Clinical Ecology*. Fort Collins, Colo.: Clinical Ecology, 1987.

——. "Human Ecology and Susceptibility to the Chemical Environment." *Annals of Allergy* 19 (1961): 518–40, 657–77, 779–99, 908–29.

——. *Human Ecology and Susceptibility to the Chemical Environment*. Springfield, Ill.: Thomas, 1962.

——. "Ingredients of Bread: Testimony in the Matter of a Definition and Standard of Identity for Bread and Related Products." Docket No. FDC-31(b), Before the Administrator, Federal Security Agency, August 3, 1949.

Randolph, Theron G., and R. W. Moss. *Allergies: Your Hidden Enemy*. Winnipeg: Turnstone Press, 1980.

Rapp, Doris J. *Allergies and the Hyperactive Child*. New York: Fireside, 1979.

Rappaport, Ben Z. "President's Address." *Journal of Allergy* 25 (1954): 274–78.

Rappaport, Helen. *Magnificent Obsession: Victoria, Albert, and the Death That Changed the Monarchy*. New York: St. Martin's Press, 2012.

Raspail, François-Vincent. *Domestic Medicine*. London: Weale, 1853.

Ratner, Bret. "Diagnosis and Management of the Allergic Child." *JAMA* 96 (1931): 570–75.

"Reagin and IgE." *Lancet* 291 (1968): 1131–32.

Richet, Charles. "An Address on Ancient Humorism and Modern Humorism." *BMJ* 2596 (1910): 921–26.

——. *L'anaphylaxie*. Paris: Librairie Félix Alcan, 1912.

——. "Foreword." In *Alimentary Anaphylaxis (Gastro-intestinal Food Allergy)*, by Guy Laroche, Charles Richet Fils, and François Saint-Girons. Translated by Mildred P. Rowe and Albert H. Rowe. Berkeley: University of California Press, 1930.

——. "Nobel Prize Lecture." December 11, 1913. http://www.nobelprize.org/nobel_prizes/medicine/laureates/1913/richet-lecture.html. Accessed July 8, 2013.

——. "Preface." In *Metapsychical Phenomena*, by J. Maxwell. London: Duckworth, 1905.

——. *Traites de métapsychique*. Paris: Librairie Félix Alcan, 1922.

Ring, J., and M. Möhrenschlager. "Allergy to Peanut Oil—Clinically Relevant?" *Journal of the European Academy of Dermatology and Venereology* 21 (2007): 452–55.

Rinkel, Herbert J. "Gastro-Intestinal Allergy: Concerning Mimicry of Peptic Ulcer Syndrome by Symptoms of Food Allergy." *Southern Medical Journal* 27 (1934): 630–63.

——. "Role of Food Allergy in Internal Medicine." *Annals of Allergy* 2 (1944): 115–24.

Rinkel, Herbert J., Theron G. Randolph, and Michael Zeller. *Food Allergy*. Springfield, Ill.: Thomas, 1951.

Rohrbacher, David. "Why Didn't Constantius II Eat Fruit?" *Classical Quarterly* 55 (2005): 323–26.

Rojido, G. Mario. "One Hundred Years of Anaphylaxis." *Allergología e immunología clínica* 16 (2001): 364–68.

Rolleston, Humphrey. *Idiosyncrasies*. London: Kegan Paul, Trench, Trumpner, 1927.

Rosenau, Milton J., and John F. Anderson. "A Review of Anaphylaxis with Especial Reference to Immunity." *Journal of Infectious Diseases* 5 (1908): 85–105.

——. *Studies upon Hypersusceptibility and Immunity*. Washington, D.C.: Government Printing Office, 1906.

Rosenberg, Charles E. *Explaining Epidemics and Other Studies in the History of Medicine*. Cambridge: Cambridge University Press, 1992.

——. "Pathologies of Progress: The Idea of Civilization at Risk." *Bulletin of the History of Medicine* 72 (1998): 714–30.

Rosenberg, E. B., S. H. Polmar, and G. E. Whalen. "Increased Circulating IgE in Trichinosis." *Annals of Internal Medicine* 75 (1971): 575–78.

Rosner, David, and Gerald Markowitz. "Industry Challenges to the Principle of Prevention in Public Health." *Public Health Reports* 117 (2002): 508–9.

Rous, Trevor, and Alan Hunt. "Governing Peanuts: The Regulation of the Social Bodies of Children and the Risks of Food Allergies." *Social Science and Medicine* 58 (2004): 825–36.

Rowe, Albert H. *Clinical Allergy Due to Foods, Inhalants, Contactants, Fungi, Bacteria, and Other Causes: Manifestations, Diagnosis, and Treatment*. London: Baillière, 1937.

——. *Elimination Diets and the Patient's Allergies: A Handbook of Allergy*. London: Kimpton, 1941.

——. "Food Allergy: Its Manifestations, Diagnosis, and Treatment." *JAMA* 91 (1928): 1623–31.

——. "Gastrointestinal Food Allergy: A Study Based on One Hundred Cases." *Journal of Allergy* 1 (1929–1930): 172–77.

Rowe, Albert H., and Albert Rowe Jr. *Food Allergy: Its Manifestations and Control and the Elimination Diets, a Compendium with Important Consideration of Inhalant (Especially Pollen), Drug, and Infectant Allergy*. 1931. Springfield, Ill.: Thomas, 1972.

Rowe, Albert H., Albert Rowe Jr., and E. James Young. "Bronchial Asthma Due to Food Allergy Alone in Ninety-Five Patients." *Allergy Abstracts* 24 (1959): 1158–62.

Roy, K. M., and M. C. Roberts. "Peanut Allergy in Children: Relationships to Health-Related Quality of Life, Anxiety, and Parental Stress." *Clinical Pediatrics* 50 (2011): 1045–51.

Royal College of Physicians/British Nutrition Foundation. "A Report on Food Intolerance and Food Aversion." *Journal of the Royal College of Physicians* (London) 18 (1984): 83–123.

Russell, William John. *Domestic Medicine and Hygiene.* London: Everett, 1878.

Ryan, Andrew. "Cheers from the (No) Peanut Gallery." June 12, 2011. Boston.com. http://articles.boston.com/2011-06-12/lifestyle/29650482_1_peanut-allergy-cracker-jack-fenway-park. Accessed March 1, 2012.

Saavedra-Delgado, Ana Maria. "François Magendie on Anaphylaxis (1839)." *Allergy Proceedings* 12 (1991): 355–56.

Sakula, Alex. "Henry Hyde Salter (1823–1871): A Biographical Sketch." *Thorax* 40 (1985): 887–88.

Salter, Henry Hyde. *On Asthma: Its Pathology and Treatment.* London: Churchill, 1860.

——. "On Some Points in the Therapeutic and Clinical History of Asthma." *Lancet* 72 (1858): 470–73.

——. "On the Aetiology of Asthma." *BMJ* 132 (1859): 538–40.

Sampson, Hugh A. "Peanut Oral Immunotherapy: Is It Ready for Clinical Practice?" *JACI: In Practice* 1 (2013): 15–21.

Sampson, Hugh A., Louis Mendelson, and James A. Rosen. "Fatal and Near-Fatal Anaphylactic Reactions to Food in Children and Adolescents." *NEJM* 327 (1992): 380–84.

Samter, Max. "On the Impossible." *Journal of Allergy* 31 (1960): 88–94.

——. "Presidential Address." *Journal of Allergy* 41 (1960): 88–94.

Samter, Max, and R. F. Beers Jr. "Concerning the Nature of Intolerance to Aspirin." *Journal of Allergy* 40 (1967): 281–93.

Satin, Morton. *Death in the Pot: The Impact of Food Poisoning in History.* New York: Prometheus Books, 2007.

Saul, Leon J. "The Relations to the Mother as Seen in Cases of Allergy." *Nervous Child* 5 (1946): 332–38.

Schleimer, Robert. "Message from the Division Chief." Northwestern University, Feinberg School of Medicine. http://www.medicine.northwestern.edu/divisions/allergy-immunology-0. Accessed September 25, 2013.

Schloss, Oscar M. "A Case of Allergy to Common Foods." *American Journal of Diseases of Children* 3 (1912): 341–62.

Schlosser, Eric. *Fast Food Nation: The Dark Side of the All-American Meal.* New York: Houghton Mifflin, 2001.

Schmeck, Harold M., Jr. "Doctors Seek Keys to Defenses of the Body." *New York Times,* December 29, 1972.

Schneider, Wilmot F. "Psychiatric Evaluation of the Hyperkinetic Child." *Journal of Pediatrics* 26 (1945): 559–70.

Schofield, Alfred T. "A Case of Egg Poisoning." *Lancet* 171 (1908): 716.

Schroeder, C. R. "Cow's Milk Protein Hypersensitivity in a Walrus." *Journal of the American Veterinary Medical Association* 83 (1933): 810–15.

Schuster, David. *Neurasthenic Nation: America's Search for Health, Happiness, and Comfort, 1869–1920.* New Brunswick, N.J.: Rutgers University Press, 2011.

Scrinis, Gyorgy. *Nutritionism: The Science and Politics of Dietary Advice.* New York: Columbia University Press, 2013.

Scull, Andrew. *Museums of Madness: The Social Organization of Insanity in Nineteenth-Century England.* London: Allen Lane, 1979.

Seale, Clive. *Media and Health.* London: Sage, 2002.

"Selfish Flyer Almost Kills Nut Allergy Girl on Plane." *Metro,* August 15, 2014, 7

Selye, Hans. *The Stress of Life.* London: Longman, Green, 1957.

Settipane, Guy A. "Anaphylactic Deaths in Asthmatic Patients." *Allergy Proceedings* 10 (1989): 271–74.

Shambaugh, George F. "Ahead of Their Time." *Archives of Otolaryngology* 79 (1964): 118–19.

Shannon, W. Ray. "Demonstration of Food Proteins in Human Breast Milk by Anaphylactic Experiments in Guinea Pigs." *American Journal of Diseases of Childhood* 22 (1921): 223–31.

——. "Neuropathic Manifestations in Infants and Children as a Result of Anaphylactic Reaction to Foods Contained in Their Dietary." *American Journal of Disease of Children* 24 (1922): 89–94.

Shemesh, Eyal, Rachel A. Annuziato, Michael A. Ambrose, Noga L. Ravid, Chloe Mullarkey, Melissa Rubes, Kelley Chuang, Mati Sicherer, and Scott H. Sicherer. "Child and Parental Reports of Bullying in a Consecutive Sample of Children with Food Allergy." *Pediatrics* 131 (2013): e10–e17.

Sherman, William B. "Presidential Address." *Journal of Allergy* 29 (1958): 274–76.

Shiekh, Aziz. "Oral Immunotherapy for Peanut Allergy." *BMJ* 341 (2010): 264.

Shore, Offley Bohun. *Domestic Medicine.* Edinburgh: Nimmo, 1866.

Shorter, Edward. *A History of Psychiatry: From the Era of the Asylum to the Age of Prozac.* New York: Wiley, 1997.

——. "Multiple Chemical Sensitivity: Pseudodisease in Historical Perspective." *Scandinavian Journal of Work, Environment, and Health* 23 (1997): 35–42.

Sicherer, Scott H., Terence J. Furlong, Anne Muñoz-Furlong, A. Wesley Burks, and Hugh A. Sampson. "A Voluntary Registry for Peanut and Tree Nut Allergy: Characteristics of the First 5149 Registrants." *JACI* 108 (2001): 128–32.

Siena, Kevin. "Introduction." In *Sins of the Flesh: Responding to Sexual Disease in Early Modern Europe,* edited by Kevin Siena, 7–29. Toronto: Centre for Reformation and Renaissance Studies, 2005.

Silverman, Chloe. *Understanding Autism: Parents, Doctors, and the Understanding of a Disorder.* Princeton, N.J.: Princeton University Press, 2013.

Silverstein, Arthur. *A History of Immunology.* 2nd ed. London: Elsevier/Academic Press, 2009.

Simon, Michele. *Appetite for Profit: How the Food Industry Undermines Our Health and How to Fight Back.* New York: Nation Books, 2006.

Simoons, Frederick J. *Eat Not This Flesh: Food Avoidances in the Old World.* 1961. Westport, Conn.: Greenwood Press, 1981.

Sinclair, John. *The Code of Health and Longevity.* Edinburgh: Constable, 1807.

Sippy, Bertram J. "The Sippy Treatment for Gastric Ulcer." *Journal of the National Medical Association* 16 (1924): 105–7.

Skoner, D., D. Gentile, R. Bush, M. B. Fasano, A. McLaughlin, and R. E. Esch. "Sublingual Immunotherapy in Patients with Allergic Rhinoconjunctivitis Caused by Ragweed Pollen." *JACI* 125 (2010): 660–66.

Smith, Andrew F. *Eating History: 30 Turning Points in the Making of American Cuisine.* New York: Columbia University Press, 2009.

——. *Peanuts: The Illustrious History of the Goober Pea.* Champaign: University of Illinois Press, 2002.

Smith, David F., and Jim Phillips. "Food Policy and Regulation: A Multiplicity of Actors and Experts." In *Food, Science, Policy, and Regulation in the Twentieth Century,* edited by David F. Smith and Jim Phillips, 1–16. London: Routledge, 2000.

Smith, Gwen, and Karen Eck. "Teen Food Allergy Deaths: Lessons from Tragedy." *Allergic Living,* Summer 2006. http://allergicliving.com/index.php/2010/07/02/food-allergy-teen-tragedies/. Accessed November 26, 2013.

Smith, Matthew. *An Alternative History of Hyperactivity: Food Additives and the Feingold Diet.* New Brunswick, N.J.: Rutgers University Press, 2011.

——. *Hyperactive: The Controversial History of ADHD.* London: Reaktion, 2012.

——. "Psychiatry Limited: Hyperactivity and the Evolution of American Psychiatry." *Social History of Medicine* 21 (2008): 541–59.

Söderqvist, Thomas. *Science as Autobiography: The Troubled Life of Niels Jerne.* Translated by David Mel Paul. New Haven, Conn.: Yale University Press, 2003.

Southgate, M. Therese. "The Cover: Victor C. Vaughan." *JAMA* 283 (2000): 848.

Spain, Will C. Review of *Food Allergy,* by Herbert J. Rinkel, Theron G. Randolph, and Michael Zeller. *Quarterly Review of Biology* 28 (1953): 97–98.

Speer, Frederic. "Allergic Tension-Fatigue in Children." *Annals of Allergy* 12 (1954): 168–71.

——. "The Allergic Tension-Fatigue Syndrome." *Pediatric Clinics of North America* 1 (1954): 1029–37.

——. "The Allergic Tension-Fatigue Syndrome in Children." *International Archives of Allergy and Applied Immunology* 12 (1958): 207–14.

——. "Food Allergy in Childhood." *Archives of Pediatrics* 75 (1958): 363–69.

——. "Historical Development of Allergy of the Nervous System." *Annals of Allergy* 16 (1958): 14–20.

——. "Is Allergy Extinct?" *Annals of Allergy* 2 (1967): 47–48.

——. "What Is Allergy?" *Annals of Allergy* 34 (1975): 49–50.

St. George, Donna. "Helen Morgan Brooks, 85, a Poet and Teacher for Many Years." *Philadelphia Inquirer,* October 19, 1989. http://articles.philly.com/1989-10-19news/26115824_1_poetry-collection-poems-family-and-love. Accessed August 8, 2013.

Strachan, D. "Hay Fever, Hygiene, and Household Size." *BMJ* 299 (1989): 1259–60.

Strain, James E. "Biographical Sketches of the First Editorial Board and Those Who Have Edited *Pediatrics*." *Pediatrics* 102 (1998): 191–93.

Strauss, Alfred A., and Heinz Werner. "Disorders of Conceptual Thinking in the Brain-Injured Child." *Journal of Nervous and Mental Disease* 96 (1942): 153–72.

"The Strawberry Season and Its Lessons." *Lancet*, June 20, 1908, 1786.

Sturdy, Steve. "Looking for Trouble: Medical Science and Clinical Practice in the Historiography of Modern Medicine." *Social History of Medicine* 24 (2011): 739–59.

Sugarman, A. A., D. L. Southern, and J. F. Curran. "A Study of Antibody Levels in Alcoholic, Depressive, and Schizophrenic Patients." *Annals of Allergy* 48 (1982): 166–71.

Sydenham, Thomas. *The Whole Works of That Excellent Practical Physician, Dr. Thomas Sydenham*. Translated by John Pechey. 9th ed. London: J. Darby, 1729.

Talbot, Fritz B. "Asthma in Children II: Its Relation to Anaphylaxis." *Boston Medical and Surgical Journal* 175 (1916): 191–95.

——. "The Relation of Food Idiosyncrasies to the Diseases of Childhood." *Boston Medical and Surgical Journal* 179 (1918): 285–88.

Tauber, Alfred I. *The Immune Self: Theory or Metaphor?* Cambridge: Cambridge University Press, 1994.

Taylor, S. L., W. W. Busse, M. I. Sachs, J. L. Parker, and J. W. Yunginger. "Peanut Oil Is Not Allergenic to Peanut-Sensitive Individuals." *JACI* 68 (1981): 372–75.

Taylor, S. L., and S. L. Hefle. "Foods as Allergens." In *Food Allergy and Intolerance*, edited by Jonathan Brostoff and Stephen J. Challacombe, 403–12. 2nd ed. London: Saunders, 2002.

"Teenage Bully Pushes the Limit at Lunch." news.com.au, June 14, 2006. http://www .childfoodallergy.com/archives/2006/06/teenage_bully_p.html. Accessed November 26, 2013.

Thomson, Spencer. *A Dictionary of Domestic Medicine and Household Surgery*. London: Griffin, 1859.

Thorpe, Susan J., Bernard Fox, Alan Heath, William Egner, and Dina Patel. "The Third International Standard for Serum IgE." World Health Organization. http://www .who.int/biologicals/BS_2220_Candidate_Preparation.pdf. Accessed October 22, 2013.

Timimi, Sami, and Begum Maitra. "ADHD and Globalization." In *Rethinking ADHD: From Brain to Culture*, edited by Sami Timimi and Jonathan Leo, 203–17. Basingstoke: Palgrave Macmillan, 2009.

Tocantins, Leandro M. "William Waddell Duke: Notes on the Man and His Work." *Blood* 1 (1946): 455–57.

Tomasi, Thomas B. "The Discovery of Secretory IgA and the Mucosal Immune System." *Immunology Today* 13 (1992): 416–18.

Tomasi, Thomas B., Jr., E. M. Tan, A. Solomon, and R. A. Pendergast. "Characteristics of an Immune System Common to Certain External Secretions." *Journal of Experimental Medicine* 121 (1965): 101–24.

Tuft, Louis. *Clinical Allergy*. Philadelphia: Saunders, 1937.

——. "Correspondence." *Journal of Allergy* 27 (1956): 293–94.

Tullman, Mark J. "Overview of the Epidemiology, Diagnosis, and Disease Prevention Associated with Multiple Sclerosis." *American Journal of Managed Care* 19 (2013): S15–20.

Turner, James S. *The Chemical Feast: The Ralph Nader Study Group Report on Food Protection and the Food and Drug Administration*. New York: Grossman, 1970.

Turner, Michelle C. "Epidemiology: Allergy History, IgE, and Cancer." *Cancer Immunology, Immunotherapy* 62 (2012): 1493–510.

Uncle Sam, M.D. "Health: Hay Fever, Asthma, Hives, Etc." *Ogden (Utah) Standard*, August 10, 1920.

"The Underprivileged Child: Where Are We in Pediatric Allergy?" *Journal of Allergy* 19 (1961): 1196–97.

Underwood, Emily. "Gut Microbes Linked to Autism-Like Symptoms in Mice." *Science Now*, December 5, 2013. http://news.sciencemag.org/biology/2013/12/gut-microbes-linked-autismlike-symptoms-mice. Accessed December 11, 2013.

Ure, D. M. "Negative Association Between Allergy and Cancer." *Scottish Medical Journal* 14 (1969): 51–54.

Van Leeuwen, W. Storm. *Allergic Diseases: Diagnosis and Treatment of Asthma, Hay Fever, and Other Allergic Diseases*. Philadelphia: Lippincott, 1925.

Van Metre, T. E., Jr., N. F. Adkinson Jr., L. M. Lichtenstein, M. R. Mardiney Jr., P. S. Norman Jr., G. L. Rosenberg, A. K. Sobotka, and M. D. Valentine. "A Controlled Study of the Effectiveness of the Rinkel Method of Immunotherapy for Ragweed Pollen Hay Fever." *JACI* 65 (1980): 288–97.

Vaughan, Victor C. "Further Studies of the Protein Poison." *JAMA* 67 (1916): 1559–62.

——. "The Protein Poison and Its Relation to Disease." *JAMA* 61 (1913): 1761–64.

Vaughan, Warren T. "Allergic Migraine." *JAMA* 88 (1927): 1383–86.

——. *Allergy: Strangest of All Maladies*. London: Hutchinson, 1942.

——. "Food Allergens: Leukopenic Index, Preliminary Report." *Journal of Allergy* (1934): 601.

——. "Minor Allergy: Its Distribution, Clinical Aspects, and Significance." *Journal of Allergy* 5 (1935): 184–96.

——. *Practice of Allergy*. 3rd ed. London: Kimpton, 1954.

——. *Strange Malady: The Story of Allergy*. New York: Doubleday, Doran, 1941.

Viner, Russell. "Putting Stress in Life: Hans Selye and the Making of Stress Theory." *Social Studies of Science* 29 (1999): 391–410.

Voorsanger, William C., and Fred Firestone. "Vaccine Therapy in Infectious Bronchitis and Asthma." *California and Western Medicine* 36 (1929): 336–40.

Wagner, Richard. *Clemens von Pirquet: His Life and Work*. Baltimore: Johns Hopkins University Press, 1968.

Waickman, Francis J. "Food Allergy/Sensitivity Diagnosed by Skin Testing." In *Food Allergy and Intolerance*, edited by Jonathan Brostoff and Stephen J. Challacombe, 831–36. 2nd ed. London: Saunders, 2002.

Waldie, Paul. "Air Canada Told to Provide Nut-Free Zones." *Globe and Mail* (Toronto), January 7, 2010.

Warner, John Harley. "From Specificity to Universalism in Medical Therapeutics: Transformation in the Nineteenth-Century United States." In *Sickness and Health in America: Readings in the History of Medicine and Public Health*, edited by Judith Walzer Leavitt and Ronald S. Numbers, 87–101. 3rd ed. Madison: University of Wisconsin Press, 1997.

Wender, Paul H. *Minimal Brain Dysfunction in Children*. New York: Wiley-Interscience, 1971.

Whalen, Elizabeth M., and Frederick J. Stare. *Panic in the Pantry: Food Facts, Fads, and Fallacies*. New York: Athenaeum, 1975.

White, Cleveland. "Acneform Eruptions of the Face: Etiologic Importance of Specific Foods." *JAMA* 103 (1934): 1277–79.

White, J. Michael. "Fatal Food Allergy." *CMAJ* 139 (1988): 8.

Wide, Leif. "Clinical Significance of Measurement of Reaginic (IgE) Antibody by RAST." *Clinical Allergy* 3 (1973): 583–95.

Willan, Robert. *On Cutaneous Diseases*. Vol. 1. Philadelphia: Kimber and Conrad, 1809.

Willis, Thomas. *Pharmaceutice Rationalis: or an Exercitation of the Operations of Medicine in Humane Bodies*. London: T. Dring, C. Harper and J. Leigh, 1679.

"With What We Must Contend." *Annals of Allergy* 19 (1961): 193–95.

Withers, Orval R. "The Allergist as a Clinician." *Journal of Allergy* 29 (1958): 277–82.

Withers, Thomas. *A Treatise on the Asthma*. London: G. G. J. and J. Robinson and W. Richardson, 1786.

Wodehouse, P. "Preparation of Vegetable Food Proteins for Anaphylactic Tests." *Boston Medical and Surgical Journal* 175 (1916): 195–96.

Woods, Angela. *The Sublime Object of Psychiatry: Schizophrenia in Clinical and Cultural Theory*. Oxford: Oxford University Press, 2011.

Worboys, Michael. *Spreading Germs: Disease Theories and Medical Practice in Britain, 1865–1900*. Cambridge: Cambridge University Press, 2000.

"A Word to the Non-Medical Public." *New York Times*, July 12, 1854.

World Health Organization. *Mental Health Atlas*. Geneva: World Health Organization, 2011.

Young, Allan. *Harmony of Illusions: Inventing Post-Traumatic Stress Disorder*. Princeton, N.J.: Princeton University Press, 1995.

Young, Michael C., Anne Muñoz-Furlong, and Scott H. Sicherer. "Management of Food Allergies in Schools: A Perspective for Allergists." *JACI* 124 (2009): 175–82.

Yunginger, J. W., K. G. Sweeney, W. Q. Sturner, L. A. Giannadrea, J. D. Teigland, M. Bray, P. A Benson, J. A. York, L. Biedrzcki, D. L. Squillace, and R. M. Helm. "Fatal Food-Induced Anaphylaxis." *JAMA* 260 (1988): 1450–52.

Yunginger, John W., and Gerald J. Gleich. "The Impact of the Discovery of IgE on the Practice of Allergy." *Pediatric Clinics of North America* 22 (1975): 3–15.

Index

allergy (*continued*)
216n.55, 221n.10, 234n.67, 238n.126;
environmental explanations for, 6,
10–15, 46–48, 58, 65, 81, 88–93, 96–101,
107–18, 122–24, 126–27, 136, 139, 142,
146, 150–51, 180–81, 187–89, 211n.86,
219n.112, 225n.65, 226n.86, 235n.86,
244n.101, 247n.2; hereditary factors
involved in, 10, 33, 35, 83, 120, 137–38,
190, 209n.58, 218n.87; legitimacy of,
6–8, 13–14, 47, 50, 69, 77, 84, 93–96, 118,
124, 126–31, 143–46, 152–53, 155, 189;
as metaphor, 20, 24, 58–59, 211n.79;
treatment of, 6–7, 9–11, 13–14, 41–42,
45, 53, 56, 63, 71–73, 79–82, 87–88, 95–
96, 100–107, 120, 141, 144–48, 170, 179,
190, 216n.55. *See also* food allergies
Allergy UK, 170
Allerteen (milk substitute), 70
almonds, 36–37, 163, 175, 204n.105
Alvarez, Walter Clement (1884–1978),
68–71, 105, 213n.10, 224n.57
American Academy of Allergy (AAA), 7,
13, 60, 72, 93–95, 126–27, 129–30, 139,
142–49, 155, 220n.38, 229n.4, 231n.20,
234n.71
American Academy of Allergy, Asthma
and Immunology (AAAAI), ix, 2, 7,
94, 155–56, 172, 183, 234n.63, 234n.71,
236n.98, 242n.57, 243n.73, 243n.76
American Academy of Allergy and
Immunology (AAAI), 138, 148–51,
154, 165, 168–72, 234n.71, 237n.114,
238n.126, 243n.76
American Academy of Environmental
Medicine (AAEM), 88, 142. *See also*
Society for Clinical Ecology
American Academy of Otolaryngology
(AAO), 148
American Board of Allergy and Immu-
nology (ABAI), 143
American Board of Medical Specialties
(ABMS), 130, 143

American College of Allergists (ACA),
7, 60, 94, 97, 102, 112, 114, 126, 130,
142, 144, 154, 167, 220n.138, 229n.4,
231n.20
American College of Allergy, Asthma and
Immunology (ACAAI), ix, 7, 94, 139
American Council on Science and Health
(ACSH), 99, 221n.10
American Medical Association (AMA),
96, 111, 146–47
American Peanut Shellers Association,
160
American Psychiatric Association (APA),
43, 114, 205n.3
anaphylactic shock, 1, 53–57, 73, 153, 162.
See also anaphylaxis
anaphylaxis, 1–4, 14, 20, 42, 46–59, 64–66,
73, 82, 96, 105, 107, 123, 125, 131–32,
140, 152–55, 160–79, 184–85, 193n.7,
201n.61, 202n.72, 206n.13, 206n.17,
208n.35, 210nn.59–60, 210n.73,
241n.49, 242n.57, 242n.61
Anaphylaxis Campaign (AC), 166,
242n.60
Anatomy of Melancholy (Burton), 107
Anderson, John (1873–1958), 95, 132,
207n.32
Anderson, McCall, 37–38, 40–41, 204n.112
Annals of Allergy (journal), 94, 102, 113–
15, 121, 141–42, 151, 161
anti-anaphylaxis, 52–53. *See also*
Besredka, Alexandre
antibiotics, 17, 162, 241n.44
antibodies, 20, 25, 46, 52–54, 75, 83, 114,
127–28, 131–41, 181–82, 209n.47
antigens, 25, 46, 54, 72, 75, 114, 131, 133,
135, 140–41, 161, 183
antihistamines, 77, 183
antiserum, 48, 52, 54
anxiety, 1, 7, 119, 135, 176. *See also* stress
appendectomy, 60, 81–82, 85
arthritis, 56, 67, 91, 145, 187
asparagus, 26

idiosyncrasy (*continued*)
200nn.46–47, 201n.63, 204n.104,
205n.120, 208n.33
immune system, 2, 8, 10, 20, 23, 25, 44–45,
57, 64–66, 74–75, 88, 123–41, 180, 183,
187–88, 206n.13
immunoglobulins: A (IgA), 133–34; D
(IgD), 133–34; E (IgE), 13–14, 125–42,
145, 151–52, 155, 163, 172, 229n.5,
232n.44, 233n.58, 233n.60, 234n.63,
234n.67; G (IgG), 133–34; M (IgM),
133–34
immunology, 7, 9, 13, 25, 44–46, 49–56,
77, 83, 122, 127–43, 151–52, 167, 188,
209n.47, 234n.41
indigestion. *See* gastrointestinal
symptoms
individuality, 15, 22–33, 37, 40, 48–57, 64,
87, 200nn.46–47, 205n.120, 208n.33,
210n.73
inductive knowledge, 7, 60, 63–66, 95–96,
122, 126. *See also* medical knowledge
industrialization, 46–47, 58, 70, 92, 108,
110, 146, 178
infant, feeding of, 9, 38–39, 105, 163, 180
infectious disease, 18, 21, 28, 45, 50, 79,
123, 133–36, 138, 180, 182
inflammation, 46, 59, 88, 134, 206n.17
ingestion test, 75–76, 81–82. *See also* food
allergies: diagnosis of
inhalant allergies, 76, 90, 101, 187,
244n.94. *See also* hay fever
inhalers. *See* bronchial inhalers
insect stings, 48, 54–55, 162, 198n.19
insurance. *See* health insurance
internal medicine, 76, 130, 143, 231n.20
International Classification of Diseases,
164
International Food Information Council
(IFIC), 149
International Life Sciences Institute
(ILSI), 169

intradermal testing, 72, 74, 214n.26. *See
also* allergy: diagnosis of; food allergies: diagnosis of
irritability, 87–88, 91, 103, 105–7, 146,
219n.111
Ishizaka, Kimishige (b. 1925), 127, 133–34
Ishizaka, Teruko (b. 1926), 127, 133–34
itching, 38, 49–50, 55, 57, 65, 81, 90, 120.
See also pruritis

Jackson, Mark, 9–12, 34, 54, 128–29, 138,
242n.60
James, Robert, 28
Jamieson, W. Allan, 39–40
Jerne, Niels (1911–1994), 9, 129
Johanssen, Gunnar (b. 1938), 127–28, 133,
136
Joint Council on Allergy and Immunol-
ogy (JCAI), 150
Journal of Allergy, 55, 70, 83, 93–94
*Journal of Allergy and Clinical Immunol-
ogy (JACI),* 147
Journal of Immunology, 55, 83
*Journal of the American Medical Associa-
tion (JAMA),* 67, 122, 164–65
Jukes, Edward, 32, 202n.72
Jungle, The (Sinclair), 108

Kallett, Arthur (1902–1972), 108–9,
224nn.56–57
Kellogg, John Harvey (1852–1943), 69, 157,
213n.13, 224n.57, 240n.25
Kessler, Walter R., 130–31
Kinnerton Confectionary (company), 175
Kitasato, Shibasaburo (1853–1931), 52
Knicker, William T., 137–38
Koch, Robert (1843–1910), 49
Koessler, Karl (1880–1925), 53
Krampner, Jon, 158, 162
Krause, Helen, 148
Küstner, Heinz (1897–1963), 132–33,
232n.37

ARTS AND TRADITIONS OF THE TABLE: PERSPECTIVES ON CULINARY HISTORY
ALBERT SONNENFELD, *SERIES EDITOR*

Salt: Grain of Life, Pierre Laszlo, translated by Mary Beth Mader

Culture of the Fork, Giovanni Rebora, translated by Albert Sonnenfeld

French Gastronomy: The History and Geography of a Passion, Jean-Robert Pitte, translated by Jody Gladding

Pasta: The Story of a Universal Food, Silvano Serventi and Françoise Sabban, translated by Antony Shugar

Slow Food: The Case for Taste, Carlo Petrini, translated by William McCuaig

Italian Cuisine: A Cultural History, Alberto Capatti and Massimo Montanari, translated by Áine O'Healy

British Food: An Extraordinary Thousand Years of History, Colin Spencer

A Revolution in Eating: How the Quest for Food Shaped America, James E. McWilliams

Sacred Cow, Mad Cow: A History of Food Fears, Madeleine Ferrières, translated by Jody Gladding

Molecular Gastronomy: Exploring the Science of Flavor, Hervé This, translated by M. B. DeBevoise

Food Is Culture, Massimo Montanari, translated by Albert Sonnenfeld

Kitchen Mysteries: Revealing the Science of Cooking, Hervé This, translated by Jody Gladding

Hog and Hominy: Soul Food from Africa to America, Frederick Douglass Opie

Gastropolis: Food and New York City, edited by Annie Hauck-Lawson and Jonathan Deutsch

Building a Meal: From Molecular Gastronomy to Culinary Constructivism, Hervé This, translated by M. B. DeBevoise

Eating History: Thirty Turning Points in the Making of American Cuisine, Andrew F. Smith

The Science of the Oven, Hervé This, translated by Jody Gladding

Pomodoro! A History of the Tomato in Italy, David Gentilcore

Cheese, Pears, and History in a Proverb, Massimo Montanari, translated by Beth Archer Brombert

Food and Faith in Christian Culture, edited by Ken Albala and Trudy Eden

The Kitchen as Laboratory: Reflections on the Science of Food and Cooking, edited by César Vega, Job Ubbink, and Erik van der Linden

Creamy and Crunchy: An Informal History of Peanut Butter, the All-American Food, Jon Krampner

Let the Meatballs Rest: And Other Stories About Food and Culture, Massimo Montanari, translated by Beth Archer Brombert

The Secret Financial Life of Food: From Commodities Markets to Supermarkets, Kara Newman

Drinking History: Fifteen Turning Points in the Making of American Beverages, Andrew F. Smith

Italian Identity in the Kitchen, or Food and the Nation, Massimo Montanari, translated by Beth Archer Brombert